SPORTS NUTRITION
FATS AND PROTEINS

SPORTS NUTRITION
FATS AND PROTEINS

Edited by
Judy A. Driskell

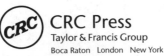

CRC Press
Taylor & Francis Group
Boca Raton London New York

CRC Press is an imprint of the
Taylor & Francis Group, an **informa** business

CRC Press
Taylor & Francis Group
6000 Broken Sound Parkway NW, Suite 300
Boca Raton, FL 33487-2742

International Standard Book Number-10: 0-8493-9079-6 (Hardcover)
International Standard Book Number-13: 978-0-8493-9079-1 (Hardcover)

Library of Congress Cataloging-in-Publication Data
Sports nutrition : fats and proteins / [edited by] Judy A. Driskell.

Sports nutrition : fats and proteins / [edited by] Judy A. Driskell.
    p. ; cm.
  Includes bibliographical references and index.
  ISBN-13: 978-0-8493-9079-1 (hardcover : alk. paper)
  ISBN-10: 0-8493-9079-6 (hardcover : alk. paper)
  1. Lipids in human nutrition. 2. Proteins in human nutrition. 3. Sports--Physiological aspects. 4. Athletes--Nutrition. I. Driskell, Judy A. (Judy Anne)
    [DNLM: 1. Nutrition. 2. Fats. 3. Proteins. 4. Sports. QU 145 S76535 2007]

QP751.S72 2007
612.3'97--dc22
                                            2006036488

**Visit the Taylor & Francis Web site at
http://www.taylorandfrancis.com**

**and the CRC Press Web site at
http://www.crcpress.com**

Dedication

I appreciate the opportunity to have worked with the chapter authors, all experts, on this book. I learned from them and dedicate this book to them.

Table of Contents

SECTION I   Introduction

SECTION II   Fats

SECTION III   Proteins

SECTION IV *Recommended Intakes of the Energy-Yielding Nutrients*

Preface

Many recreational, collegiate, and professional athletes in the U.S. and other developed countries consume more fat, saturated fat, and cholesterol in their diets than is recommended. Many of these athletes consume more than the minimal amount of protein to meet their needs. This book addresses the recommendations for fat and protein intakes for athletes and the general population that have been published by organizations and professionals. Critical reviews of these topics that are of upmost importance to athletes and professionals working with athletes are included in this book.

The quantity and types of fats in the diet have an influence on energy intake, health, and physical performance. Certain quantities of omega-3 and omega-6 fatty acids are needed for good health. High intakes of total fat, saturated fats, and to a lesser extent cholesterol have been reported to increase the risk of obesity, coronary heart disease, diabetes, and perhaps other chronic diseases such as cancer.

The quantity and quality of proteins in the diet also influence energy intake, health, and physical performance. Many athletes take protein or amino acid supplements, and evidence exists that some of these supplements may be or are beneficial to physical performance.

Fats, proteins, and carbohydrates are all energy-yielding nutrients. What is the appropriate amount of each of these energy-yielding nutrients that athletes should consume for optimal physical performance and overall health?

This volume includes a collection of chapters written by scientists from several academic disciplines that have expertise in an area of fat or protein nutrition as it relates to exercise and sports. The introductory chapter is followed by chapters on:

- Various dietary fats (lipids) and fatty acids: total fats, saturated fats, and cholesterol; medium-chain triglycerides; omega-3 and omega-6 fatty acids; conjugated linoleic acid (CLA); and wheat germ oil and octacosanol
- Protein quality, various protein supplements, and selected amino acid supplements: protein — quantity and quality; whey, casein, and soy proteins; creatine; glucosamine and chrondroitin sulfate; carnitine; β-hydroxy-β-methylbutyrate (HMB); branched-chain amino acids (BCAAs); glutamine; and other individual amino acids
- Recommended proportions of carbohydrates to fats to proteins in the diet

Sports nutritionists, sports medicine and fitness professionals, researchers, students, dietitians and other health practitioners, and the well-informed layman will find this book timely and informative.

Judy A. Driskell, Ph.D., R.D.
University of Nebraska

The Editor

Judy A. Driskell, Ph.D., R.D., is professor of nutrition and health sciences at the University of Nebraska. She received her B.S. degree in biology from the University of Southern Mississippi in Hattiesburg. Her M.S. and Ph.D. degrees were obtained from Purdue University. She has served in research and teaching positions at Auburn University, Florida State University, Virginia Polytechnic Institute and State University, and the University of Nebraska. She has also served as the nutrition scientist for the U.S. Department of Agriculture/Cooperative State Research Service and as a professor of nutrition and food science at Gadjah Mada and Bogor universities in Indonesia.

Dr. Driskell is a member of numerous professional organizations, including the American Society for Nutrition, the American College of Sports Medicine, the International Society of Sports Nutrition, the Institute of Food Technologists, and the American Dietetic Association. In 2005 she received the Research Award of the Nebraska chapter of Gamma Sigma Delta, the honor society in agriculture. In 1993 she received the Professional Scientist Award of the Food Science and Human Nutrition Section of the Southern Association of Agricultural Scientists. In addition, she was the 1987 recipient of the Borden Award for Research in Applied Fundamental Knowledge of Human Nutrition. She is listed as an expert in B-complex vitamins by the Vitamin Nutrition Information Service.

Dr. Driskell co-edited the CRC book *Sports Nutrition: Minerals and Electrolytes* with Constance V. Kies. In addition, she authored the textbook *Sports Nutrition* and co-authored an advanced nutrition textbook, *Nutrition: Chemistry and Biology*, both published by CRC. She co-edited *Sports Nutrition: Vitamins and Trace Elements*, 1st and 2nd editions; *Macroelements, Water, and Electrolytes in Sports Nutrition*; *Energy-Yielding Macronutrients and Energy Metabolism in Sports Nutrition*; *Nutritional Applications in Exercise and Sport*; *Nutritional Assessment of Athletes*; and *Nutritional Ergogenic Aids*, all with Ira Wolinsky. She has published over 150 refereed research articles and 13 book chapters as well as several publications intended for lay audiences and has given numerous presentations to professional and lay groups. Her current research interests center around vitamin metabolism and requirements, including the interrelationships between exercise and water-soluble vitamin requirements.

Contributors

John J.B. Anderson, Ph.D.
Department of Nutrition
University of North Carolina
Chapel Hill, North Carolina

Martha A. Belury, Ph.D., R.D.
Department of Human Nutrition
Ohio State University
Columbus, Ohio

Wayne E. Billon, Ph.D., R.D.
Department of Health Sciences
Western Carolina University
Cullowhee, North Carolina

Sara Chelland Campbell, M.S.
Department of Nutrition, Food and
  Exercise Sciences
Florida State University
Tallahassee, Florida

Michael Gleeson, Ph.D.
School of Sport and Exercise Sciences
Loughborough University
Loughborough, Leicestershire,
  United Kingdom

Mark D. Haub, Ph.D.
Department of Human Nutrition
Kansas State University
Manhattan, Kansas

Catherine G.R. Jackson, Ph.D.
Department of Kinesiology
California State University, Fresno
Fresno, California

Satya S. Jonnalagadda, Ph.D., R.D.
Novartis Nutrition Corporation
St. Louis Park, Minnesota

Celeste G. Koster, M.A. Ed.
Department of Human Nutrition
Ohio State University
Columbus, Ohio

**Richard B. Kreider, Ph.D.,
  F.A.C.S.M., F.I.S.S.N.**
Department of Health, Physical
  Education and Recreation
Baylor University
Waco, Texas

Ji-Young Lee, Ph.D.
Department of Nutrition and Health
  Sciences
University of Nebraska
Lincoln, Nebraska

**Nancy M. Lewis, Ph.D., R.D.,
  F.A.D.A., L.M.N.T.**
Department of Nutrition and Health
  Sciences
University of Nebraska
Lincoln, Nebraska

Karina R. Lora, M.S.
Department of Nutrition and Health
  Sciences
University of Nebraska
Lincoln, Nebraska

Henry C. Lukaski, Ph.D.
Grand Forks Human Nutrition Research
  Center
U.S. Department of Agriculture
Grand Forks, North Dakota

Susan H. Mitmesser, Ph.D., R.D.
Mead Johnson Nutritionals
Evansville, Indiana

Robert J. Moffatt, Ph.D.
Department of Nutrition and Exercise
Florida State University
Tallahassee, Florida

Steven L. Nissen, Ph.D.
Department of Animal Science
Iowa State University
Ames, Iowa

Heather E. Rasmussen, M.S., R.D.
Department of Nutrition and Health
  Sciences
University of Nebraska
Lincoln, Nebraska

Brian S. Snyder, M.S.
Department of Human Nutrition
Kansas State University
Manhattan, Kansas

Neal F. Spruce
Apex Fitness Group
Camarillo, California

**Mark A. Tarnopolsky, M.D., Ph.D.,
  F.R.C.P.C.**
Departments of Pediatrics and Medicine
McMaster University
Hamilton, Ontario, Canada

Brian W. Timmons, Ph.D.
Department of Pediatrics
McMaster University
Hamilton, Ontario, Canada

C. Alan Titchenal, Ph.D., C.N.S.
Department of Human Nutrition, Food
  and Animal Sciences
University of Hawaii at Manoa
Honolulu, Hawaii

Section I

Introduction

1 Introduction to Sports Nutrition: Fats and Proteins

John J.B. Anderson

CONTENTS

1.1 INTRODUCTION

The focus of this text is on both recreational and more advanced athletes who deserve up-to-date information on meeting their nutritional needs for fats and proteins. A flurry of publications over the last several years has provided new science for achieving optimal nutrient intake for maximizing muscle and other tissue functions demanded by athletic performance. This chapter attempts to introduce the essence of our basic knowledge of the optimal intakes of fats and proteins and their tissue utilization in sports. Keep in mind that fat intake provides a major portion of our dietary energy (calories), but not the only source, and that fat intake must be considered in the context of carbohydrate intake, the other major source of dietary calories. Calories provided by dietary protein are not insignificant, but they definitely are minor compared to the energy provided by carbohydrates and fats. Keep in mind also that nutrient needs differ in a major way between athletes who perform more aerobic activities and those who perform more resistive types of exercise.

1.1.1 ATHLETES' NEEDS FOR ENERGY

The energy breakdown in U.S. diets is typically given as 50% from carbohydrates, 35% from fats, and 15% from proteins, but this pattern can vary considerably if carbohydrates partly substitute for fats, with proteins remaining at approximately 15% of total energy consumption. Thus, a 10% increase in carbohydrates would necessitate a 10% decrease in fats, so that the mix of the two major energy components would be 60% and 25%. The latter percentage breakdown of energy is more consistent with the actual intakes of many elite athletes, especially endurance athletes, whereas the typical U.S. pattern is more common for recreational athletes and some athletes who need to bulk up for their sports (Table 1.1). Requirements vary according to the two major types of activities, aerobic exercise or resistive exercise.[1] In fact, some of the powerful heavy athletes, such as sumo wrestlers, may have a diet higher than 35% in fat and lower than 50% in carbohydrate.

Recommended Dietary Allowances (RDAs) for energy for adult males and females are 3100 and 2400 kcal/day, respectively, but these amounts are generally exceeded by active competitive athletes, though not necessarily by recreational athletes.[2] RDAs, of course, depend on body size, and many athletes have high body mass indices (BMIs) without being obese; so the highly muscled athlete may need much more than the RDA, while the endurance-type, more aerobic athlete may need more than the RDA but not as much as the high BMI well-muscled types.

Some endurance athletes increase their intakes of energy and protein through the use of supplemental powders that may also contain micronutrients, i.e., vitamins and minerals. These athletes can greatly increase their intakes, especially while participating in their sports by diluting these powders in water and carrying their

---

TABLE 1.1
Approximate Energy Distribution of Macronutrients

Macronutrient	General Diet	Endurance Athletes	Power Athletes
Carbohydrates	50%	65%	55%
Fats	35%	20%	25%
Proteins	15%	15%	20%

bags on their backs. Supplements are generally considered to help these athletes, who may be on the road or trail for hours at a time. Almost all other athletes do not need to go to such lengths to meet their energy and protein needs, but they may need breaks from time to time to consume an energy drink or bar.

In general, trained athletes do not wish to gain or lose weight, but rather to stay at their weight of optimal performance. These athletes typically consume foods with high nutrient density, i.e., fairly rich in micronutrients per total amount of energy in a serving, and they commonly take a nutrient supplement of one type or another, depending on their specific sport or activity. Recreational athletes should also try to include more nutrient-rich foods in their diets, and they may also wish to take a daily supplement of vitamins and minerals appropriate for age and gender.

1.1.2 ATHLETES' NEEDS FOR PROTEIN

Proteins are special types of essential nutrients, and they are equally important with energy for supporting optimal function of the body in sports. Proteins provide the following: amino acids, about half of which are essential because humans cannot make them; nitrogen (N), from all the amino acids, used for the synthesis of other molecules essential to life; and energy, from the hydrocarbon backbone of amino acids. Thus, proteins have three important roles in satisfying the needs of cells and tissues throughout our bodies, not simply skeletal muscle.

Foods rich in proteins are traditionally animal products such as meats, eggs, and dairy foods, but soybeans and other legumes are also good protein sources, especially when mixed with animal sources or with cereal grains and a few vegetables if the athlete is a vegan (strict vegetarian).

In general, adult males should consume roughly 80 to 120 g of protein a day if they are involved in athletic or recreational competition, depending on their sport, whereas females should ingest approximately 65 to 95 g a day, again depending on their sport.[3] Because the RDAs for adult males and females are only 56 and 44 g per day,[2] respectively, the actual intakes of protein in the U.S. are much greater than the RDAs, and recommendations for some types of athletes actually are twice as great.

1.1.3 ATHLETES' NEEDS FOR ESSENTIAL FATTY ACIDS

Athletes, like others, need essential fatty acids (EFAs) to support many functions of the body. The two types of EFAs are omega-6 and omega-3 fatty acids. Typical U.S. diets provide more of the omega-6 FAs and less of the omega-3 FAs than needed to maintain a healthy balance between the two types, which are used for eicosanoid synthesis. Eicosanoid is a general term that includes the prostaglandins, the original name given to this class of lipid molecules. Recommendations for healthy intakes of each type exist, but few in the U.S. consume enough omega-3 FAs because of low intakes of fish, fish oils, and a few other food sources. A small percentage take fish oil supplements that help restore the balance between the two types of EFAs.

1.1.4 ATHLETES' NEEDS FOR MICRONUTRIENTS AND WATER

Micronutrients, including water, are also needed by athletes in order to function. Foods should provide these nutrients if we consume enough servings from the different food groups, but athletes, like many others, do not consume sufficient amounts of fruits and vegetables on a daily basis. So, they typically need a vitamin–mineral supplement to try to maximize their athletic functions. In general, many of these micronutrients help metabolize carbohydrates, fats, and proteins, and therefore play roles that may be directly involved with exercise and sport, whereas others have functions that support life, cell renewal, and other activities at a more basic level.

1.2 SPECIFIC ASPECTS OF FAT NEEDS

Fats have one property that distinguishes them from other macronutrients, i.e., carbohydrates and proteins: they are not water soluble but rather fat or lipid soluble. This property means that the body must have specific mechanisms to handle the fat in digestion, transport across membranes, and transport in blood serum. Many different types of molecules in cells and body fluids must contain fatty acids in order to function. A few definitions are necessary first to elucidate the importance of the dietary fats.

Most fats are triglycerides, which consist of three fatty acids linked or bonded to one glycerol molecule. Glycerol is actually a small carbohydrate, but when it is linked to fatty acids the glyceride product is classified as a fat. So, monoglycerides, diglycerides, and triglycerides are all considered fat molecules. Lipid is another broader term used to include the fats or triglycerides, cholesterol, phospholipids, and many other fat-soluble molecules in foods or synthesized in our bodies.

A special class of the lipids is known as eicosanoids or prostaglandins. These molecules take on importance when consideration is given to unsaturated fatty acids, including both the omega-3 and omega-6 fatty acids, which serve as precursors of the eicosanoids, as discussed below.

1.2.1 TOTAL FAT

The 35% or so of energy provided by dietary fat refers only to the triglycerides found in our foods. High-performing athletes typically consume 20 to 25% fat, but they make certain that they get enough unsaturated fats because these fats, especially the omega-3 fatty acids, are generally thought to support immune function and keep athletes from catching common colds and nagging infections.

1.2.2 POLYUNSATURATED FATS AND EICOSANOIDS

Of the 35% of energy consumed by most in the U.S. population, the recommended percentage contributions of the specific types of fatty acids, i.e., saturated (SFAs), monounsaturated (MFAs), and polyunsaturated (PFAs), are roughly 10% each. Actual intakes of SFAs in the U.S. tend to be the highest at 13% or more, whereas

MFAs approximate 10% and PFAs are typically less than 10%. The mix of PFAs has also been estimated to have a ratio of 5–10 to 1 of omega-6 FAs to omega-3 FAs. Consumers of mostly animal foods may have an even greater ratio, and vegetarians may have ratios less than 5 to 1, depending on their food selection. High fish eaters, especially those who consume deep-sea fish, have ratios near 5 to 1. More will be covered below on the ratio of these PFAs and their impact on eicosanoid synthesis in reference to athletes.

MFAs have important roles in health, such as in protecting, at least in part, against elevations of serum total cholesterol, but they have limited utility compared to PFAs.

Under the umbrella of the DRIs, the omega-3 and omega-6 PFAs actually have recommendations that are categorized as Adequate Intakes (AIs) because of an insufficient knowledge base, i.e., mean requirements, to assign RDAs.[2]

1.2.2.1 Omega-6 Fatty Acids (n-6)

Examples of dietary omega-6 FAs are linoleic acid ($C_{18:2}$) and arachidonic acid ($C_{20:4}$). The major dietary sources of linoleic acid are vegetable oils, and linoleic acid may be converted to arachidonic acid in diverse cells prior to its conversion to prostaglandins of the 2 series.

1.2.2.2 Omega-3 Fatty Acids (n-3)

Examples of dietary omega-3 FAs are α-linolenic acid (ALA; $C_{18:3}$), eicosapentaenoic acid (EPA; $C_{20:5}$), and docosahexaenoic acid (DHA; $C_{22:6}$). α-linolenic acid is found primarily in soybean oil and flaxseed oil, but we are more likely to obtain EPA and DHA from fish oils. The latter molecules are converted to prostaglandins (PG3) of the 3 series and leukotrienes (LT5) of the 5 series.

The two series of eicosanoids are illustrated in Table 1.2. The products, depending on their local serum concentrations or amounts secreted, have effects on neighboring cells and tissues. It is the actions of these eicosanoids of one type or another that may have important effects on athletic performance, almost exclusively in the highly trained competitive athletes (see below).

TABLE 1.2
The Two Series of Eicosanoids

	Omega-6 Series	Omega-3 Series
Essential fatty acid precursors	Linoleic acid (C18:2)[a]	α-Linolenic acid (C18:3)[a]
Product PFAs	Arachidonic acid (C20:4)[a]	Eicosapentaenoic acid (C20:5)[a]
Eicosanoids	Prostaglandin 2 (PG2)	Prostaglandin 3 (PG3)
		Leukotriene (LT5)
Roles in athletes	Heart, arterial constriction, lungs	Blood clotting, immune defense

[a] The number of carbon atoms and number of double bonds (after the colon) are given in parentheses.

1.2.2.3 Balance of Polyunsaturated Fatty Acids

The balance between the two types of essential PFAs is best assessed by determining the dietary ratio of these PFAs because the ratio drives the syntheses of the different eicosanoids in the tissues. Low intakes of omega-3 FAs result in an increase in the formation of omega-6 FAs that feed into eicosanoids of this series.[4] This balance has important consequences for athletes because greater production of one type of eicosanoid may impact immune defense, tissue healing, heart function, and other organ functions that affect athletic performance — primarily of top-level competitors rather than of recreational athletes.

The amounts of the types of eicosanoids generated, i.e., PG2 vs. PG3 and LT5, depend on the dietary precursors or, for some individuals, the supplements of these two types of PFAs. Except for total vegetarians, i.e., vegans, most individuals cannot consume enough omega-3 fatty acids from foods; they can only get enough if they take a supplement of fish oil or another source rich in omega-3 fatty acids. Even the consumption of deep-sea fish a couple of times a week does not provide enough omega-3 fatty acids to balance the usual intake.

1.3 SPECIFIC ASPECTS OF PROTEIN NEEDS

Protein recommendations for active athletes and recreational participants are typically a little higher than for less active individuals (see above), in order to support tissue repair and renewal, including muscle, defense against infectious diseases, and generally the recycling of cellular proteins, including enzymes, membrane proteins, and export proteins. In an energy-balanced diet rich in carbohydrates and fats, dietary proteins are used mainly for their specific roles in tissues and cells rather than for energy.

1.3.1 TOTAL PROTEIN

As mentioned in the introduction, protein from a variety of food sources provides a balance of amino acids, both essential and nonessential, to support cellular and tissue functions. Although intakes of proteins almost invariably exceed RDAs, the 15% or so of protein in the total diet of the entire U.S. population is also much higher than the gender-specific RDAs for protein.[2]

Athletes who are building muscle through strength activities probably need protein during these growth periods, but not much more than is recommended — because the recommendations are generally on the high side. Recreational athletes typically will not need additional protein because they will have needs only for tissue repair and renewal.

1.3.2 ANIMAL PROTEIN

In general, animal proteins have fairly high quality, i.e., highly absorbable, essential amino acids, so that single sources of protein supply almost all the essential amino acids in reasonable amounts. Mixing animal and plant proteins together in the same meal also typically provides high protein quality (see below). The main concern about animal proteins, however, is that they are also rich in SFAs, but not in PFAs. They may also contain cholesterol. The low-fat animal meats and low-fat dairy products are considered healthier because they have less saturated fat and cholesterol.

One animal protein woefully incomplete in essential amino acids, and therefore of poor protein quality, is collagen that is found in gelatins. This protein must be consumed with one or more other proteins in a meal in order to obtain a mix of all the amino acids.

1.3.3 PLANT PROTEIN

Plant proteins generally are limited to one or two essential amino acids, which make them of low or poor protein quality. An exception to this rule is soy protein. Soy protein has a protein quality equivalent to that of beef. Other legumes, peas and beans, also have fairly high protein quality. Mixing two or more servings of legumes and grains, such as wheat, rice, or corn, provides a fairly high quality protein meal. Vegetarian diets rich in plant proteins are considered to provide sufficient amounts of all amino acids needed by competitive athletes as long as a variety of protein foods are consumed and adequate energy is ingested.[5]

Another view is that plant-based diets may limit physical development to some extent, and therefore reduce the potential capacity of certain individual athletes in sports that require large body size and strength, i.e., power-type athletes.[6] The flip side of this argument, however, is that power-type athletes can get overly large in body size, i.e., BMIs that exceed 30, and these athletes thereby place themselves at risk for obesity, diabetes mellitus type 2, and elevated lipoproteins and blood pressure.[7] Power athletes typically consume excessive amounts of animal protein and, therefore, also saturated fat and cholesterol.

1.4 LINKING THE ENERGY CONTRIBUTIONS OF FATS AND PROTEINS

The provision of adequate fat, i.e., triglycerides (TGs), is important for exercising individuals to meet their energy needs and to provide EFAs, i.e., both omega-6 and omega-3 FAs. With the typical fat intake of 35% of total energy, however, it is almost impossible to consume enough of the omega-3 FAs. Therefore, the optimal balance between omega-3 FAs and omega-6 FAs cannot be achieved without a supplement, e.g., fish oil rich in omega-3 FAs. The energy from fat is sufficient, but not the specific omega-3 FAs.

As for protein, a diet providing about 15 to 18% energy from protein should be more than adequate. Such a diet supplies 100 to 150 g of protein, depending on the total caloric intake. With 35% of the total energy being derived from fat and 15% or so from protein, the remainder of energy, or 50% of calories, would be provided by carbohydrates, both starches and sugars. No recommendation is made for alcohol, which may provide from 1 to 3% of total calories in the general population. The actual energy distributions may vary quite a bit for competitive athletes in endurance sports, who typically have higher intakes of carbohydrates (60% or more) and protein (20% or higher). In this scenario, fat intake would be approximately 20% or so.

1.4.1 UNDER CONDITIONS OF ENERGY BALANCE

Competitive athletes need to maintain energy balance, i.e., a state of equilibrium between energy intake and energy expenditure on a daily basis, in order to perform at or near their personal best times or other criteria. Recreational athletes may fluctuate more in their energy intakes as well as in their body weights, depending on the season of the year and other factors. Energy balance is considered a good outcome, if lean body mass (LBM) is maintained through regular programs of activity. If LBM is not maintained, especially as verified by dual-energy x-ray absorptiometry (DXA) measurements, then fat mass has increased and exercise has been diminished. The direct relationship of exercise to LBM is extremely important in athletes who are at optimal fitness.

1.4.2 UNDER CONDITIONS OF INSUFFICIENT ENERGY INTAKE

The condition of insufficient energy consumption occurs much more often among female athletes who want a slim body composition — low in body fat — in order to optimize performance in their sport or activity. Underconsumption may lead to an eating disorder, a far too common occurrence in competitive female athletes. Although the etiology of eating disorders is complex, i.e., female athlete triad,[8] prevention of these disorders in athletes requires careful counseling and guidance; otherwise, the women will no longer be able to compete. The likelihood of eating disorders among recreational female athletes is far less likely.

1.4.3 UNDER CONDITIONS OF EXCESSIVE ENERGY INTAKE

This situation occurs among some professional football players, sumo wrestlers, and a few other types of power athletes. Excessive energy consumption for greater BMIs is desirable in these sports because of the association of mass and strength. Down-linemen in football have been reported to have BMIs in the obese range (BMI > 30).[7] The "obese" body weights and excess fat place these athletes at increased risk of diabetes mellitus type 2, hypertension, and cardiovascular and other diseases.

1.5 FAT AND PROTEIN INTAKES FOR OPTIMAL FUNCTION

As already highlighted, the typical breakdown of energy distribution of carbohydrates, fats, and proteins depends to a major extent on the types of activities in which athletes participate — and to a lesser degree on body size and composition. Endurance athletes — runners, skiers, skaters, and others — typically need a high carbohydrate and protein intake to meet their high energy demands and tissue repair and replacement needs. Power athletes — lifters, track throwers, football down-linemen, sumo wrestlers, and others — require a high total energy intake, including fats. It is speculated that practically all of these two broad classes of high-level competitive athletes consume adequate amounts of energy, but not enough EFAs, especially the omega-3 PFAs, unless they take a daily supplement. Recreational athletes have no specific recommendations for their athletic participation, but they should be consuming nutrients as recommended for the general U.S. population.[2]

1.6 SUMMARY

This introductory chapter has tried to capture the state-of-the-art knowledge about what high-level athletes should be consuming in order to maintain optimal performance in their specific sports. Two types of athletes, endurance and power, have been used to model the general recommendations for energy, especially from fats and carbohydrates and protein. Because proteins also serve other important cellular needs, emphasis has been placed on achieving intakes of the essential amino acids to meet cellular and tissue needs, especially muscle tissue. Finally, some emphasis has been given to the intakes of EFAs, especially the omega-3 FAs, which are used in eicosanoid synthesis for many specific functions of the body. The needs of high-level athletes have been much more detailed than the needs of recreational athletes, who need to follow the general nutrient recommendations for the U.S. adult population. The nutrient needs of growing children who are athletes are not covered in this chapter, but of course the nutritional concerns of children and adolescents should first be on meeting the needs for continuing growth and then on the needs for athletic participation.

REFERENCES

1. Evans, W.J. Exercise. In Bowman, B.A. and Russell, R.M., Eds. *Present Knowledge in Nutrition*, 8th ed. ILSI Press, Washington, DC, 2001.
2. Food and Nutrition Board, Institute of Medicine. *Dietary Reference Intakes for Energy, Carbohydrate, Fiber, Fat, Fatty Acids, Cholesterol, Protein, and Amino Acids.* National Academy Press, Washington, DC, 2005.
3. Young, V.R. Protein and amino acids. In Bowman, B.A. and Russell, R.M., Eds. *Present Knowledge in Nutrition*, 8th ed. ILSI Press, Washington, DC, 2001.
4. Jones, P.J.H. and Papamandjaris, A.A. Lipids: cellular metabolism. In Bowman, B.A. and Russell, R., Eds. *Present Knowledge in Nutrition*, 8th ed. ILSI Press, Washington, DC, 2001.
5. Nieman, D.C. Physical fitness and vegetarian diets: is there a relation? *Am J Clin Nutr* 70: 570S–575S, 1999.
6. Anderson, J.J.B. Plant-based diets and bone health: nutritional implications. *Am J Clin Nutr* 70 (Suppl. 3): 539S–542S, 1999.
7. Harp, J.B. and Hecht, L. Obesity in the National Football League. *JAMA* 293: 1061–1062, 2005.
8. Thrash, L. and Anderson, J.J.B. Female athlete triad. *Nutr Today* 35: 168–173, 2000.

Section II

Fats

2 Total Fats, Saturated Fats, and Cholesterol

Heather E. Rasmussen and Ji-Young Lee

CONTENTS

2.1 INTRODUCTION/CLASSIFICATION

2.1.1 CHEMICAL STRUCTURE AND GENERAL PROPERTIES

2.1.1.1 Total Fats

Lipids are a group of insoluble organic compounds that often encompass simple lipids, phospholipids, sphingomyelins, and sterols. Simple lipids include free fatty acids and triglycerides that contain a combination of three fatty acids esterified to a glycerol backbone. Approximately 95% of lipids are consumed in the form of triglycerides, whereas monoglycerides and diglycerides consisting of one and two fatty acids esterified to a glycerol backbone, respectively, exist in smaller amounts within the body. Properties of fatty acids depend on both carbon chain length and degree of saturation. Triglycerides containing short-chain fatty acids (two to eight carbons in length) and unsaturated fatty acids tend to be a liquid (i.e., oil) at room temperature, whereas those containing long-chain saturated fatty acids exist as solid fats at room temperature. At the cellular level, fats play an important role in cell membrane composition, fluidity, peroxidation, prostaglandin and leukotriene synthesis, and cellular metabolic processes. In addition to being essential for absorption and transport of fat-soluble vitamins (e.g., A, D, E, and K), fatty acids are implicated in the mechanisms of brain development, inflammatory processes, atherosclerosis, carcinogenesis, aging, and cell renewal.[1] As fats are the most energy dense of the nutrients and are efficiently stored in adipose tissue, they are the primary source of energy both at rest and during physical exercise.

2.1.1.2 Saturated Fats

Saturated fats are fatty acids, or are comprised of fatty acids, that contain no double bonds on their hydrocarbon backbone. The length of the carbon chains of saturated fatty acids varies from 4 to 24 carbon atoms. The most common saturated fatty acids found in nature are lauric acid (12:0), myristic acid (14:0), palmitic acid (16:0), and stearic acid (18:0), ranging in chain length from 12 to 18 carbons, as indicated. Saturated fats mainly exist in a solid state at room temperature, with several exceptions, such as coconut oil and palm kernel oil, which are liquid at room temperature. Saturated fats can exist naturally, or can be produced by a processing method called hydrogenation, creating a saturated fat from unsaturated fatty acids. The partially hydrogenated fats provide a desirable structure and texture, long shelf life, and stability during deep-frying in a variety of manufactured food products. However, health concerns have been raised over hydrogenation due to the by-product formation of *trans* fats, *trans* isomers of unsaturated fats, during this process. Studies have shown that *trans* fats increase the risk of coronary heart disease.[2] Therefore, the Food and Drug Administration (FDA) ordered that, as of January 1, 2006, food manufacturers have to indicate the contents of *trans* fats in the nutrition labels for all conventional foods and supplements.

2.1.1.3 Cholesterol

Sterols are a class of lipids that consist of a steroid and an alcohol. The most physiologically abundant sterol in humans is cholesterol, which is an integral part of the plasma membranes, conferring the fluidity of the lipid bilayer. Due to its amphipathic nature, cholesterol is an important structural component of cell membranes and the outer layer of plasma lipoproteins. Cholesterol plays an essential role both in the structure of cells and as a precursor to corticosteroids, mineral corticoids, bile acids, vitamin D, and sex hormones such as testosterone, estrogen, and progesterone. As excess free cholesterol has cytotoxicity in cells, it is esterified to a fatty acid to become a cholesteryl ester, a neutral form of cholesterol. Cholesteryl esters can be stored in the lipid droplets of cells without cytotoxicity, and therefore cholesterol esterification is increased when free cholesterol content in cells becomes excessive.

While cholesterol is exclusively an animal sterol, over 40 plant sterols have been identified. Similar to cholesterol, plant sterols serve to maintain the structural integrity of a cell. The most abundant plant sterols are sitosterol, campesterol, and stigmasterol, which differ from cholesterol by the presence of an extra methyl or ethyl group within the sterol side chain. This addition of the methyl or ethyl group on the sterol side chain results in poor intestinal absorption of plant sterols in humans,[3] with only 1.5 to 5.0% of sitosterol absorbed when typical amounts of sterols are consumed (240 to 320 mg).[4] Clinical studies have demonstrated a direct role of dietary plant sterols in reducing cholesterol absorption.[5] According to the FDA, ingestion of plant sterols (0.8 g/day) and plant sterol esters (1.3 g/day), along with a diet low in saturated fat and cholesterol, may reduce the risk of coronary heart disease.

2.2 LIPID METABOLISM

2.2.1 DIGESTION AND TRANSPORT

The lipid component of the typical Western diet consists of triglycerides, phospholipids, and cholesterol. Triglycerides constitute the majority of dietary lipid intake, reaching approximately 150 g/day. Digestion of triglycerides is initiated by lingual lipase, which is secreted by glands in the mouth, contributing to limited digestion in the stomach. In order for lingual lipase to exert its effect on triglycerides, emulsification must take place by a combination of stomach contraction and acid milieu. The partially digested lipid emulsion exits the stomach and is introduced to bile, composed mostly of bile acids and salts, in the proximal small intestine. In the fasting state, bile acids are concentrated in the gallbladder.

After food consumption, bile enters the duodenum in response to cholecystokinin-pancreozynim.[6] Bicarbonate from the pancreas creates a favorable pH for emulsification and hydrolysis of triglycerides and, in conjunction with bile, creates an optimal environment for pancreatic lipase. Hydrolysis of triglycerides by pancreatic lipase results in a mixture of monoglycerides, diglycerides, and free fatty acids. Only a small portion of triglycerides are completely hydrolyzed to glycerol and free fatty acids. Bile acids and salts, along with phospholipids, aid in lipid absorption by forming micelles. This aggregation of molecules in a colloidal system allows for the solubility of the hydrophobic molecules by positioning the polar portions of bile salts, bile acids, and phospholipids outward. This outward polarity allows the micelle to penetrate the unstirred water layer, allowing for absorption into the intestinal mucosal cells, or enterocytes. The lipid contents of the micelles then enter the enterocytes by several mechanisms, i.e., simple diffusion, facilitated diffusion, and active transport involving membrane transporters. For fatty acids longer than 10 to 12 carbons in length, an intracellular re-formation of triglycerides then occurs. Shorter-chained fatty acids (up to 10 to 12 carbons in length) are directly shuttled into the portal blood and transported to the liver.

After absorption and reassembly of the long-chain fatty acids into triglycerides in the intestine, the triglycerides are packaged into chylomicrons. Chylomicrons are lipoprotein particles containing approximately 90% triglyceride, with the remaining 10% consisting of cholesterol, phospholipids, and protein.[7] Several apolipoproteins, protein components in lipoprotein particles, are present in chylomicrons, including apoB-48, apoAs of intestinal origin, apoCs, and apoE. After dietary intake of lipids, chylomicrons are generated in intestinal mucosal cells and play a role in the post-prandial transport of exogenous (dietary) cholesterol and triglycerides to other tissues. Triglyceride hydrolysis occurs in the circulation by the action of lipoprotein lipase, an extracellular enzyme that resides on the capillary walls, predominantly in adipose tissue and cardiac and skeletal muscle, releasing free fatty acids and diglycerides to be absorbed into the tissues for energy. The remaining lipoprotein particle, termed a chylomicron remnant, travels through the bloodstream to be taken into the liver by endocytosis mediated by a specific receptor for apoE.[8]

2.2.2 BODY RESERVES

Fatty acids introduced to the tissues are either utilized for energy or stored for later use, depending on the energy state of the body. In a fed state, fatty acids are primarily used for the synthesis of triglycerides in subcutaneous and deep visceral adipose tissue. While only approximately 450 g of glycogen can be stored in the body at one time, a nearly unlimited capacity for fat storage exists. Fat storage depends on the individual. For nonobese males, average triglyceride storage ranges between 9 and 15 kg, translating into a total energy storage of 80,000 to 140,000 kcal.[9] While trained athletes have less fat reserves, ample amounts remain to provide energy in times of prolonged periods of insufficient energy intake. Not only in caloric deprivation, but in states of high energy expenditure, carbohydrate availability may be limited and utilization of fat stores may be warranted.

In addition to the fat storage in adipose tissue, a small amount of fat is present as lipid droplets in muscle tissues, or in circulation as free fatty acids associated with albumin or as part of a lipoprotein particle. The amount of fat both in the plasma and stored in muscle varies according to several factors, including energy state, fitness level, and dietary fat intake. Within the muscle cells, free fatty acids are primarily oxidized for energy.

2.2.3 FAT METABOLISM DURING EXERCISE: FROM ADIPOSE, FROM INTRAMUSCULAR TRIGLYCERIDES (IMTG)

Triglycerides in the body are continuously being hydrolyzed and esterified, depending on the body's energy status, i.e., a fed or fasting state. When the body is in an energy-deficient state, as occurs with exercise, increased hydrolysis of triglyceride stores and resultant liberation of fatty acids from adipose and muscle tissue occur. During exercise, fat and carbohydrate metabolism are tightly coupled, both controlled by nervous and hormonal mechanisms. At rest, total energy provision is greatly supplemented by fat oxidation, whereas a majority of the energy is obtained from glycogen stores during intense, short-term exercise. As exercise continues, the use of carbohydrate as a fuel source decreases while the utilization of fat via oxidation of muscle and adipose triglyceride stores increases. The proportion of each substrate utilized depends on factors such as the duration and intensity of exercise, the fitness level of the individual, and the meal prior to exercise.

Specific hormones increase during exercise, stimulating fat mobilization, transport, and oxidation. Lipolysis is initiated in the adipocytes, stimulated by epinephrine and norepinephrine, which can activate hormone-sensitive lipase (HSL). The release of epinephrine and norepinephrine also inhibits pancreatic insulin secretion, decreasing its inhibition of HSL. The free fatty acids produced by lipolysis are transported across the adipocyte plasma membrane either passively or via transport proteins such as fatty acid binding protein and fatty acid translocase.[10] Once the free fatty acids reach circulation, they are bound to albumin and transported to muscle tissue. Since exercise-induced energy deficiency is occurring, reesterification of fatty acids to triglycerides is suppressed and lipolysis is accelerated, increasing blood levels of free fatty acid bound to albumin during exercise.[11]

Once the fatty acids are in the cytoplasm of the muscle cells, they are transported across the mitochondrial membrane by carnitine palmityol transferases I and II for β-oxidation and energy production. During exercise, total fat oxidation rates can increase more than ten-fold during the transition from rest to moderate-intensity exercise.[9] The availability of glucose, rather than that of fatty acids, controls the rate of fatty acid oxidation because glucose can decrease the oxidation of long-chain fatty acids by inhibiting their transport into the mitochondria.[12]

In addition to the use of fatty acids liberated from adipocytes, or obtained from the plasma as albumin-bound long-chained fatty acids or in very low-density lipoproteins (VLDLs), research indicates that the intramuscular triglyceride (IMTG) pool can serve as a dynamic fuel source during physical activity. Because no blood transport is required, intramuscular fatty acids can be readily used for energy in exercising muscle. A detailed discussion on IMTG can be found in Section 2.4.1.

2.3 CHOLESTEROL METABOLISM

While many mechanisms regulate cholesterol homeostasis within the body, limited means of cholesterol input and output exist. Cholesterol input into the body pool is derived from two sources: cholesterol synthesized in the body and cholesterol from the diet. Cholesterol is not an energy-providing nutrient and cannot be broken down by the body. To remove cholesterol from the body, it must be excreted in the form of free cholesterol or bile acids through the liver.

2.3.1 CHOLESTEROL BIOSYNTHESIS

The average North American diet provides approximately 300 to 500 mg of cholesterol per day,[13] ingested as either free cholesterol or cholesteryl esters. A feedback system exists in which cholesterol synthesis decreases as the ingestion of dietary cholesterol is increased. Endogenous supplies originating from newly synthesized cholesterol, bile, and intestinal mucosal epithelium are about 1000 to 1600 mg/day.[14] Synthesis of cholesterol is a multistep process regulated by 3-hydroxy-3-methylglutaryl-CoA (HMG-CoA) reductase, the rate-limiting enzyme in cholesterol biosynthesis. When an increase in dietary cholesterol occurs, a reduction in hepatic cholesterol synthesis is observed, while synthesis in peripheral tissues may not be altered.[15] In this way, hepatic synthesis is the primary regulator of cholesterol balance in the body, despite the human liver accounting for only 10% of whole-body synthesis.[16] In hamsters fed a diet containing 2% cholesterol (wt/wt), cholesterol feeding induced hypercholesterolemia and inhibited cholesterol synthesis.[17] In addition to feedback inhibition as a result of dietary cholesterol intake, cholesterol synthesis is regulated by other forms of feedback inhibition, hormonal regulation, and sterol-mediated regulation of transcription.[18]

2.3.2 CHOLESTEROL ABSORPTION

Cholesterol absorption efficiency normally shows great variation among individuals, ranging from 30 to 80% with an average of ~50%.[13,19] Cholesterol feeding studies have shown that cholesterol absorption efficiency is unchanged up to a relatively large intake of cholesterol, where it reaches a saturation level with poor maximal absorption capacity.[19,20] Young male Syrian hamsters fed a lithogenic diet containing high cholesterol for 7 weeks showed a reduction in dietary cholesterol absorption efficiency of 26%.[21] In rhesus monkeys, cholesterol absorption and fecal excretion are suggested to play a major role in regulating plasma cholesterol concentrations.[22]

Recently, several transporters have been identified to be involved in cholesterol absorption, including ATP-binding cassette transporters G5 (ABCG5) and G8 (ABCG8) and Niemann-Pick C1 Like 1 (NPC1L1). ABCG5 and ABCG8, transmembrane proteins functioning as a heterodimer, have been shown to play pivotal roles in biliary cholesterol secretion from the liver as well as cholesterol absorption in the intestine.[23,24] NPC1L1 is required for the intestinal uptake of cholesterol and works as a modulator of whole-body cholesterol homeostasis.[25] Because a positive relationship exists between the fractional absorption of cholesterol and plasma cholesterol levels,[26] NPC1L1 may be a target for the treatment of hypercholesterolemia.[27]

2.3.3 CHOLESTEROL TRANSPORT

With the notable exception of free fatty acids that circulate through the body attached to albumin, lipids are transported in the circulation as a component of lipoprotein particles. A lipoprotein is a spherical particle consisting of a surface monolayer of phospholipids, apolipoproteins, and free cholesterol, and an inner core of triglycerides and cholesteryl esters. The phospholipids are arranged so that their hydrophilic heads are on the outside, allowing the lipoproteins to be dissolved in the circulation. Apolipoproteins, the protein component of lipoproteins, contribute to the regulation of lipoprotein metabolism as well as lipid emulsification. The functions of lipoproteins include maintaining lipid solubility and providing an efficient transport mechanism for lipids in the body.

Several classes of lipoproteins exist, characterized by the various amounts of triglycerides, cholesterol, phospholipids, and protein with which they are composed. The lipoproteins are commonly classified based on their density and are as follows: chylomicrons, VLDLs, low-density lipoproteins (LDLs), and high-density lipoproteins (HDLs). Individual lipoprotein class exerts differential physiological function in the body.

Chylomicrons are the largest of the lipoproteins and have the lowest density at 0.95 g/ml. As mentioned earlier, a major role of chylomicrons is to transport lipids originating from dietary sources from the small intestine to other tissues and ultimately to the liver. After triglycerides are deposited in peripheral tissues by the action of lipoprotein lipase, the chylomicron remnants are transferred to the liver, where they are endocytosed. As the remnant is hydrolytically degraded, the cholesterol released from the chylomicron regulates the rate of biosynthesis of cholesterol in the liver.

VLDLs, which have a density range of 0.95 to 1.006 g/ml, are produced in the liver and function as transporters for endogenous triglycerides and cholesterol to peripheral tissues.[28] The primary apolipoprotein constituents of VLDLs are apolipoproteins B-100, Cs, and E. Apolipoprotein E present in VLDL plays an important role in plasma lipoprotein metabolism through its high binding affinity to cell surface LDL receptors, which could reduce plasma VLDL and LDL concentration as well as the atherosclerotic process.[29]

After VLDL loses its triglyceride molecules by lipopoprotein lipase primarily in adipose and muscle tissues, the resulting smaller and denser particles become LDL. LDL particles contain a large quantity of cholesteryl esters, and the apolipoprotein constituent is mostly apolipoprotein B-100.[30] LDL particles are normally taken up by the liver and extrahepatic tissues, mainly by an LDL receptor-mediated endocytosis.[8] LDL receptors are cell surface glycoproteins and their primary function is to take up LDL particles from the circulation in response to cellular cholesterol status.[31] In doing so, they maintain cellular cholesterol homeostasis and modulate plasma LDL cholesterol concentrations, ultimately affecting atherogenesis. Once LDLs enter the tissues through these receptors, their components are hydrolyzed, producing cholesterol, amino acids, fatty acids, and phospholipids.

Of the lipoproteins, HDLs contain the highest amount of protein and make up approximately 20 to 30% of the total serum cholesterol. Though numerous apolipoproteins, including As, E, and Cs, are present in HDL particles, apolipoproteins A-I and A-II represent approximately 80 to 90% of the total apolipoprotein content of HDL. Two clinically defined fractions of HDL exist, i.e., HDL_2 and HDL_3, which have density ranges of 1.016 to 1.125 g/ml and 1.125 to 1.210 g/ml, respectively. Nascent HDL is produced mainly in the liver and intestine by the function of ABCA1, a cholesterol transport protein that plays a key role in cholesterol and phospholipid efflux.[32,33] Nascent HDL particles are short-lived in plasma, becoming mature HDL particles when they acquire cholesterol. Lecithin: cholesterol acyltransferase (LCAT) plays a critical role in esterifying free cholesterol from cells, particularly in the extrahepatic tissues, to cholesteryl ester. Numerous studies have shown that HDL protects against cardiovascular disease due, in part, to its participation in reverse cholesterol transport. In this process, excess cholesterol from extrahepatic tissues, including cells in the artery wall, is transported by HDL to the liver for excretion from the body.

2.4 FUNCTION AND EFFECT OF LIPIDS

2.4.1 FATS/SATURATED FATS AND PHYSICAL PERFORMANCE

The impact of fat intake on substrate utilization, exercise training, and performance depends on several factors, including time of ingestion and quantity of fat ingested. Consuming a diet higher in fat prior to exercise has been shown to enhance the body's capacity to oxidize fatty acid.[34] However, how diets affect a recovery period after exercise is also important when considering the efficacy of fat intake on physical performance.

Though the benefits of high carbohydrate intake before exercise are well documented, the benefit of a high-fat diet before exercise is not clearly understood. A high-fat/low-carbohydrate diet lowers glycogen stores in the liver and muscle, in part by increasing the utilization of fat stores for energy. While consuming a high-fat/low-carbohydrate diet for a short period of time (1 to 3 days) can actually decrease one's exercise endurance and capacity, a longer period of consumption (>7 days) may enhance fat oxidation during exercise, compensating for the reduced carbohydrate availability. Marked carbohydrate sparing occurs with a longer period of fat adaptation (5 days), with 1 day of carbohydrate intake for glucose normalization without any alteration in exercise performance.[35,36]

As previously mentioned, triglycerides may be stored within striated muscle cells, i.e., IMTG, and provide an important energy source for exercise. At the cellular level, muscle cells have machinery for esterification and hydrolysis of IMTG depending on cellular energy status. As in adipose tissue, when muscle cells have excess energy, fatty acids and glycerols are esterified to form triglycerides for storage, which can be used to supply energy when needed by the cells. Muscle contraction during exercise requires energy so that it triggers hydrolysis of triglycerides primarily by hormone-sensitive lipase, whose products are further metabolized to generate energy.

Given that IMTG is present in muscle cells, it has been presumed that it provides energy to the cells during exercise. However, the degree of contribution of IMTG to exercise as an energy source is still controversial.[37] Several factors, including exercise intensity, exercise duration, pre-exercise IMTG level, training status, and gender, can affect use of IMTG during exercise.[37] It is likely that IMTG is utilized during moderate-intensity exercise, whereas little or no IMTG is used during low- or high-intensity exercise. During moderate-intensity exercise such as continuous bicycling at 65% VO_2 peak, i.e., oxygen uptake peak, the whole-body IMTG oxidation rate reached maximum during the first hour and declined during the second hour of exercise.[38] IMTG content in the vastus lateralis muscle decreased at the first 2 hours of bicycle exercise at 60% VO_2 without further reduction for 2 hours.[39] These studies suggest that IMTG provides energy during an early stage of moderate exercise. Compared with men, IMTG appears to be quantitatively important for women during prolonged moderate-intensity exercise, partly due to higher basal IMTG levels in women than in men.[40]

Because of the potential role of IMTG as an energy source during exercise, replenishment by post-exercise nutrition, such as increased fat intake, has been explored. Studies have shown that high fat intake (35 to 57% of energy) replenishes IMTG stores faster than low fat intakes (10 to 24%) following prolonged exercise.[41,42] With a fat intake of 35% after exercise, IMTG recovery time is only 22 hours.[42] A concern exists for the adequacy of replacing glycogen stores by carbohydrate intake when fat intake is substantially increased. It is possible that post-exercise diets moderate in fat will be adequate for repletion of IMTG stores. Additional studies examining fat intake before and after exercise need to be performed to recommend an optimal fat intake to improve athletics' performance.

2.4.2 CHOLESTEROL AND PHYSICAL ACTIVITY

Physical activity has beneficial effects on both plasma HDL cholesterol and triglyceride concentrations as well as LDL and HDL particle size.[43] A meta-analysis on the effects of aerobic exercise on lipid profiles of adults at the age of 50 years and older reported that aerobic exercise increased plasma HDL cholesterol, creating a more favorable ratio of plasma total cholesterol to HDL cholesterol concentration.[44] The magnitude of increased plasma HDL cholesterol concentration following aerobic exercise training may partially depend on exercise intensity, frequency, duration of the individual exercise session, and the length of the training period. It is suggested that changes in plasma HDL cholesterol levels occur incrementally and reach statistical significance around a distance of 7 to 10 miles of moderate-intensity exercise per week, or equivalent to 1200 to 1600 kcal.[45] Resistance exercise has been shown to reduce plasma LDL cholesterol concentration.[43]

In addition to physical activity independently affecting plasma lipid levels, a combination of interventions, including diet and exercise regimens, has been shown to be effective at positively altering plasma lipid profiles. Decreased saturated fat intake and exercise incorporation induce complementary effects on plasma lipid levels, the combination of which shows a more optimal plasma lipid profile than either intervention alone.[46] The modification in dietary lipid intake complements the reduced levels of plasma HDL cholesterol and triglycerides often seen by an increase in physical activity. Therapies involving both a low-saturated-fat diet and exercise incorporation lowered plasma total cholesterol, LDL cholesterol, and triglyceride concentrations by 7 to 18, 7 to 15, and 4 to 18%, respectively, whereas plasma HDL cholesterol concentration was increased by 5 to 14%. Specifically, when diet alone, exercise alone, and a combination of diet and exercise were compared with the control, the diet group (total fat and saturated fat limited to 30 and 7%, respectively) showed the greatest reduction in total cholesterol (7.9%) and LDL cholesterol (7.3%), and the exercise group (trained three times per week for 60 minutes) showed the greatest increases in HDL cholesterol levels (2.3%) and total cholesterol levels (12.2%). The combination group with identically altered diet and exercise as the previous two groups showed favorable results within all four lipid groups.[47] The greatest plasma lipid-altering effects have been seen in long-term trials,[46] suggesting the significance of the length of treatment to obtain health benefits from diet and exercise intervention.

2.4.3 HEALTH EFFECTS OF FAT AND CHOLESTEROL ON DISEASES

2.4.3.1 Obesity and Diabetes

Obesity, often resulting from chronic excess of dietary energy, is strongly linked to both increased inflammatory status and type 2 diabetes.[48] Visceral obesity, dyslipidemia, and insulin resistance are all conditions that, when they occur simultaneously, comprise what is termed the metabolic syndrome, increasing the risk for both diabetes and cardiovascular disease. Weight loss has been shown to decrease insulin concentration and increase insulin sensitivity.[49]

Obesity can be influenced by a variety of factors, including genetics, metabolism, environment, and socioeconomic status. Obesity is positively correlated to excess energy intake and low levels of physical activity. In addition, both the degree of total fat consumption and the type of fat consumed play a role in obesity. Dietary fat intake is a significant predictor of sustained weight reduction and progression of type 2 diabetes in high-risk subjects.[50] Short-term studies suggest that very high intakes of fat (>35% of calories) may modify metabolism and potentially promote obesity.[51] Cross-cultural studies have also shown an increase in body mass index (BMI) in countries with higher intakes of fat.[52] In part, the dietary intake of both saturated and total fat is related to the risk of developing diabetes, primarily through its association with a higher BMI.[53] An upward trend in overweight has occurred since 1980, including an increase in adults 20 to 74 years of age who are obese, as well as an increase in overweight seen in children. The National Center of Health Statistics reports that the age-adjusted prevalence of overweight increased from 55.9% (1988 to 1994) to 65.1% (1999 to 2002) in adults.[54] During this same period, the prevalence of obesity (BMI of 30 or higher) also increased from 22.9% to 30.4%, while extreme obesity (BMI of 40.0 or higher) increased from 2.9% to 4.9%. Modest reductions in total fat intake are suggested to facilitate a decrease in caloric intake, leading to better weight control and potential improvement in metabolic syndrome.[55]

2.4.3.2 Coronary Heart Disease (CHD)

Atherosclerosis, the underlying pathological process of CHD, is characterized by an accumulation of plaque and fatty material within the intima of the coronary arteries, cerebral arteries, iliac and femoral arteries, and the aorta. It is the atherosclerotic development in the coronary arteries that leads to CHD and its manifestations. The deposition and buildup of cholesterol and inflammation create reduced blood flow to the heart and possible thrombosis, and are the principle causes of myocardial and cerebral infarction.

Of all cardiovascular diseases, CHD is the leading cause of death for both men and women in the U.S., causing one in five deaths in 2003. Approximately every 29 seconds someone in the U.S. suffers from a CHD-related event, and approximately every minute someone dies from such an event. In addition, it is predicted that 1.2 million Americans will have a new or recurrent coronary attack in 2006, and the estimated direct and indirect cost of CHD for 2006 is $142.5 billion. After the age of 40, the lifetime risk of having coronary heart disease is 49% for men and 32% for women.[56] Risks for CHD include both modifiable and nonmodifiable factors, including male gender, increasing age, overweight/obesity, saturated fat intake, and elevated plasma cholesterol levels.

One of the major risk factors for CHD is dyslipidemia, encompassing increases in plasma concentrations of total and LDL cholesterol, along with a decrease in HDL cholesterol concentration. A direct correlation exists between human deaths caused by CHD and plasma cholesterol concentrations.[57,58] In particular, a positive correlation between death from CHD and total cholesterol levels exceeding 200 mg/dl prompted the National Cholesterol Education Program to recommend serum cholesterol levels to remain at 200 mg/dl or lower for the general population. Two thirds of CHD-related mortality occurs in individuals who had plasma total cholesterol concentrations higher than 200 mg/dl when they were young adults.[58] Between the years of 1999 and 2002, 17% of adults at the age of 20 and more in the U.S. possessed high serum cholesterol levels of 240 mg/dl or higher.[54] Elevated plasma LDL cholesterol has been shown to play a major role in the formation of atherosclerotic plaque, making it a common target for prevention strategies.[59] According to the 2006 American Heart Association statistical update, approximately 40% of individuals in the U.S. have plasma LDL cholesterol concentrations greater than 130 mg/dl, above the recommendation for individuals with a moderate risk (two or more risk factors and a 10-year risk of developing CHD of <10%) or moderately high risk (two or more risk factors and a 10-year risk of developing CHD of 10 to 20%).[60] The risk of CHD falls as concentrations of plasma HDL cholesterol increase, especially to levels of >40 mg/dl.

Contrary to previous beliefs, altering the amount of cholesterol ingested has only a minor effect on total plasma cholesterol concentration in most people. A study performed on over 80,000 female nurses found that increasing cholesterol intake by 200 mg for every 1000 calories in the diet did not appreciably increase the risk for heart disease.[61] Because the body is well equipped with compensatory mechanisms to maintain cholesterol homeostasis, if a decrease in dietary cholesterol intake occurs, the biosynthesis of cholesterol increases, almost to a level to fully compensate for the decrease in cholesterol intake; in contrast, when body has excess cholesterol, cholesterol biosynthesis decreases with a concomitant increase in cholesterol excretion pathways through biliary cholesterol and bile acids.

Plasma cholesterol concentrations are more subject to regulation by dietary fat than dietary cholesterol. As previously noted, short-term studies indicate that very high intakes of fat (>35% of calories) may have the ability to modify metabolism and potentially promote obesity.[51] The Women's Health Initiative Dietary Modification Trial, a long-term dietary intervention study on approximately 49,000 women, was designed to investigate the effect of dietary intervention on the risk of cancer and CHD. The 8.1-year follow-up showed trends toward greater reductions in CHD risk, i.e., reduction in LDL cholesterol levels in individuals consuming lower intakes of saturated fat (2.9% decrease by year 6), but found nearly identical rates of heart attacks, strokes, and other forms of cardiovascular disease.[62] Findings from the study are similar to both the Nurses' Health Study and the Health Professionals Follow-Up Study, indicating no link between the overall percentage of calories from fat and several health outcomes, including cancer, heart disease, and weight gain.

A majority of saturated fatty acids appear to have a negative effect on plasma cholesterol profiles, i.e., increases in LDL cholesterol level and LDL:HDL ratio and a decrease in HDL cholesterol level, which can enhance the risk of CHD. Hypercholesterolemic effects of saturated fatty acids are attributed, in part, to their abilities to alter the secretion of bile acids, to regulate gene expression, to enhance LDL formation, and to inhibit the reverse cholesterol transport pathway by retarding the activity of lecithin:cholesterol acyltransferase, a plasma protein important for reverse cholesterol transport pathway. Therefore, recent clinical trials replacing saturated fatty acids with monounsaturated fatty acids showed an improvement in plasma lipid profiles, as well as beneficial effects on insulin sensitivity.[63–65] Decreasing saturated fat intake from 12% to 8% has been shown to decrease plasma LDL cholesterol by 5 to 7 mg/dl, based upon equations from Hegsted et al.[66] and Mensink and Katan.[67] While most of the saturated fatty acids, such as lauric (12:0), myristic (14:0), and palmitic (16:0) acids, are all considered hypercholesterolemic, researchers have shown that stearic acid (18:0) actually has a neutral or mild hypocholesterolemic effect on plasma total and LDL cholesterol.[68–73] In addition, 18:0 was as effective as 18:1 in lowering plasma cholesterol levels when it replaced 16:0 in the diet.[74]

2.4.3.3 Cancer

According to the American Cancer Society, little evidence currently exists that implicates cholesterol itself as causing the increased risk of certain cancers associated with eating foods from animal sources. In contrast to cholesterol, increased risk of cancer has been associated with the intake of saturated fats, with varying evidence in regard to the effect of total fat consumption on the risk of various cancers. However, diets high in fat are often correlated with those high in calories, potentially contributing to obesity and overweight, a risk factor linked to the incidence of multiple cancers such as pancreas, kidney, colon, and esophagus.[75,76]

A report of the National Cholesterol Education Program (NCEP) indicates that the percentage of total fat in the diet, independent of caloric intake, has not been documented to be related to cancer risk in the general population.[77] The Women's Health Initiative Dietary Modification Trial, involving approximately 49,000 subjects, showed that those exposed to dietary intervention including an 8.1% lower fat intake than the control group developed colon cancer at the same rate as the control.[78] As with colon cancer, the study showed similar rates of breast cancer risk in women eating a low-fat diet (8.1% decrease from comparison) and in those without diet modification. The Nurses' Health Study also reported no association between total fat intake or specific types of fat and breast cancer risk.[79] In contrast, a higher risk of prostate cancer progression is seen in men with a high fat intake, with fat of animal origin correlating to the highest risk of prostate cancer.[80,81]

Various clinical, experimental, and epidemiologic studies have suggested that colorectal cancer is related to diets high in total fat, protein, calories, alcohol, and meat, and low in calcium and folate. A literature search on dietary fat and breast cancer risk involving published articles from January 1990 through December 2003 found a positive association between increased total and saturated fat intake and the development of breast cancer.[82] The review acknowledges that not all epidemiological studies provided a strong positive association between dietary fat and breast cancer risk, but a moderate association does exist.[82,83]

Research has shown a correlation between saturated fat intake and cancer risk. A recent prospective cohort study performed by the European Prospective Investigation into Cancer project found no association between breast cancer and saturated fat intake measured by a food-frequency questionnaire, but when using a food diary, a daily intake of 35 g of saturated fat doubles the risk of breast cancer in comparison to women who had a daily intake of 10 g or less.[84] A greater intake of saturated fat may increase the risk of esophageal adenocarcinoma and distal stomach cancer.[85] In addition, a meta-analysis of the association between dietary fat intake and breast cancer found significant summary relative risks for saturated fat.[86]

While cholesterol intake is not correlated with cancer risk, intake of both fat and saturated fat has been implicated in the risk of cancer. In general, total fat intake may not be positively correlated with cancer risk, while saturated fat intake may possess a positive correlation with various cancers.

2.5 LIPID INTAKES

2.5.1 DIETARY SOURCES OF CHOLESTEROL AND FATS

Only food of animal origin contains cholesterol. Organ meats and egg yolks are especially high in cholesterol, with moderate levels in meat, seafood, poultry, dairy products, and animal fats. According to the U.S. Department of Agriculture National Nutrient Database Standard Reference, Release 17,[87] foods with the highest content of cholesterol per common measure, listed in descending order, are poultry giblets (419 to 641 mg/cup), beef liver (324 mg/3 oz), and one whole egg (245 mg/egg). Other foods considered high in cholesterol commonly eaten are shrimp and butter.

Dietary fat can be found in nearly all foods in varying amounts. Individual foods with high amounts of fat per common measure include all oils, meats such as pork and duck, nuts, and cheeses.[87] Saturated fat, similar to cholesterol, mainly comes from animal sources. Foods with high amounts of saturated fat are red meat, poultry, butter, and whole milk. In addition to animal food sources, tropical oils such as coconut and palm kernel oil also contain considerable amounts of saturated fat, approximately 87 and 50% of total fatty acids, respectively. As for individual fatty acids, butyric acid (4:0) is contained in butter, lauric acid (12:0) in coconut oil, palm oil, and cocoa butter, myristic acid (14:0) in cow's milk and dairy products, and palmitic acid (16:0) and stearic acid (18:0) in meat.

2.5.2 COMMON FAT INTAKES

From 1971 to 2000, an increase in mean energy intake of calories, with a decrease in the mean percentage of calories from total fat and saturated fat, has occurred in the U.S. In the 1999 to 2000 National Health and Nutrition Examination Survey (NHANES), the daily mean percentage of calories from total fat and the percentage of calories from saturated fat were decreased from 36.9% to 32.8% and 13–13.5% to 11%, respectively, compared with those in 1971 to 1974.[88] While a decrease in the percentage of total fat and saturated fat consumed was seen between 1971 and 2000, when total fat intake was assessed, the absolute level of fat intake actually increased from the time periods 1989–1991 (73.4 g) to 1994–1996 (76.4 g).[89]

Mean dietary cholesterol levels declined from the 1970s to 1988–1994, leveling off between 1988–1994 and 1999–2000. For adults aged 20 to 74, mean dietary cholesterol intake decreased from 487 to 341 mg in men and 313 to 242 mg in women.[90] Possible reasons for this decrease include improved measurements of the cholesterol content of foods and a decreased consumption of whole eggs.[91]

2.5.3 RECOMMENDED FAT INTAKES

2.5.3.1 Adults

In 2002, the Institute of Medicine (IOM) of the National Academies released new dietary reference intakes for fat and cholesterol.[92] The IOM recommends cholesterol intake to be as low as possible within a nutritionally adequate diet. Specifically, it recommends an intake of less than 300 mg of dietary cholesterol when plasma LDL cholesterol is <130 mg/dl, and an intake of less than 200 mg/dl when plasma LDL cholesterol is greater than or equal to 130 mg/dl. This is supported by the NCEP Expert Panel, recommending that less than 200 mg of cholesterol per day be consumed as a part of the Therapeutic Lifestyle Changes (TLC) diet to achieve maximal plasma LDL cholesterol lowering.[51]

For adults, based on the Acceptable Macronutrient Distribution Range, the IOM recommends a range of 20 to 35% of total calorie intake to be ingested as fat. Low intake of fats may increase the risk of inadequate intakes of essential fatty acids such as linoleic acid and α-linolenic acid, and vitamin E. In addition, low-dietary-fat intake may have a potential adverse affect on lipid profiles due to increased carbohydrate intake often associated with low-fat diets.[93] Therefore, the NCEP recommends a lower limit of 25% for individuals with elevated plasma cholesterol concentrations, established cardiovascular disease, and more than one major risk factor. On the other hand, an upper level intake of total fat, i.e., approximately 35% of total calories, is associated with increased calorie and saturated fat intake. In individuals with lipid or metabolic disorders, total fat intakes should not be extreme because very high levels of fat intake could aggravate lipid and nonlipid risk factors common in metabolic syndrome.

Due to the dose–response relationship between saturated fat and plasma LDL cholesterol levels, the IOM recommends saturated fat consumption to be as low as possible, while maintaining the recommended 20 to 35% of total calories from fat. More specifically, adults with plasma LDL cholesterol concentrations below 130 mg/dl should consume less than 10% of calories from saturated fat, while adults with elevated LDL cholesterol (greater than or equal to 130 mg/dl) should consume less than 7% of their total calories from saturated fat.[92] As previously mentioned, not all saturated fat raises plasma LDL cholesterol levels, exemplified by stearic acid (18:0) exerting a neutral or hypocholesterolemic effect. Despite strong evidence that individual fatty acids have independent effects on plasma cholesterol levels, no recommendations for individual fatty acid consumption have been made.

Only 20% of approximately 14,000 individuals with hypercholesterolemia reported intakes of fat, saturated fat, and cholesterol consistent with the NCEP guidelines.[94] Therefore, while the recommended intakes of total fat, saturated fat, and cholesterol are nearly identical among expert groups, a potential disparity exists between expert recommendations and population compliance. It is necessary to continue with public education to increase their compliance to the dietary recommendation.

2.5.3.2 Adult Athletes

The recommended intakes of total fat, saturated fat, and cholesterol are the same for both power and endurance athletes as they are for nonathletes. As previously discussed, differing levels of fat intake can have modest effects on energy sources utilized during exercise. Overall, recommendations for fat, saturated fat, and cholesterol specific for sports nutrition do not differ from those recommended to the general population.

2.6 SUMMARY

Dietary sources of fat and cholesterol are well established and their digestion and metabolism is a complex process. Fatty acid metabolism may be altered by energy status and exercise training. While cholesterol intake does not reflect exercise training or performance, studies indicate that fat ingestion pre- and post-exercise may increase IMTG stores and enhance fatty acid oxidation. IMTG stores play a role in energy availability during exercise, and altering fat intake pre- and post-exercise may affect IMTG stores.

The effects of total fats, saturated fats, and cholesterol on health and disease have been well documented. While increased amounts of total fat and saturated fat in the diet have largely shown to be detrimental to personal health, i.e., increased risk of coronary heart disease, some contradicting evidence exists concerning their impact on certain diseases, such as various cancers. Plasma cholesterol levels have been positively correlated with the risk of coronary heart disease, as well as diabetes.

Despite this correlation, it is the intake of saturated fat that has an unfavorable effect on plasma cholesterol.

The recommended intakes of total fat, saturated fat, and cholesterol have been established and were recently addressed by the IOM. Recommended intakes of total fat, saturated fat, and cholesterol mirror those of the general population. Further research is warranted before definitive recommendations are made concerning the effect of total fat, saturated fat, and cholesterol intake on exercise and physical performance.

REFERENCES

1. Thomson, A.B., Schoeller, C., Keelan, M., Smith, L., and Clandinin, M.T., Lipid absorption: passing through the unstirred layers, brush-border membrane, and beyond. *Can. J. Physiol. Pharmacol.* 71, 531–555, 1993.
2. Mozaffarian, D., Katan, M.B., Ascherio, A., Stampfer, M.J., and Willett, W.C., Trans fatty acids and cardiovascular disease. *N. Engl. J. Med.* 354, 1601–1613, 2006.
3. Subbiah, M.T. and Kuksis, A., Differences in metabolism of cholesterol and sitosterol following intravenous injection in rats. *Biochim. Biophys. Acta* 306, 95–105, 1973.
4. Kritchevsky, D., Phytosterols. *Adv. Exp. Med. Biol.* 427, 235–243, 1997.
5. Ostlund, R.E., Jr., Phytosterols in human nutrition. *Annu. Rev. Nutr.* 22, 533–549, 2002.
6. Farkkila, M. and Miettinen, T.A., Lipid metabolism in bile acid malabsorption. *Ann. Med.* 22, 5–13, 1990.
7. Havel, R.J., Lipid transport function of lipoproteins in blood plasma. *Am. J. Physiol.* 253, E1–E5, 1987.
8. Salter, A.M. and Brindley, D.N., The biochemistry of lipoproteins. *J. Inherit. Metab Dis.* 11 (Suppl. 1), 4–17, 1988.
9. van Loon, L.J., Use of intramuscular triacylglycerol as a substrate source during exercise in humans. *J. Appl. Physiol.* 97, 1170–1187, 2004.
10. Hui, T.Y. and Bernlohr, D.A., Fatty acid transporters in animal cells. *Front Biosci.* 2, d222–d231, 1997.
11. Jeukendrup, A.E., Saris, W.H., and Wagenmakers, A.J., Fat metabolism during exercise: a review. Part II. Regulation of metabolism and the effects of training. *Int. J. Sports Med.* 19, 293–302, 1998.
12. Wolfe, R.R., Metabolic interactions between glucose and fatty acids in humans. *Am. J. Clin. Nutr.* 67, 519S–526S, 1998.
13. Grundy, S.M., Absorption and metabolism of dietary cholesterol. *Annu. Rev. Nutr.* 3, 71–96, 1983.
14. Wilson, M.D. and Rudel, L.L., Review of cholesterol absorption with emphasis on dietary and biliary cholesterol. *J. Lipid Res.* 35, 943–955, 1994.
15. Spady, D.K., Woollett, L.A., and Dietschy, J.M., Regulation of plasma LDL-cholesterol levels by dietary cholesterol and fatty acids. *Annu. Rev. Nutr.* 13, 355–381, 1993.
16. Ferezou, J., Rautureau, J., Coste, T., Gouffier, E., and Chevallier, F., Cholesterol turnover in human plasma lipoproteins: studies with stable and radioactive isotopes. *Am. J. Clin. Nutr.* 36, 235–244, 1982.
17. Jackson, B., Gee, A.N., Martinez-Cayuela, M., and Suckling, K.E., The effects of feeding a saturated fat-rich diet on enzymes of cholesterol metabolism in the liver, intestine and aorta of the hamster. *Biochim. Biophys. Acta* 1045, 21–28, 1990.

18. Hua, X., Sakai, J., Ho, Y.K., Goldstein, J.L., and Brown, M.S., Hairpin orientation of sterol regulatory element-binding protein-2 in cell membranes as determined by protease protection. *J Biol Chem* 270, 29422–29427, 1995.
19. Quintao, E., Grundy, S.M., and Ahrens, E.H., Jr., An evaluation of four methods for measuring cholesterol absorption by the intestine in man. *J. Lipid Res.* 12, 221–232, 1971.
20. Connor, W.E. and Lin, D.S., The intestinal absorption of dietary cholesterol by hypercholesterolemic (type II) and normocholesterolemic humans. *J. Clin. Invest.* 53, 1062–1070, 1974.
21. Khallou, J., Riottot, M., Parquet, M., Verneau, C., and Lutton, C., Biodynamics of cholesterol and bile acids in the lithiasic hamster. *Br. J. Nutr.* 66, 479–492, 1991.
22. Bhattacharyya, A.K., Factors regulating plasma cholesterol concentration. *Artery* 16, 84–89, 1989.
23. Yu, L., Hammer, R.E., Li-Hawkins, J., Von Bergmann, K., Lutjohann, D., Cohen, J.C., and Hobbs, H.H., Disruption of Abcg5 and Abcg8 in mice reveals their crucial role in biliary cholesterol secretion. *Proc. Natl. Acad. Sci. U.S.A.* 99, 16237–16242, 2002.
24. Yu, L., Li-Hawkins, J., Hammer, R.E., Berge, K.E., Horton, J.D., Cohen, J.C., and Hobbs, H.H., Overexpression of ABCG5 and ABCG8 promotes biliary cholesterol secretion and reduces fractional absorption of dietary cholesterol. *J. Clin. Invest.* 110, 671–680, 2002.
25. Hui, D.Y. and Howles, P.N., Molecular mechanisms of cholesterol absorption and transport in the intestine. *Semin. Cell Dev. Biol.* 16, 183–192, 2005.
26. Kesaniemi, Y.A. and Miettinen, T.A., Cholesterol absorption efficiency regulates plasma cholesterol level in the Finnish population. *Eur. J. Clin. Invest.* 17, 391–395, 1987.
27. Davis, H.R., Jr., Zhu, L.J., Hoos, L.M., Tetzloff, G., Maguire, M., Liu, J., Yao, X., Iyer, S.P., Lam, M.H., Lund, E.G., Detmers, P.A., Graziano, M.P., and Altmann, S.W., Niemann-Pick C1 Like 1 (NPC1L1) is the intestinal phytosterol and cholesterol transporter and a key modulator of whole-body cholesterol homeostasis. *J. Biol. Chem.* 279, 33586–33592, 2004.
28. Miller, N.E., Hammett, F., Saltissi, S., Rao, S., van Zeller, H., Coltart, J., and Lewis, B., Relation of angiographically defined coronary artery disease to plasma lipoprotein subfractions and apolipoproteins. *Br. Med. J. (Clin. Res. Ed.)* 282, 1741–1744, 1981.
29. Yamada, N., Shimano, H., and Yazaki, Y., Role of apolipoprotein E in lipoprotein metabolism and in the process of atherosclerosis. *J. Atheroscler. Thromb.* 2 (Suppl. 1), S29–S33, 1995.
30. Dixon, J.L. and Ginsberg, H.N., Regulation of hepatic secretion of apolipoprotein B-containing lipoproteins: information obtained from cultured liver cells. *J. Lipid Res.* 34, 167–179, 1993.
31. Schneider, W.J., Beisiegel, U., Goldstein, J.L., and Brown, M.S., Purification of the low density lipoprotein receptor, an acidic glycoprotein of 164,000 molecular weight. *J. Biol. Chem.* 257, 2664–2673, 1982.
32. Brunham, L.R., Kruit, J.K., Iqbal, J., Fievet, C., Timmins, J.M., Pape, T.D., Coburn, B.A., Bissada, N., Staels, B., Groen, A.K., Hussain, M.M., Parks, J.S., Kuipers, F., and Hayden, M.R., Intestinal ABCA1 directly contributes to HDL biogenesis *in vivo*. *J. Clin. Invest.* 116, 1052–1062, 2006.

33. Timmins, J.M., Lee, J.Y., Boudyguina, E., Kluckman, K.D., Brunham, L.R., Mulya, A., Gebre, A.K., Coutinho, J.M., Colvin, P.L., Smith, T.L., Hayden, M.R., Maeda, N., and Parks, J.S., Targeted inactivation of hepatic Abca1 causes profound hypoalphalipoproteinemia and kidney hypercatabolism of apoA-I. *J. Clin. Invest.* 115, 1333–1342, 2005.

34. Burke, L.M., Hawley, J.A., Angus, D.J., Cox, G.R., Clark, S.A., Cummings, N.K., Desbrow, B., and Hargreaves, M., Adaptations to short-term high-fat diet persist during exercise despite high carbohydrate availability. *Med. Sci. Sports Exerc.* 34, 83–91, 2002.

35. Burke, L.M., Hawley, J.A., Angus, D.J., Cox, G.R., Clark, S.A., Cummings, N.K., Desbrow, B., and Hargreaves, M., Adaptations to short-term high-fat diet persist during exercise despite high carbohydrate availability. *Med. Sci. Sports Exerc.* 34, 83–91, 2002.

36. Carey, A.L., Staudacher, H.M., Cummings, N.K., Stepto, N.K., Nikolopoulos, V., Burke, L.M., and Hawley, J.A., Effects of fat adaptation and carbohydrate restoration on prolonged endurance exercise. *J. Appl. Physiol.* 91, 115–122, 2001.

37. Roepstorff, C., Vistisen, B., and Kiens, B., Intramuscular triacylglycerol in energy metabolism during exercise in humans. *Exerc. Sport Sci. Rev.* 33, 182–188, 2005.

38. Romijn, J.A., Coyle, E.F., Sidossis, L.S., Gastaldelli, A., Horowitz, J.F., Endert, E., and Wolfe, R.R., Regulation of endogenous fat and carbohydrate metabolism in relation to exercise intensity and duration. *Am. J. Physiol.* 265, E380–E391, 1993.

39. Watt, M.J., Heigenhauser, G.J., Dyck, D.J., and Spriet, L.L., Intramuscular triacylglycerol, glycogen and acetyl group metabolism during 4 h of moderate exercise in man. *J. Physiol.* 541, 969–978, 2002.

40. Steffensen, C.H., Roepstorff, C., Madsen, M., and Kiens, B., Myocellular triacylglycerol breakdown in females but not in males during exercise. *Am. J. Physiol. Endocrinol. Metab.* 282, E634–E642, 2002.

41. Decombaz, J., Schmitt, B., Ith, M., Decarli, B., Diem, P., Kreis, R., Hoppeler, H., and Boesch, C., Postexercise fat intake repletes intramyocellular lipids but no faster in trained than in sedentary subjects. *Am. J. Physiol. Regul. Integr. Comp. Physiol.* 281, R760–R769, 2001.

42. van Loon, L.J., Koopman, R., Stegen, J.H., Wagenmakers, A.J., Keizer, H.A., and Saris, W.H., Intramyocellular lipids form an important substrate source during moderate intensity exercise in endurance-trained males in a fasted state. *J. Physiol.* 553, 611–625, 2003.

43. Szapary, P.O., Bloedon, L.T., and Foster, G.D., Physical activity and its effects on lipids. *Curr. Cardiol. Rep.* 5, 488–492, 2003.

44. Kelley, G.A., Kelley, K.S., and Tran, Z.V., Exercise, lipids, and lipoproteins in older adults: a meta-analysis. *Prev. Cardiol.* 8, 206–214, 2005.

45. Kokkinos, P.F. and Fernhall, B., Physical activity and high density lipoprotein cholesterol levels: what is the relationship? *Sports Med.* 28, 307–314, 1999.

46. Varady, K.A. and Jones, P.J., Combination diet and exercise interventions for the treatment of dyslipidemia: an effective preliminary strategy to lower cholesterol levels? *J. Nutr.* 135, 1829–1835, 2005.

47. Stefanick, M.L., Mackey, S., Sheehan, M., Ellsworth, N., Haskell, W.L., and Wood, P.D., Effects of diet and exercise in men and postmenopausal women with low levels of HDL cholesterol and high levels of LDL cholesterol. *N. Engl. J. Med.* 339, 12–20, 1998.

48. Browning, L.M. and Jebb, S.A., Nutritional influences on inflammation and type 2 diabetes risk. *Diabetes Technol. Ther.* 8, 45–54, 2006.
49. Potteiger, J.A., Jacobsen, D.J., Donnelly, J.E., and Hill, J.O., Glucose and insulin responses following 16 months of exercise training in overweight adults: the Midwest Exercise Trial. *Metabolism* 52, 1175–1181, 2003.
50. Lindstrom, J., Peltonen, M., Eriksson, J.G., Louheranta, A., Fogelholm, M., Uusitupa, M., and Tuomilehto, J., High-fibre, low-fat diet predicts long-term weight loss and decreased type 2 diabetes risk: the Finnish Diabetes Prevention Study. *Diabetologia* 49, 912–920, 2006.
51. Third Report of the National Cholesterol Education Program (NCEP) Expert Panel on Detection, Evaluation, and Treatment of High Blood Cholesterol in Adults (Adult Treatment Panel III), final report. *Circulation* 106, 3143–3421, 2002.
52. Bray, G.A. and Popkin, B.M., Dietary fat intake does affect obesity! *Am. J. Clin. Nutr.* 68, 1157–1173, 1998.
53. van Dam, R.M., Willett, W.C., Rimm, E.B., Stampfer, M.J., and Hu, F.B., Dietary fat and meat intake in relation to risk of type 2 diabetes in men. *Diabetes Care* 25, 417–424, 2002.
54. National Center for Health Statistics, Health, United States. DHHS Publication 2004-1232. 2004.
55. Grundy, S.M., Abate, N., and Chandalia, M., Diet composition and the metabolic syndrome: what is the optimal fat intake? *Am. J. Med.* 113 (Suppl. 9B), 25S–29S, 2002.
56. Thom, T., Haase, N., Rosamond, W., Howard, V.J., Rumsfeld, J., Manolio, T., Zheng, Z.J., Flegal, K., O'Donnell, C., Kittner, S., Lloyd-Jones, D., Goff, D.C., Jr., Hong, Y., Members of the Statistics Committee and Stroke Statistics Subcommittee, Adams, R., Friday, G., Furie, K., Gorelick, P., Kissela, B., Marler, J., Meigs, J., Roger, V., Sidney, S., Sorlie, P., Steinberger, J., Wasserthiel-Smoller, S., Wilson, M., and Wolf, P., Heart disease and stroke statistics — 2006 update: a report from the American Heart Association Statistics Committee and Stroke Statistics Subcommittee. *Circulation* 113, e85–e151, 2006.
57. Kjelsberg, M.O., Cutler, J.A., and Dolecek, T.A., Brief description of the Multiple Risk Factor Intervention Trial. *Am. J. Clin. Nutr.* 65, 191S–195S, 1997.
58. Stamler, J., Daviglus, M.L., Garside, D.B., Dyer, A.R., Greenland, P., and Neaton, J.D., Relationship of baseline serum cholesterol levels in 3 large cohorts of younger men to long-term coronary, cardiovascular, and all-cause mortality and to longevity. *JAMA* 284, 311–318, 2000.
59. Grundy, S.M., Primary prevention of coronary heart disease: selection of patients for aggressive cholesterol management. *Am. J. Med.* 107, 2S–6S, 1999.
60. Grundy, S.M., Cleeman, J.I., Merz, C.N., Brewer, H.B., Jr., Clark, L.T., Hunninghake, D.B., Pasternak, R.C., Smith, S.C., Jr., and Stone, N.J., Implications of recent clinical trials for the National Cholesterol Education Program Adult Treatment Panel III guidelines. *Circulation* 110, 227–239, 2004.
61. Hu, F.B., Stampfer, M.J., Rimm, E.B., Manson, J.E., Ascherio, A., Colditz, G.A., Rosner, B.A., Spiegelman, D., Speizer, F.E., Sacks, F.M., Hennekens, C.H., and Willett, W.C., A prospective study of egg consumption and risk of cardiovascular disease in men and women. *JAMA* 281, 1387–1394, 1999.

62. Howard, B.V., Van Horn, L., Hsia, J., Manson, J.E., Stefanick, M.L., Wassertheil-Smoller, S., Kuller, L.H., LaCroix, A.Z., Langer, R.D., Lasser, N.L., Lewis, C.E., Limacher, M.C., Margolis, K.L., Mysiw, W.J., Ockene, J.K., Parker, L.M., Perri, M.G., Phillips, L., Prentice, R.L., Robbins, J., Rossouw, J.E., Sarto, G.E., Schatz, I.J., Snetselaar, L.G., Stevens, V.J., Tinker, L.F., Trevisan, M., Vitolins, M.Z., Anderson, G.L., Assaf, A.R., Bassford, T., Beresford, S.A., Black, H.R., Brunner, R.L., Brzyski, R.G., Caan, B., Chlebowski, R.T., Gass, M., Granek, I., Greenland, P., Hays, J., Heber, D., Heiss, G., Hendrix, S.L., Hubbell, F.A., Johnson, K.C., and Kotchen, J.M., Low-fat dietary pattern and risk of cardiovascular disease: the Women's Health Initiative Randomized Controlled Dietary Modification Trial. *JAMA* 295, 655–666, 2006.
63. Lovejoy, J.C., Smith, S.R., Champagne, C.M., Most, M.M., Lefevre, M., DeLany, J.P., Denkins, Y.M., Rood, J.C., Veldhuis, J., and Bray, G.A., Effects of diets enriched in saturated (palmitic), monounsaturated (oleic), or trans (elaidic) fatty acids on insulin sensitivity and substrate oxidation in healthy adults. *Diabetes Care* 25, 1283–1288, 2002.
64. Perez-Jimenez, F., Lopez-Miranda, J., Pinillos, M.D., Gomez, P., Paz-Rojas, E., Montilla, P., Marin, C., Velasco, M.J., Blanco-Molina, A., Jimenez Pereperez, J.A., and Ordovas, J.M., A Mediterranean and a high-carbohydrate diet improve glucose metabolism in healthy young persons. *Diabetologia* 44, 2038–2043, 2001.
65. Vessby, B., Unsitupa, M., Hermansen, K., Riccardi, G., Rivellese, A.A., Tapsell, L.C., Nalsen, C., Berglund, L., Louheranta, A., Rasmussen, B.M., Calvert, G.D., Maffetone, A., Pedersen, E., Gustafsson, I.B., and Storlien, L.H., Substituting dietary saturated for monounsaturated fat impairs insulin sensitivity in healthy men and women: the KANWU Study. *Diabetologia* 44, 312–319, 2001.
66. Hegsted, D.M., Ausman, L.M., Johnson, J.A., and Dallal, G.E., Dietary fat and serum lipids: an evaluation of the experimental data. *Am. J. Clin. Nutr.* 57, 875–883, 1993.
67. Mensink, R.P. and Katan, M.B., Effect of dietary fatty acids on serum lipids and lipoproteins. A meta-analysis of 27 trials. *Arterioscler. Thromb.* 12, 911–919, 1992.
68. Ahrens, E.H., Jr., Insull, W., Jr., Blomstrand, R., Hirsch, J., Tsaltas, T.T., and Peterson, M.L., The influence of dietary fats on serum-lipid levels in man. *Lancet* 272, 943–953, 1957.
69. Hegsted, D.M., McGandy, R.B., Myers, M.L., and Stare, F.J., Quantitative effects of dietary fat on serum cholesterol in man. *Am. J. Clin. Nutr.* 17, 281–295, 1965.
70. Keys, A., Effects of different dietary fats on plasma-lipid levels. *Lancet* 17, 318–319, 1965.
71. Grundy, S.M. and Mok, H.Y., Determination of cholesterol absorption in man by intestinal perfusion. *J. Lipid Res.* 18, 263–271, 1977.
72. Grundy, S.M., Influence of stearic acid on cholesterol metabolism relative to other long-chain fatty acids. *Am. J. Clin. Nutr.* 60, 986S–990S, 1994.
73. Hassel, C.A., Mensing, E.A., and Gallaher, D.D., Dietary stearic acid reduces plasma and hepatic cholesterol concentrations without increasing bile acid excretion in cholesterol-fed hamsters. *J. Nutr.* 127, 1148–1155, 1997.
74. Bonanome, A. and Grundy, S.M., Effect of dietary stearic acid on plasma cholesterol and lipoprotein levels. *N. Engl. J. Med.* 318, 1244–1248, 1988.
75. Lagergren, J., Controversies surrounding body mass, reflux, and risk of oesophageal adenocarcinoma. *Lancet Oncol.* 7, 347–349, 2006.
76. Morita, T., Tabata, S., Mineshita, M., Mizoue, T., Moore, M.A., and Kono, S., The metabolic syndrome is associated with increased risk of colorectal adenoma development: the Self-Defense Forces health study. *Asian Pac. J. Cancer Prev.* 6, 485–489, 2005.

77. Third Report of the National Cholesterol Education Program (NCEP) Expert Panel on Detection, Evaluation, and Treatment of High Blood Cholesterol in Adults (Adult Treatment Panel III), final report. *Circulation* 106, 3143, 2002.

78. Beresford, S.A., Johnson, K.C., Ritenbaugh, C., Lasser, N.L., Snetselaar, L.G., Black, H.R., Anderson, G.L., Assaf, A.R., Bassford, T., Bowen, D., Brunner, R.L., Brzyski, R.G., Caan, B., Chlebowski, R.T., Gass, M., Harrigan, R.C., Hays, J., Heber, D., Heiss, G., Hendrix, S.L., Howard, B.V., Hsia, J., Hubbell, F.A., Jackson, R.D., Kotchen, J.M., Kuller, L.H., LaCroix, A.Z., Lane, D.S., Langer, R.D., Lewis, C.E., Manson, J.E., Margolis, K.L., Mossavar-Rahmani, Y., Ockene, J.K., Parker, L.M., Perri, M.G., Phillips, L., Prentice, R.L., Robbins, J., Rossouw, J.E., Sarto, G.E., Stefanick, M.L., Van Horn, L., Vitolins, M.Z., Wactawski-Wende, J., Wallace, R.B., and Whitlock, E., Low-fat dietary pattern and risk of colorectal cancer: the Women's Health Initiative Randomized Controlled Dietary Modification Trial. *JAMA* 295, 643–654, 2006.

79. Holmes, M.D., Hunter, D.J., Colditz, G.A., Stampfer, M.J., Hankinson, S.E., Speizer, F.E., Rosner, B., and Willett, W.C., Association of dietary intake of fat and fatty acids with risk of breast cancer. *JAMA* 281, 914–920, 1999.

80. Whittemore, A.S., Kolonel, L.N., Wu, A.H., John, E.M., Gallagher, R.P., Howe, G.R., Burch, J.D., Hankin, J., Dreon, D.M., and West, D.W., Prostate cancer in relation to diet, physical activity, and body size in blacks, whites, and Asians in the United States and Canada. *J. Natl. Cancer Inst.* 87, 652–661, 1995.

81. Optenberg, S.A., Thompson, I.M., Friedrichs, P., Wojcik, B., Stein, C.R., and Kramer, B., Race, treatment, and long-term survival from prostate cancer in an equal-access medical care delivery system. *JAMA* 274, 1599–1605, 1995.

82. Binukumar, B. and Mathew, A., Dietary fat and risk of breast cancer. *World J. Surg. Oncol.* 3, 45, 2005.

83. Prentice, R.L., Caan, B., Chlebowski, R.T., Patterson, R., Kuller, L.H., Ockene, J.K., Margolis, K.L., Limacher, M.C., Manson, J.E., Parker, L.M., Paskett, E., Phillips, L., Robbins, J., Rossouw, J.E., Sarto, G.E., Shikany, J.M., Stefanick, M.L., Thomson, C.A., Van Horn, L., Vitolins, M.Z., Wactawski-Wende, J., Wallace, R.B., Wassertheil-Smoller, S., Whitlock, E., Yano, K., Adams-Campbell, L., Anderson, G.L., Assaf, A.R., Beresford, S.A., Black, H.R., Brunner, R.L., Brzyski, R.G., Ford, L., Gass, M., Hays, J., Heber, D., Heiss, G., Hendrix, S.L., Hsia, J., Hubbell, F.A., Jackson, R.D., Johnson, K.C., Kotchen, J.M., LaCroix, A.Z., Lane, D.S., Langer, R.D., Lasser, N.L., and Henderson, M.M., Low-fat dietary pattern and risk of invasive breast cancer: the Women's Health Initiative Randomized Controlled Dietary Modification Trial. *JAMA* 295, 629–642, 2006.

84. Gonzalez, C.A., The European Prospective Investigation into Cancer and Nutrition (EPIC). *Public Health Nutr.* 9, 124–126, 2006.

85. Chen, H., Tucker, K.L., Graubard, B.I., Heineman, E.F., Markin, R.S., Potischman, N.A., Russell, R.M., Weisenburger, D.D., and Ward, M.H., Nutrient intakes and adenocarcinoma of the esophagus and distal stomach. *Nutr. Cancer* 42, 33–40, 2002.

86. Boyd, N.F., Stone, J., Vogt, K.N., Connelly, B.S., Martin, L.J., and Minkin, S., Dietary fat and breast cancer risk revisited: a meta-analysis of the published literature. *Br. J. Cancer* 89, 1672–1685, 2003.

87. U.S. Department of Agriculture National Nutrient Database Standard Reference, Release 17. http://www.nal.usda.gov/fnic/foodcomp/Data/SR17/sr17.html. Accessed April 25, 2006.

88. Briefel, R.R. and Johnson, C.L., Secular trends in dietary intake in the United States. *Annu. Rev. Nutr.* 24, 401–431, 2004.

89. Chanmugam, P., Guthrie, J.F., Cecilio, S., Morton, J.F., Basiotis, P.P., and Anand, R., Did fat intake in the United States really decline between 1989–1991 and 1994–1996? *J. Am. Diet. Assoc.* 103, 867–872, 2003.

90. Wright, J.D., Want, C.-Y., Kennedy-Stephenson, J., and Ervin, R.B., Dietary intake of ten key nutrients for public health, United States: 1999–2000. *Vital Health Statistics*, 334, 1–4, 2003.

91. Enns, C.W., Goldman, J.D., and Cook, A., Trends in food and nutrient intake by adults: NFCS 1977–78, CSFII 1989–91. *Family Econ. Nutr. Rev.* 10, 2–15, 1997.

92. Dietary Reference Intakes for Energy, Carbohydrate, Fiber, Fat, Fatty Acids, Cholesterol, Protein, and Amino Acids. http://www.iom.edu/CMS/3788/4576/4340.aspx. Accessed May 1, 2006.

93. Mamo, J.C., James, A.P., Soares, M.J., Purcell, K., Griffiths, D., and Schwenke, J.L., Carbohydrate rich diets exacerbate postprandial lipaemia in moderately dyslipidemic subjects, whereas red meat protein-enriched diets have no adverse effects. *Asia Pac. J. Clin. Nutr.* 13, S52, 2004.

94. Hsia, J., Rodabough, R., Rosal, M.C., Cochrane, B., Howard, B.V., Snetselaar, L., Frishman, W.H., and Stefanick, M.L., Compliance with National Cholesterol Education Program dietary and lifestyle guidelines among older women with self-reported hypercholesterolemia. The Women's Health Initiative. *Am. J. Med.* 113, 384–392, 2002.

3 Medium-Chain Triglycerides

Wayne E. Billon

CONTENTS

3.1 INTRODUCTION

In a brief discussion that appeared in the Mayo Clinic Bulletin, Dr. Wilder reported on progress made by Dr. Geyelin in preventing epileptic seizures by prolonged fasting. Dr. Wilder suggested that the positive results may not have been the fast itself, but the resulting ketonemia that occurs from fasting. He mentioned that "as has long been known, it is possible to provoke ketogenesis by feeding diets which are very rich in fat and very low in carbohydrate." This article appeared in 1921.[1] The promotion of ketogenic diets, by reason of consumption of high fat and low carbohydrate, are nothing new. When medium-chain triglycerides (MCTGs) were recognized as dietary components that promoted ketosis, they were incorporated into the ketogenic diet. MCTGs have been used effectively for years, orally and in tube feedings, for the treatment of malabsorption syndromes or wasting disease syndromes.[2–4]

The purpose of this chapter is to provide a brief description of the digestion, absorption, and metabolism of MCTGs, their similarities and differences with long-chain triglycerides (LCTGs), the dietary sources of MCTGs, and a review of human studies on the usefulness of MCTGs as an ergogenic aid.

3.2   OVERVIEW OF METABOLISM

3.2.1   CHEMICAL AND PHYSICAL PROPERTIES

Fatty acids (FAs) consist of a carbon chain of varying lengths with a hydrocarbon tail and a carboxyl group for a head. Upon ionization of the carboxyl group, a negative charge is created. By means of an ester bond, an FA is attached to a molecule of glycerol forming a molecule of water and a monoglyceride. A triglyceride (TG) consists of three FAs attached to a molecule of glycerol by means of ester bonding. FAs can be classified according to the number of carbons they contain (chain length), their level of saturation (number of double bonds), or the orientation of their double bonds (omega 3, omega 6, or omega 9). FAs can be short-chain (SCFA), medium-chain (MCFA), or long-chain (LCFA). The chain length, number of double bonds, and location of the double bonds determine the biological activity and physical characteristics of FAs and ultimately of TGs. A TG does not have to consist of three identical FAs but may have a mixture of FAs. Medium-chain triglycerides (MCTGs) consist predominately of MCFAs, and long-chain triglycerides (LCTGs) consist predominately of LCFAs. Figure 3.1 indicates a unit of glycerol and an MCTG. Not all FAs in nature exist as TGs, but most of them do.

The naming of FAs according to the chain length is arbitrary. There is not total agreement in the literature as to the exact dividing line between classifications of FAs by chain length. Some reports indicate that SCFAs are 2, 3, 4, or 6 carbons long, while others classify caproic, a 6-carbon FA, as an MCFA. Likewise, some classify MCFAs as 6 (or 8) carbons to 12 (or 14) carbons. In most cases, MCFAs are considered to be 6 to 12 carbons long and LCFAs are from 14 to 24 carbons.[5-7] In his book *Nutritional Biochemistry*, Brody indicates SCFAs as less than 8 carbons, MCFAs as 8 to 12 carbons, and LCFAs as 16 to 24 carbons. He mentions that some

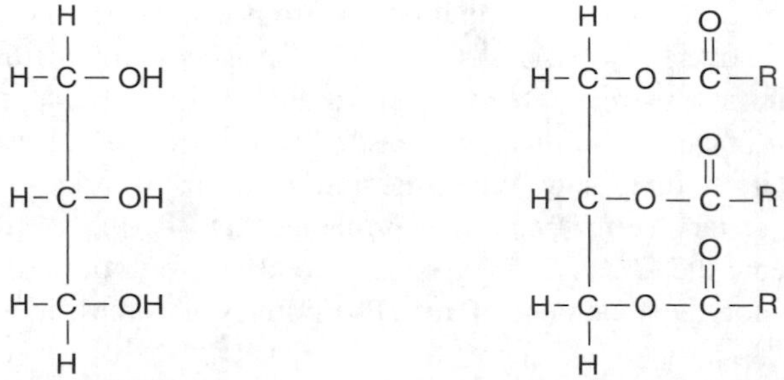

FIGURE 3.1   Chemical structure of glycerol and the chemical structure of a medium-chain triglyceride where the R represents a medium-length fatty acid.

TABLE 3.1
Names, Characteristics, and Dietary Sources of Some Fatty Acids Found in Nature

Fatty Acid Common Name and Formula	Chemical or Systematic Name	Carbon Atoms: Double Bonds	Melting Point, °C	Solubility in Water, g/100 g at 20°C	Common Food Source
Medium-Chain					
Caproic $CH_3(CH_2)_4CO_2H$	Hexanoic	6:0	−3.24	30.9	Palm kernel, cow's milk (butter fat)
Caprylic $CH_3(CH_2)_6CO_2H$	Octanoic	8:0	16.3	0.068	Coconut oil
Capric $CH_3(CH_2)_8CO_2H$	Decanoic	10:0	31.0	0.015	Coconut oil
Lauric $CH_3(CH_2)_{10}CO_2H$	Dodecanoic	12:0	44.2	0.0055	Coconut, palm kernel
Long-Chain					
Myristic $CH_3(CH_2)_{12}CO_2H$	Tetradecanoic	14:0	54.4	0.0020	Coconut oil
Palmitic $CH_3(CH_2)_{14}CO_2H$	Hexadecanoic	16:0	62.9	0.00072	Animal fat
Palmitoleic $CH_3(CH_2)_5CH=CH$ $(CH_2)_7CO_2H$	9-Hexadecenoic	16:1	0.5		Mackerel, avocado
Stearic $CH_3(CH_2)_{16}CO_2H$	Octadecanoic	18:0	69.6	0.00029	Animal fat, cocoa butter
Oleic $CH_3(CH_2)_7CH=CH$ $(CH_2)_7CO_2H$	9-Octadecanoic	18:1	16.3	—	Olive oil, avocado oil
Linoleic $CH_3(CH_2)_4CH=CHC$ $H_2CH=CH(CH_2)_7$ CO_2H	9,12-Octadecadienoic	18:2	−5	—	Safflower oil
Linolenic $CH_3CH_2CH=CHCH_2$ $CH=CHCH_2CH=$ $CH(CH_2)_7CO_2H$	9,12,15-Octadecatrienoic	18:3	−10	—	Rapeseed oil (flaxseed oil)

Modified from Ralston, A.W.J. and Hoerr, C.W., *J. Organ. Chem.*, 7, 546–555, 1942;[9] Westergaard, H. and Dietschy, J.M., *J. Clin. Invest.*, 58, 97–108, 1976.[13]

12- and 14-carbon FAs are considered "in between" MCFAs and LCFAs.[8] Most others classify 14-carbon FAs as LCFAs.

Table 3.1 lists some of the common FAs along with their main dietary source and some of their physical and chemical characteristics. Note that as the carbon chain length increases, the melting point increases and the solubility decreases.[9] This is a noteworthy and striking difference between MCFAs and LCFAs. The greater the solubility, the faster the rate of digestion and absorption of the FA. The mechanism of absorption is also different. Observe that as the number of double bonds increases, the melting point decreases dramatically. For those who classify lauric acid (a 12-carbon FA) and myristic acid (a 14-carbon FA) as being between MC and LC, it may be noted that they do appear to be in a separate classification when comparing their characteristics to the SCFAs and LCFAs, particularly the solubility constants.

3.2.2 FAT CONSUMPTION

Fat consumption refers to the ingestion of all types of TGs, regardless of their size or saturation factor. In 1997 the U.S. Department of Agriculture (USDA) reported that fat consumption by humans in the U.S. can exceed 100 g/day.[10] A more recent report indicates that Americans consumed an average of 65 g of fat per capita per day in 2000. This represents a 34% increase in fat consumption since the 1970 to 1974 survey.[11] In 2003 another survey found the average daily intake of total fat for adults aged 19 to 64 to be 86.5 g for males and 61.4 g for females. Some individuals consumed over 140 g of fat per day.[12] A fat is generally considered to be a solid at room temperature, while an oil is generally considered to be a liquid at room temperature.

3.2.3 FAT DIGESTION AND ABSORPTION

Most fat is consumed in the form of TGs. Digestion of TGs, both MC and LC, begins in the stomach with lingual lipase and gastric lipase,[14] but most digestion of TGs takes place in the small intestines with pancreatic lipase.[15] Lingual and gastric lipase become more important with infants[16] and those with malabsorption syndromes secondary to conditions such as cystic fibrosis and alcoholic pancreatitis.[15–18]

    Lingual lipase activity varies with species. Lingual lipase in humans originates from the serous secretions of von Ebner glands on the tongue.[19] Gastric lipase is secreted from the glands in the fundus of the stomach.[8] Lingual lipase is present in humans in trace amounts, but gastric lipase dominates in preduodenal enzymatic digestion.[20] In rats and newborn infants, lingual lipase hydrolyzed MCTGs five to eight times faster than LCTGs. The optimum pH for lingual lipase in humans is 3.5 to 6.0. This means it would still have some activity when in the upper small intestines. This would be particularly true during the neonatal period when the pH in the lumen of the small intestine is close to 6.5.[21] Lingual and gastric lipase digests TGs by removing the *sn*-3 FA (third FA) from glycerol. The remaining diglyceride and the free FAs pass to the small intestines where pancreatic lipase continues the digestion process by cleaving fatty acids from the *sn*-1 (first FA) position, leaving a monoglyceride with an attached FA at the *sn*-2 position.[20,22] Pancreatic lipase, like gastric lipase, can also remove FAs from the *sn*-3 position. Reports vary, but it has been suggested that lingual and gastric lipases can hydrolyze FAs from 10 to 30% of the dietary TGs while in the stomach.

Lingual and gastric lipase and the remaining diglycerides pass to the small intestines where they continue to cleave FAs along with pancreatic lipase.[15,21,23]

The effectiveness of digestion and absorption of LCTGs is increased by the secretion of bile acids from the gall bladder. Bile acts as an emulsifying agent that forms a micelle with LCFAs and, in addition to keeping fats separated, allows for greater surface area and facilitates their passage through the unstirred water layer that surrounds the epithelial surface of the small intestines.[24] A major difference occurs at this point between MCFAs and LCFAs. Since LCFAs have a low solubility, they have a difficult time penetrating this aqueous unstirred water layer. On the other hand, MCFAs with a much higher solubility can penetrate this layer and be absorbed much quicker, even with pancreatic insufficiency.[25] Thus, bile salts and pancreatic lipase are absolutely essential for efficient digestion and absorption of LCTGs.

Under normal conditions, the gastrointestinal tract can absorb greater than 95% of the TGs ingested. If greater than 5% of the ingested fat is not digested, but instead lost in the feces, steatorrhea (a form of diarrhea caused by fat malabsorption) can result.[26] Most of the LCFAs and MCFAs are absorbed in the proximal small intestines,[27] but can be absorbed in the ileum,[28] the large intestines,[29] possibly the rectum,[26,30] and even the stomach.[18] About half of the MCFAs in human milk can be absorbed in the stomach.[31]

The exact method of absorption of FAs is still under investigation, but it is believed that, for the most part, LCFAs are carried across the intestinal mucosa by a protein-mediated mechanism,[32] while MCFAs can be more easily absorbed through the aqueous unstirred water layer[33] and enter the intestinal mucosa by diffusion.[24] It is well established that once the LCFAs are absorbed, they are incorporated into chylomicrons (CMs) in the intestinal mucosa and transported via the lymphatic system to the circulatory system and eventually to the liver.[8,33,34] Most of these CMs undergo some degree of hydrolysis in extrahepatic tissue before reaching the liver and release most of the attached LCFAs as a result of hydrolysis.[35] This is usually not the case with MCFAs, which can bypass the lymphatic system, be absorbed directly into the portal vein, and go straight to the liver. The percentage of FAs that are incorporated into CMs and transported via the lymphatic system vs. those that are transported via the portal vein depends on the total amount of fat ingested, the chain length of the FAs ingested, and their degree of saturation. Lymph is the major means of transporting LCFAs, while the portal blood is the major transport mechanism of MCFAs. However, some LCFAs are absorbed into the portal system and some MCFAs are reassembled into TGs and thus end up in CMs and are transported via the lymphatic system.[26,36–40] MCTGs do not require bile acids for absorption, and large amounts can be absorbed in patients who are even deficient in pancreatic lipase.[25] For this reason, MCTGs have been used for over 50 years to provide an enteral source of kilocalories in the treatment of fat malabsorption syndromes.[41]

MCFAs are usually found in adipose tissue in only trace amounts, but can be found in larger amounts after supplementation in the diet.[42,43] TGs deposited in adipose tissue consist predominately of LCFAs.[35] The amount and kind of FAs fed will have an effect on the transit time through the small intestines. To determine the effects of transit time, eight healthy subjects participated in a study that was designed so each subject was his own control. Four treatments were used. One LCTG treatment

TABLE 3.2
Transit Time through the
Small Bowel

Treatment	Transit Time[a]
Low dose of MCTGs	56 ± 6 min
High dose of MCTGs	69 ± 9 min
LCTGs	105 ± 13 min
Normal saline	101 ± 9 min

[a] Compiled from Ledeboer, M. et al., *JPEN*, 19, 58, 1995.

was administered in a dose of 15 mmol/h, which was equal to 125 kcal/h. Two MCTG treatments were administered. One was in equimolar amounts compared to the LCTG treatment at 15 mmol/h (56 kcal/h). The second treatment contained 113 kcal/h (30 mmol/h), nearly isocaloric with LCTG treatment. Since the molecular weight of MCTGs is about half that of the LCTGs, the caloric values would be different if equimolar amounts were used. Thus, the MCTG treatment was completed twice, once as equimolar and once as equicaloric with the LCTG treatment. The fourth treatment was a control and consisted of saline solution administered at 15 ml/h. Each treatment was infused into the duodenum for 360 min followed by at least 7 days of rest. Each subject that received MCTGs complained of abdominal cramps and diarrhea. The subjects on the high dose of MCTGs experienced diarrhea until the day after the experiment. The subjects receiving the low dose of MCTGs experienced abdominal cramps and diarrhea only during the day of treatment. Because of this discomfort, only five subjects were subjected to the high-dose treatment of MCTGs. None of the subjects receiving the LCTGs experienced cramps or diarrhea. The effects on transit time can be found in Table 3.2. The transit time was significantly reduced ($p < 0.05$) during the administration of MCTGs, compared to the control. Also, MCTGs did not stimulate cholecystokinin (CCK) release but LCTGs did.[44] In a very similar experiment conducted with intraduodenal administration of MCTGs, LCTGs, and a control at similar equimolar doses, the same results were found. The MCTG treatment significantly ($p < 0.05$) accelerated the small bowel transit time. CCK's secretion was significantly ($p < 0.05$) increased with the administration of LCTGs, but no significant alterations were observed during the MCTGs treatment or control.[45] Increased transit time means increased bowel movements that would take place sooner after ingestion than usual. This would be an important consideration when using MCTGs as an ergogenic aid for athletic performance.

Most MCFAs reach the liver bound to albumin without being incorporated into CMs like LCFAs, but about 8% of the MCTGs were found in CMs 3 h after consuming a meal that contained MCTGs.[41] Some propose that MCTGs be consumed in greater quantities to promote weight loss without the MCTGs being incorporated into adipose tissue. Others propose increased consumption of MCTGs for a quick source of energy that may benefit athletes. These proposals are based on assumptions that MCTGs are utilized very rapidly for energy without being converted into adipose tissue. These assumptions may not be true. Studies have shown that the liver does not utilize all MCTGs for rapid oxidation into ketone bodies for energy,[35,41,46] but may reesterify some MCFAs into LCFAs after elongation.[47,48] This is particularly true when the percentage of MCFAs consumed in the diet is high.[48] It has been demonstrated in preterm infants that octanoic acid (an 8-carbon FA), fed in a standard formula, was detected in plasma as myristic acid (a 14-carbon FA) and palmitic acid (a 16-carbon FA).[47]

3.2.4 FATTY ACID UTILIZATION

CMs are synthesized in the small intestine mucosa and are transported to the circulatory system via the thoracic duct.[49] They can appear in the circulatory system in a matter of minutes.[50-52] The circulating CMs are enzymatically attacked by lipoprotein lipase on the luminal side of blood vessels. TGs attached to the CMs are hydrolyzed, releasing FAs. These FAs are able to be utilized by muscle for energy or can be incorporated into adipose tissue for storage.[50] The fate of the hydrolyzed FAs depends on the amount of total fat ingested, total kilocalories ingested, and the energy demands on the body. If the body is at rest and consumes an excess of fat, or an excess of kilocalories that are converted to fat, then excessive amounts of FAs will be deposited in adipose tissue as TGs. If the body is at work or does not consume an excess of fat or kilocalories, more of the FAs will be utilized by the muscle for energy. During a fasting period, the energy utilized from free FAs is produced by the hybridization of TGs stored in adipose tissue. Signaling mechanisms activate hormone-sensitive lipase, an enzyme that hydrolyzes intracellular tri- and diglycerides, releasing FAs into circulation in the blood (usually in the form of LCFAs). The FAs are carried by albumin to muscle tissue where they are utilized for energy.[53]

Higher than normal intakes of MCTGs have become attractive to the athlete since the MCFAs that make them up can be absorbed faster, go into portal circulation, and enter the mitochondria without carnitine. It is well known that increased consumption of MCTGs can increase circulation of ketone bodies.[1,54,55] Provided the liver has ample calories, the rapid metabolism of MCFA can result in the production of ketone bodies (β-hydroxybutyrate, acetoacetate, and acetone) or an increase in free fatty acids (FFAs) in circulation. These ketones and FFAs can then be used by the muscles for energy.[56] How well this works will be discussed in Section 3.4.

FAs are in a more reduced state than glucose. The oxidation of FAs requires more oxygen than glucose, but more energy is released in the process. Fats yield 9 kcal/g, while glucose yields 4. MCTGs provide 8.2 kcal/g.[57] The oxidation of FAs takes place under aerobic conditions in the mitochondria of cells. First, LCFAs must migrate through the cytoplasm and enter the mitochondria by means of a carrier, carnitine.[58] Once in the mitochondria, the LCFAs undergo beta-oxidation and enter the Krebs cycle and produce ATP. This mechanism requires enzymes and transporters inside the cell that accrue carnitine. A deficiency in any of the transporters or any of the enzymes results in an increased excretion of carnitine in the urine and an inability of LCFAs to enter the mitochondria, resulting in hypoketotic hypoglycemia and hepatic encephalopathy. Another advantage to MCFA ingestion is their ability to enter into the mitochondria without carnitine. Thus, treatment for carnitine deficiency includes a low-fat diet supplemented with MCTGs.[59] Since a large percentage of ingested MCTGs can bypass the lymphatic system, enter the mitochondria directly, and be oxidized, they make an attractive alternative to a quick energy source, but ingestion of large amounts of MCTGs can have drawbacks in that they may cause gas, abdominal cramps, diarrhea, and may stimulate an elongation process and cause additional fat deposition, or may contribute to cardiovascular disease. Each of these possibilities will be discussed later.

To summarize, MCTGs are hydrolyzed faster and more completely than LCTGs and are absorbed more quickly into the small intestine mucosa. A greater percentage goes directly into portal circulation to the liver, where they can enter the mitochondria without carnitine and preferentially enter into the Krebs cycle.[60] However, a large intake of MCTGs can cause gas, cramps, bloating, and diarrhea,[45] and the elongation of MCFAs resulting in deposits in adipose tissue, along with the possibilities of promoting cardiovascular disease, is still under investigation.

3.3 DIETARY AND SUPPLEMENTAL SOURCES

To select a natural diet that is high in MCFAs and low in LCFAs would be very difficult, boring, and unhealthy. While MCFAs appear in several natural foods, there is not a class of foods that is high in MCFAs while being low in LCFAs and balanced in other nutrients. While some foods are higher in one FA than another, both groups of FAs are intermingled in a variety of natural foods. Also, MCTGs do not contain the essential fatty acids (EFAs) linoleic and linolenic. Both EFAs are long-chain FAs with 18 carbons. Linoleic has two double bonds and linolenic has three. A diet without EFAs would cause severe deficiencies incompatible with life. It can be noted in Table 3.3 that MCFAs are not found in abundance in most foods. Coconut oil and palm kernel oil are two plant oils that are high in MCFAs, but note that these FAs are also saturated. The lack of MCFAs in everyday foods creates an argument for taking supplements containing MCFAs, if there is sufficient reason for increasing intake. "Sufficient reason" is a topic of considerable interest in the sports and dieting research arenas. Commercial preparations that contain nothing but MCFAs are available. The MCFAs used in these preparations are usually called MCT oil, which was developed in the 1950s by V.K. Babayan.[65] MCT oil has been used since then for clinical treatment of fat malabsorption and routinely in tube and intravenous feedings. Since MCTGs (MCT oil) are listed on the Generally Recognized As Safe (GRAS) list by the U.S. Food and Drug Administration, they can legally be added to food products. Recently, there has been a new wave of claims that MCTGs are useful in weight reduction and as an energy source for athletes. MCTG products containing MCT oil are abundant in health food and other stores in various forms, including powders, liquids, and incorporated into foods. The research concerned with some of these claims will be discussed in the next section.

3.4 ERGOGENIC BENEFITS

3.4.1 PERFORMANCE

Typically, a low-fat, high-carbohydrate diet has been the diet of choice for many athletes. The competitive athlete, however, demands a more productive routine. Out of a quest for excellence, numerous nutritional protocols have been examined. Among them are included methods to elevate plasma FFA concentration and thus, as discussed earlier, deliver more FAs or ketones to skeletal muscle for oxidation during exercise. Some of the procedures researched include fasting, the ingestion of MCTGs, LCTGs, or combinations of the two, L-carnitine, caffeine, and even intravenous infusions of lipid emulsions. From these studies have emerged suggestions that a high-fat diet, particularly high in MCTGs, may increase VO_{2max}, endurance, and glycogen sparing. Following are brief summaries of some of the research conducted to determine the accuracy of these claims.

Misell et al. completed a study to assess the effects of daily consumption of MCT oil for 2 weeks on the performance of endurance runners. The subjects consumed dietary supplements containing either 56 g of LCTGs (corn oil) or 60 g of MCT oil for 14 days. At the end of 14 days, there was a 3-week washout period and a second crossover trial of 14 days. After each of the two trial periods, subjects completed a maximal treadmill test followed by an endurance treadmill test. The subjects ran at 85% VO_{2max} for 30 min proceeded by 75% VO_{2max} until exhaustion. VO_{2max} and endurance time did not differ ($p > 0.05$) between MCT oil and LCTGs trials, nor were any differences found ($p > 0.05$) in lactate, glucose, FFA, glycerol, or TGs between the trials. Respiratory exchange ratio (REP) was higher ($p < 0.05$) at 15 min for the MCT oil. The REP was similar between trials at other time points measured.[66]

The effects of three levels of fat on performance and metabolism were evaluated by Horvath et al.[67] A low-fat diet (16% of total kcal) and a medium-fat diet (31% of total kcal) were compared by feeding the diets to 12 males and 13 females for approximately 30 days. Six males and 6 females completed a second phase of the trial by increasing their fat consumption to a high-fat diet (44% of total kcal) for approximately another 30 days. Protein percentages in the diet remained about the same as percent fat increased and carbohydrate (CHO) percentage decreased. CHO was never below 250 g/day for the females and 325 g/day for the males. Body weight or percent body fat was not affected by the different diets. Additionally, VO_{2max}, expiratory gas exchange, maximum heart rates, peak power and average power, plasma lactate, pyruvate, and triglycerides were not affected by the different diets.[68]

Endurance time increased between the low-fat and the medium-fat diet by an average of 14% for all subjects, but there was no significant difference between the medium-fat and high-fat diets. The authors concluded that runners on a low-fat diet consumed fewer calories and thus had less endurance. The runners on a high-fat diet, with adequate calories, did not compromise anaerobic power or endurance.[67]

Another study was conducted with cyclists to examine the effectiveness of CHO vs. CHO + MCTGs on metabolism and performance. Eight endurance-trained men completed a 35 kJ/kg time trial as quickly as possible while consuming 250 ml/15

TABLE 3.3
Fatty Acid Composition of Some Popular Fats and Oils

| | Type of FA | | | | | | | | | | |
| | Medium-Chain Fatty Acids | | | | | | Long-Chain Fatty Acids | | | | |
Name of FA Food Source	Caproic 6:0	Caprylic 8:0	Capric 10:0	Lauric 12:0	Myristic 14:0	Palmitic 16:0	Palmitoleic 16:1	Stearic 18:0	Oleic 18:1	Linoleic 18:2	Linolenic 18:3
Almond oil[1]	—	—	—	—	—	7	—	2	69	17	—
Avocado[2]	—	—	—	—	—	19.5	7.5	<2	58	12	2.5
Cocoa butter[3]	—	—	—	—	—	25.6	—	34	35.4	3.4	—
Coconut[3]	.04	7	8	48	16	9.5	—	2	6.5	<2.5	<2
Corn[3]	—	—	—	—	<1	13.5	—	2.25	34.5	48	1.1
Cotton seed[3]	—	—	—	—	1.25	23	—	2.5	28.5	45.5	1.1
Olive[3]	—	—	—	—	tr	13.5	—	3.1	69.3	11.55	0.7
Linseed (flax)[2]	—	—	—	<1.2	—	7	<0.5	5	15	18	37.5
Palm[3]	<1.5	—	—	—	3.2	45.5	—	4.75	39.5	9.5	<1.5
Palm kernel[3]	—	4	5	46	16	8	—	2	15	1.25	—
Rapeseed[3]	—	—	—	—	1.05	5.25	—	1.8	54.5	20.4	10.05
Safflower[4]	—	—	—	—	0.1	4.3	0.1	1.9	14.4	74.6	0.4
Soy[3]	—	—	—	—	<0.5	9.5	—	3.75	24.5	53	8.05
Sunflower[3]	—	—	—	—	<0.5	6.5	—	5.5	39.5	47.5	<0.7
Walnut[2]	—	—	—	—	—	7	—	2	17	60	12
Beef tallow[3]	—	—	—	—	3.85	28.5	4.75	23	38	2.75	<2.5
Chicken fat[4]	—	—	—	0.1	0.9	21.6	5.7	6.0	37.3	19.5	1.0
Lard[3]	—	—	—	—	1.5	26	3.35	14.5	48.5	9.5	<1.5
Cod fish[3]	—	—	—	—	1.4	19.6	3.5	3.8	13.8	0.7	0.1
Haddock[3]	—	—	—	—	1.5	20.0	4.0	6.1	14.2	2.2	0.4
Mackerel[3]	—	—	—	—	8.6	17.6	10.0	2.2	14.8	1.0	0.8

Rainbow trout[3]	—	—	—	3.5	13.3	4.8	3.8	18.7	5.5	5.9
Cow's milk[3]	1.6	3.0	3.1	9.5	26.3	2.3	14.6	29.8	2.4	0.8
Goat's milk[1]	—	7	3	9	25	—	12	27	3	1
Human milk[5]	—	—	4.6	6.4	23.4	3.7	8.6	33.3	12.0	1.8

Note: Modified from:

1 = Fats, Oils, Fatty Acids, Triglycerides: Chemical Structure, *ScientificPsychic* website, http://www.scientificpsychic.com/fitness/fattyacids1.html, 2006.[61]

2 = Fatty Acid Composition of Plant Oils Used in Pharmacy and Cosmetic, Cyberlipid Center website, http://www.cyberlipid.org/glycer/glyc0065.htm#top, 2006.[62]

3 = Gordon, M.H., in *Encyclopedia of Human Nutrition*, 2nd ed., Vol. 2, Caballero, B., Ed., Elsevier/Academic Press, Amsterdam, 2005, pp. 2274–2276.[63]

4 = USDA/ARS Nutrient Data Laboratory website [no longer available], 2004.[64]

5 = Babayan, V.K., *Lipids*, 22, 417–420, 1987.[65]

min of either a 6% CHO solution, a 6% CHO + 4.2% MCTG solution, or a sweet placebo. The time trials were completed faster for both of the treatments than for the placebo, 7% and 5%, respectively ($p < 0.01$). The study suggested that CHO ingestion during exercise improves performance compared with a sweet placebo, but the addition of MCTGs does not provide any further performance enhancement.[68]

Another study was conducted to determine whether ~25 g of MCTGs consumed 1 h prior to exercise would reduce the rate of muscle glycogen use during high-intensity exercise. The subjects consumed either 0.72 g of sucrose/kg of body weight or 0.36 g of tricaprin (C10:0) 1 h before exercise. There was no change in muscle glycogen concentration for either trial, and the calculated glycogen oxidation was also similar. Glucose uptake at rest was increased.[69]

Still another study tested the effect of pre-exercise meals on metabolism and the performance of cyclists. The meals consisted of high fat, high CHO, or high protein 90 min before a weekly exercise test. A CHO supplement was ingested throughout the exercise. The fat oxidation peak rate on the high-carbohydrate meal was half that of the other meals and reduced the fat oxidation across all workloads. However, meal composition did not have a clear effect on performance.[70]

The effects of ingesting different amounts of MCTGs and CHO on gastric symptoms, fuel metabolism, and exercise performance were measured in nine endurance-trained cyclists by Goedecke et al. During exercise, the cyclists ingested 400 ml of 10% glucose, 10% glucose + 1.72% MCTGs, or 10% glucose + 3.44% MCTGs solutions at the start of exercise and 100 ml every 10 min thereafter. Gastrointestinal symptoms were not a problem. MCTGs raised serum FFAs and β-hydroxybutyrate concentrations but did not affect fuel oxidation or the time trial performance.[71] Hawley also reported that an increase in serum FFAs did not effect exercise capacity.[72,73] In yet another review, Hawley included long-term adaptation to high-fat diets (>7 days) and concluded that high-fat, low-CHO diets can prolong endurance time at fixed, submaximal work rates, but pointed out that this is relevant to only a small group of competitive athletes. With or without an effect on performance, high-fat diets can considerably alter substrate utilization during submaximal exercise. The adaptation to a high-fat diet from a high-CHO diet does not appear to amend glycogen utilization in working muscle during prolonged exercise of moderate intensity.[74]

Another study with cyclists was completed to investigate the effect of MCTG intake during time trial cycling performance. During the trials, subjects ingested either a 10% CHO solution, a 10% CHO–electrolyte solution with 5% MCTGs, a 5% MCTGs solution, or a placebo consisting of artificially colored and flavored water. There was no difference between the CHO or the CHO + MCTGs ingestion, but the ingestion of MCTGs had a negative effect on performance.[75]

Satabin et al. completed a study in which nine subjects participated in three exercise tests on a bicycle ergometer 1 h after ingestion of one of three different isocaloric meals (total of 400 kcal). The meals were calculated to theoretically contain 20% of the total energy expenditure of the exercise and consisted of a drink that contained glucose, MCTGs (78% C6 to C8), or LCTGs. A fourth test was performed after an overnight fast. Significant differences were found in the hormones insulin, epinephrine, and norepinephrine. As would be expected, insulin concentration was increased by the CHO diet ($p < 0.001$). Norepinephrine concentration increased after 30 min of exercise ($p < 0.05$), while the epinephrine concentration did not increase until after 1 h of exercise. When at rest 30 min after ingestion of MCTGs or LCTGs, respiratory exchange ratio (RER) was significantly decreased ($p < 0.05$) compared to the CHO diet or the fasting state. At the end of exercise, 80% of the glucose was oxidized from the glucose-containing drink compared to 45% for the MCTGs and 9% for the LCTGs. The authors concluded that their research suggested both MCTG and LCTG ingestion act on epinephrine secretion. This questions the relationship between the digestive tract and sympathetic activity.[76]

Lambert et al. found a positive effect of MCTGs when they examined the effects of a high-fat diet vs. a usual diet prior to CHO loading on fuel metabolism and cycling time trial performance. Five well-trained male subjects with an average age of 22.4 years were selected. The subjects had been cycling on a regular basis for at least 3 years. Two randomized crossover trials were conducted in which subjects consumed either a high-fat diet (>65% MJ from fat) or their usual diet (30 ± 5% MJ from fat) for 10 days. After 10 days they ingested a high-CHO loading diet (CHO > 70% MJ) for 3 days. The subjects ingested 400 ml of a 3.44% MCTG solution 1 h before each exercise trial. During the trial, they ingested 600 ml/h of a 10% glucose + 3.44% MCTG solution. None of the treatments altered weight, body fat, or lipid profile, nor were there changes in circulating glucose, lactate, FFA, or β-hydroxybutyrate concentrations during exercise. However, the high-fat diet CHO treatment was associated with improved time trials. The high-fat diet for 10 days prior to CHO loading was associated with an increased reliance on fat, a decreased reliance on muscle glycogen, and improved time trial performance after prolonged exercise.[77] Note that the tests involved subjects that were well trained before the trials began and only five subjects were used. Lipid profiles were not altered, but they should not be expected to be altered in 13 days. The authors mention a previous trial by Helge et al. that found an opposite effect.[78] In Helge's research, 10 untrained men were used to test the effects of a high-CHO diet compared to 10 similar untrained men on a high-fat diet. This trial lasted 7 weeks. In the eighth week all subjects were converted to a high-CHO diet. Since all of the 20 subjects were untrained at the start of the trials, all improved in the parameters measured as the trials progressed. After 8 weeks, endurance was the same in the high-CHO diet as it was at 7 weeks, while endurance continued to improve with those that were on the high-fat diet. However, the endurance of the subjects on the high-fat diet was still significantly less than the endurance of those on the high-CHO diet ($p < 0.05$). Muscle glycogen rate of breakdown was halved by endurance training but not significantly different between groups. Also, muscle glycogen stores were not depleted by either group at exhaustion. The RER was the same in the high-CHO group throughout the trial when compared to the pretrial value, but the RER decreased for the group on the high-fat diet ($p < 0.05$). After including high CHO in the eighth week, all subjects on both trials had similar RERs. The authors concluded that ingesting a high-fat diet during an endurance training program is detrimental to improvement of performance.[78]

Differences between the two trials mentioned above should be noted. That conflicting results were obtained between these two studies could be due to the fact that either the length of time the subjects were on the high-fat diet was greatly different or the subjects in the first study were well trained at the beginning of the study while the others were not trained at all. Also, none of the subjects were worked to exhaustion. If they had been, different results may have been obtained. Additional research is needed to reproduce these studies with varying lengths of fat consumption, degree of training of the subjects, and workload.

In a review article, Hawley noted that even though it has been reported that acute increases in FAs delivered to working muscle have decreased muscle glycogenolysis by 15 to 48% during whole-body exercise at 65 to 90% of VO_{2max}, the overall effects of the elevated FFAs are vague. Even with substantial muscle glycogen sparing, exercise capacity is not systematically improved with the increase in FFA availability.[73] Many researchers are trying to identify exactly what happens with chronic feeding of MCTGs. The liver produces ketones but does not utilize them for energy. Instead, they diffuse into circulation and can be utilized by the muscle and other tissue for energy. FAs are made available by hormone-sensitive lipase catabolism of TGs stored in adipocytes.[79] Theoretically, a chronic intake of MCTGs could cause an increase in plasma FAs and increase the liver's production of ketones. These FAs and ketones could be used by muscle for readily available energy and thus spare glycogen. It may be important to consider that glucose transport into cells can be inhibited by FA oxidation. Increases in PFK1 (an alpha subunit of heterooctameric phosphofructokinase involved in glycolysis) is primarily responsible for this inhibition. As increased oxidation of FAs occurs in the mitochondria, an increase in citrate and ATP occurs in the cytosol and inhibits PFK1. This prohibits glucose 6-phosphate from being utilized. Glucose 6-phosphate then blocks hexokinase by a feedback mechanism.[79]

MCTGs are less dense than LCTGs, but they produce a greater thermic effect following ingestion. Hill and co-workers hypothesized that the previously observed high rate of thermogenesis produced by MCTGs with overfeeding was due to hepatic *de novo* synthesis of LCFAs from the excess MCFAs fed in the diet. To determine this, a randomized crossover design was used whereby 10 nonobese males were overfed (150% of estimated energy requirements) two formula diets for 6 days each. All diets were liquid and were cholesterol- and fiber-free. The only difference in the diets was the composition of the kind of fat. One contained 40% of energy as MCTGs, and the other contained 40% of energy as LCTGs (soybean oil). The MCTG overfeeding resulted in nearly a threefold increase in fasting TG levels, whereas the LCTGs did not produce a change. About 10% of the TGs recovered were MCFAs (8:0 to 12:0) on the MCTG diet, while only 1% of MCFAs were found in the TGs on the LCTG diet. The MCTG diet also resulted in greater concentrations (14:0, 16:0, and 16:1) than the LCFA diet (18:1, 18:2, and 20:4). Total cholesterol (TC) was reduced significantly with the LCTG diet but did not change with the MCTG diet. High-density lipoprotein cholesterol (HDL-C) was not significantly altered by either diet but was slightly decreased by the MCTG diet. There were no significant differences noted in insulin or glucose concentrations on either diet. The authors reported a reduction in low-density lipoprotein cholesterol (LDL-C) with both diets, but LDL-C was predicted and not measured.[80] Important considerations of these results include the fact that the diet was only 6 days long; this should not be interpreted to mean that the same results would be obtained if the diet were long term. Also, the diet was not a practical daily diet in that it was all liquids, was cholesterol- and fiber-free, and the subjects were overfed 150%. These are not normal conditions and would not be usual for athletes.

Jeukendrup et al.[81] found that when MCTGs were ingested in combination with CHO, 72% of the ingested MCTGs were oxidized. This compared to 33% being oxidized when MCTGs were ingested alone. The data confirmed that due to the high metabolic availability of MCTGs during exercise, MCTGs could serve as an energy source in addition to glucose. However, other studies did not find that a high rate of MCTG oxidation significantly changed the total rate of fat oxidation.[82]

Jeukendrup et al. looked at CHO utilization in subjects receiving CHO or CHO + MCTG supplements. Plasma FFAs were comparably elevated in all trials, but plasma ketones were significantly increased after MCTG ingestion when compared to the CHO trial. However, they concluded that the MCTGs co-ingested (29 g) with CHO during the exercise period (180 min) did not influence CHO utilization or glycogen breakdown.[83]

In another study, Jeukendrup and colleagues also reviewed the effects of fat metabolism during exercise. Their summary of the effects of short-term high-fat diets included an increase in the availability of lipid substrate but a decrease in the storage of glycogen. This allows for an increase in fat oxidation during exercise, but fatigue resistance and exercise performance may be decreased. Most of the effects of long-term fat diets were significantly detrimental to performance and to recovery when reverting back to a high-carbohydrate diet. The authors point out that high-fat diets are associated with increased obesity and cardiovascular disease, but most of the studies in those areas were performed on nonathletes. The authors conclude that since high-fat diets are associated with obesity, insulin resistance, and cardio-vascular disease, and since little is known of the effects of high-fat diets on athletes, it would be prudent for athletes to exercise caution when using such a diet.[84]

Another study attempted to determine if MCTGs in combination with CHO would alter substrate metabolism and improve ultra-endurance cycling performance. Eight endurance-trained cyclists took part in this study in which on two separate occasions they cycled for 270 min at 50% of peak power output. The tests were interspersed with four 75-kJ sprints at 60-min intervals, followed immediately by a 200-kJ time trial. One hour prior to the trials, the subjects ingested one of two treatments, either 75 g of CHO or 32 g of MCTGs. These were followed by 200 ml of a 10% CHO solution or a 4.3% MCTGs + 10% CHO solution every 20 min during both trials. No differences were found in VO_2 or RER between the MCTGs and CHO trials ($p = 0.40$). The interspersed sprints ($p = 0.03$ for trial × time interaction) and trial times ($p < 0.001$) were slower in the MCTG ingestion. The authors concluded that MCTGs ingested prior to exercise and co-ingested with CHO during exercise did not alter substrate metabolism and significantly compromised sprint performance during prolonged ultra-endurance cycling exercise. The authors also noted that previous studies found that the ingestion of small boluses (25 to 30 g) of MCTGs increased serum ketone concentrations, but did not alter overall rate of fat or CHO oxidation.[85]

In a study using male endurance runners, a low-fat diet was fed with approxi-mately 15% of energy coming from fat and an additional consumption of either supplemental MCT oil, 30 g twice a day, or LCTGs (corn oil), 28 g twice a day, for 14 days. Each dietary trial was separated by at least 3 weeks. Concentrations of TC were significantly higher ($p = 0.004$), LDL-C was significantly higher ($p = 0.033$), and TGs were significantly higher ($p = 0.006$) with the MCT oil. The concentration of HDL-C was not significantly different between the trials. All of the blood lipids were still within desirable ranges, but the test results suggest that consumption of MCT oil for 2 weeks negatively alters the blood lipid profile of athletes.[86]

In summary, it can be concluded that trials testing the consumption of MCTGs for the purpose of improving athletic performance or endurance during an athletic event have not produced evidence that MCTG ingestion is effective. Some studies suggested a negative effect. The one study that produced a positive result was completed with elite well-trained endurance athletes and needs to be investigated further. The health concerns of MCTGs also need to be further investigated.

3.4.2 MCTGs AND HEALTH

Health concerns are an important issue with high-fat diets and diets high in MCTGs. Considering that it has been claimed that MCFAs do not increase plasma cholesterol, Tholstrup et al. compared the effects of a diet rich in either MCFAs or oleic acid on fasting blood lipids, lipoproteins, glucose, insulin, and lipid transfer protein activities in healthy men. The trial employed a double-blind, randomized, crossover design, with 17 healthy young men. The treatments consisted of replacing part of their usual dietary fat intake with 70 g of MCTGs (66% 8:0 and 34% 10:0) or high-oleic acid sunflower oil (89.4%18:1). Intervention periods lasted for 21 days. After completing one of the diets, there was a 2-week washout period. Blood was obtained before and after the intervention periods. Compared with the intake of high-oleic sunflower oil, MCTG intake resulted in 11% higher plasma TC ($p = 0.0005$), 12% higher LDL-C ($p = 0.0001$), 32% higher very low density lipoprotein cholesterol (VLDL-C) ($p = 0.080$), a 12% higher ratio of LDL-C to HDL-C ($p = 0.002$), 22% higher plasma total TG ($p = 0.0361$), and higher plasma glucose ($p = 0.033$). Plasma HDL-C, insulin concentrations, and activities of cholesterol ester transfer protein and phospholipids transfer protein did not differ significantly between the diets. The authors concluded that compared with the high-fat oleic acid diet, the MCTG diet unfavorably affected lipid profiles in healthy young men by increasing plasma LDL-C and TG.[87]

The changes in FA composition of TGs when fed MCTGs are another concern, as mentioned previously. It has been hypothesized that excess dietary MCTGs cause an increase in hepatic synthesis of MCFAs through *de novo* synthesis or chain elongation and desaturation. The elongation process is costly energy-wise and may account for the increase in energy expenditure when MCTGs were overfed. The authors cited another study that is consistent with this finding[88] in which case an increase in postprandial thermogenesis was theorized to be due to hepatic *de novo* lipogenesis.[80] Since the writing of this article, additional work supports this theory.[89]

Nine middle-aged men with mild hypercholesterolemia were studied to determine the effects of a natural food diet supplemented with MCTGs, palm oil, or high-oleic acid sunflower oil on blood lipids. TC and LDL-C concentrations obtained on the MCTG diet and the palm oil diet were not significantly different, but they were significantly higher than those produced by a high-oleic acid (sunflower oil) diet. The MCTG diet resulted in nonsignificant increases in TG concentrations when compared to the palm oil or high-oleic acid diet. No differences were found in the HDL-C concentrations. The authors concluded that, on the basis of percent of energy in the diet, the study suggested MCTGs are cholesterol-raising FAs that can raise TC and LDL-C similar to palm oil and also have the tendency to raise TGs.[90]

Naohisa et al. completed a study to investigate the effects of dietary MCTGs on serum lipid levels, liver function, and hepatic fat accumulations in healthy men. Eleven men consumed diets between 2200 and 2600 kcal daily. The diets consisted of 70 to 80 g of fat and included either 40 g of MCTGs or 40 g of LCTGs as blended vegetable oil. The FA content of the oil was predominately unsaturated. The diet was administered for 4 weeks. No significant differences were found between the diets for serum TC, VLDL-C, LDL-C, HDL-C, or TGs. No other blood, urine, or liver tests indicated a problem from the ingestion of 40 g of MCTGs for 4 weeks.[91] Note that the subjects were not athletes.

A single-blind, randomized, crossover study to test the effects of a single dose feeding was completed whereby 20 healthy men were fed a single dose of 71 g of either MCT oil or canola oil. Blood was drawn at baseline before the participants ingested the oils. The dose of 71 g of oil was chosen because it was equivalent to a large order of French fries or a salad with oil-based dressing and a cookie. Blood was drawn at 1, 2, 3, 4, and 5 h postingestion and analyzed for TGs. Two weeks later, the project was repeated with the oils consumed being reversed, that is, those who received the canola received the MCT oil and vice versa. The canola oil caused a 47% increase in TGs above baseline ($p < 0.001$) and the MCT oil caused a 15% decrease in TGs below the baseline. Remember that these results are based on lipid profiles just hours after ingestion of the test oils, and the authors point out that the effect of long-term usage of MCT oil on TGs is yet to be established.[92] This finding is in disagreement with the work of Hill et al.[80] and Swift et al.[93] It should also be remembered that with a trial such as this, where the amount of oil used was equivalent to the oil in a large order of French fries or a salad with an oil-based dressing and a cookie, the French fries, the salad, or the cookie were not consumed. Had they been consumed, there could possibly have been a difference in the postprandial TG levels. Thus, it would not be correct to assume that eating a large order of French fries would produce exactly the same results as reported here, and it was not the authors' intention to imply such. The subjects in this trial also were not athletes.

A study was conducted to observe the effects of MCTGs and corn oil on plasma lipids in patients with primary hypertriglyceridemia. Ten subjects ate a low-fat diet for 2 weeks followed by different proportions of corn oil and MCTGs for 12 weeks. Fasting plasma TC, TGs, and HDL-C concentrations were measured at the end of each period. Compared with corn oil, MCTGs were associated with an increased mean for fasting TC concentration ($p < 0.05$) and non-HDL cholesterol concentrations were also higher with MCTGs than with corn oil ($p < 0.005$). It was concluded that MCTGs can raise TC concentrations in primary hypertriglyceridemic subjects.[94] Again, since these subjects were not athletes, these results should not be assumed necessarily to be true for athletes, but this should be thoroughly investigated with athletes before recommendations for increasing fat or MCTGs in the diet are made.

The effects of MCT oil, myristic acid (14:0), and oleic acid (18:1) on serum lipoproteins were studied. The test fats were incorporated into solid foods. All subjects, 37 women and 23 men, were fed an initial diet high in oleic acid for 3 weeks. At the end of the initial diet, the subjects were divided into three groups. One group received a diet high in MCT oil, the second a diet high in myristic acid, and the third group continued on the oleic diet. The results indicated that the subjects on the diet high in myristic acid had LDL-C levels that were 0.37 mmol/l higher than those of the oleic acid diet ($p = 0.0064$). Those on the MCT oil diet had increased LDL-C levels, but not significantly higher than the oleic acid diet. HDL-C concentrations increased with the myristic acid diet by 0.10 mmol/l ($p = 0.02$), but there was no difference with the MCT oil diet. The MCT oil diet slightly elevated TG concentrations, but there was no significant difference between the diets. There was a significant decrease in the apoA-I-to-apoB ratio in the MCT oil diet compared to both of the other diets ($p < 0.02$). The authors concluded that MCT oil raises LDL-C concentrations slightly and affects the apoA-I-to-apoB ratio unfavorably compared with oleic acid. Myristic acid is hypercholesterolemic and raised both LDL-C and HDL-C concentrations compared with oleic acid.[95]

Thomas et al. conducted a study to evaluate the effect of MCTGs with and without exercise on postprandial lipemia (PPL). Twenty-five young men and women were chosen. Each subject had to perform three trials: (1) a control group ate a meal with only 1.5 g of fat/kg of body weight; (2) MCT oil was substituted for 30% of the fat calories; and (3) MCT oil was consumed as in trial 2, but 12 h of exercise was completed before the meal. ANOVA indicated that the substitution of MCT oil to the control meal did not affect the PPL. However, the PPL was significantly lower after the MCT oil + exercise vs. the other trials. The results suggest that MCT oil does not affect the TG response to a fat meal.[96]

On a different note, considering atherosclerosis as a result of the aging process and not due to the lipid theory, Kaunitz reviewed the research completed prior to 1986 and concluded that MCTGs could possibly prevent or slow down atherosclerosis.[57]

In summary, it can be noted that most of the research concerning health effects of acute and chronic ingestion of MCTGs has been completed with nonathletes and has involved nonpractical diets that have not been tested over the long term. Until long-term health effects of chronic practical ingestion of MCTGs can be adequately reported, athletes should exercise caution when using MCTGs as an ergogenic aid.

3.4.3 Structured Lipids

In the past decade, chemically defined structured lipids have become popular research items. These lipids were originally produced by mixing pure MCTGs and LCTGs and allowing hydrolysis to produce FFAs. This was followed by random transesterification of the FAs into mixed triglyceride molecules. This results in a TG containing combinations of short-, medium-, and long-chain fatty acids on a single glycerol backbone. The resulting TGs have unique chemical, physical, and physiological properties. Today the use of 1,3-specific or 2-specific lipases can be used to synthesize 1,3-specific or 2-specific triglycerides containing MC and LCTG on the same glycerol.[97]

A study was conducted to test performance after consumption of specific structured TGs consisting of a mixture of MCFAs and LCFAs (MLM), in an attempt to prevent the adverse effects observed by feeding larger doses of MCTGs (i.e., gastrointestinal distress and elevated plasma lipids). Seven well-trained cyclists worked 3 h at 55% of maximum O_2 uptake. During this time, they ingested CHO or CHO plus the MLM. Immediately after the constant-load cycling, the subjects performed a time trial of ~50 min duration. Treatments did not significantly affect performance. Plasma FA concentrations were significantly higher after 3 h of cycling compared to the resting stage, but no differences in the sum total between groups was noted. No gastrointestinal disturbances were noted. The MLM consisted of M = 8:0 (caprylic) and L = 18:2 (linoleic). Breath and blood samples revealed no plasma 8:0 FAs, but the amount of phospholipid FAs was significantly higher after CHO + MLM than with CHO intake. The fact that 8:0 did not appear in the plasma when large doses were consumed may indicate the MLM treatment was not glycogen sparing. Possible explanations by the authors for a lack of 8:0 in the plasma include possible elongation of the 8:0 FAs to 14:0 FAs and longer, or possibly the 8:0 FAs were metabolized so fast they were not detected. In any case, the treatments did not improve performance.[98] Kasai et al. found structured lipids to cause a reduction in body fat and to lower TC.[99] Mu and Hoy reported that structured TGs are absorbed by the same mechanism as conventional LCTGs.[100]

Carvajal et al. found a difference in the fecal excretion of FAs in rats when they were fed diets containing different types of structured TGs.[101] The future of structured lipids' use in diets remains to be seen, but most of the current research results are positive.

3.4.4 MCTGs AND WEIGHT REDUCTION

While weight reduction is usually not a goal for athletes, exercise, along with dieting, is a necessary component of any weight loss regimen. Researchers concerned with obesity have noted that MCTGs seem to promote an increase in energy expenditure, and thus a chronic intake of MCTGs may be a possible means of weight loss. Developments in this area could be of interest to athletes. For example, St.-Onge and Jones reported on a review of the literature concerning MCTGs and weight reduction. In their summary they state that diets with elevated levels of MCTGs cause an increase in energy expenditure, a depression of food intake, and a lower body mass. While these results should be of some interest to athletes, the authors point out that most of the research completed with MCTGs and weight reduction were done over short testing periods. The longest test period reported was 14 days. Clinical trials of longer duration need to be conducted before specific recommendations can be made.[102] Others have shown that MCTGs in a diet help reduce body weight when compared to LCTGs[103] and increase thermogenesis in humans[104,105] and rats.[106] This is also true for structured TGs.[99] The future of MCTGs and structured lipids in weight reduction diets is also yet to be decided.

3.5 TOXICITY

As a food additive in the U.S., MCTGs are found on the GRAS list and are well tolerated but are not without side effects if consumed in large enough quantities. Recommended daily intake ranges from 30 to 100 g, so long as the intake is not over 40% of the daily energy requirement.[35] In a thorough review, Traul et al. report on numerous studies and conclude that human dietary consumption is safe at 1 g/kg.[107] However, that is not to say that 75 kg/day for a 75-kg man would be well tolerated. Gas, cramps, bloating, and diarrhea have all been reported. This is in agreement with side effects commonly reported and includes nausea, vomiting, bloating, abdominal cramps, or osmotic diarrhea.[35,45,107] Extended trials with humans to determine possible long-term effects on reproduction, cardiovascular complications, or carcinogenicity have not been completed.

3.6 SUMMARY AND RECOMMENDATIONS

Numerous studies have investigated the use of MCTGs as an ergogenic aid prior to exercise, during exercise, and as a training aid. From these studies there are no convincing arguments that MCTGs have a significantly positive effect on muscle glycogen concentration, endurance, RER, or overall performance. In fact, there are reports of negative effects of MCTG ingestion on athletic performance and lipid profiles. When taken with CHO, results are improved over MCTGs taken alone; however, the overall performance is still not an improvement over CHO alone. If MCTGs are taken in larger doses, gastrointestinal disturbances can inhibit performance. In addition, when MCTGs are ingested in larger quantities than needed, there is the question of possible elongation of MCFAs into LCFAs and deposited as such in adipocytes. There is also the question of possible cardiovascular complications with chronic ingestion of MCTGs. Until future research indicates a definite safe advantage of MCTGs, the current suggestions of adequate CHO ingestion and loading seem to be the safest and most reliable training method. Research with specially structured TGs appears to have an interesting future, particularly with weight control, but to date has not provided evidence for improvement of athletic performance. In addition, it should be noted that anyone with a tendency to produce ketones, such as diabetics, or anyone who has compromised liver function should avoid MCTG ingestion as a means of improving athletic performance. A final note that was not discussed in this chapter but should also be a practical consideration is the financial cost of MCTG supplements when there are no significant benefits indicated.

REFERENCES

1. Wilder, R.M. The effect of ketonemia on the course of epilepsy. *Mayo Clinic Bull.* 2, 1, 1921.

2. Kuo, P.T. and Huang, N.N. The effect of medium chain triglyceride upon fat absorption and plasma lipid and depot fat of children with cystic fibrosis of the pancreas. *J. Clin. Invest.* 44, 1924–1933, 1965.

3. Nebeling L.C. and Lerner, E. Implementing a ketogenic diet based on medium-chain triglyceride oil in pediatric patients with cancer. *J. Am. Diet. Assoc.* 95, 693–697, 1995.

4. Craig, G.B., Darnell, B.E., Weinsier, R.L., Saag, M.S., Epps, L., Mullins, L., Lapidus, W.I., Ennis, D.M., Akrabawi, S.S., Cornwell, P.E., and Sauberlich, H.E. Decreased fat and nitrogen losses in patients with AIDS receiving medium-chain-triglyceride-enriched formula vs. those receiving long-chain-triglyceride-containing formula. *J. Am. Diet. Assoc.* 97, 605–611, 1997.

5. Pond, C.M. *The Fats of Life*, Cambridge University Press, Cambridge, U.K., 1998, pp. 8–11.

6. Leonard, A.E., Pereira S.L., Sprecher H., and Huang, Y.S. Elongation of long-chain fatty acids. *Prog. Lipid Res.* 43, 35–54, 2004.

7. Pehowich, D.J., Gomes, A.V., and Barnes, J.A. Fatty acid composition and possible health effects of coconut constituents. *West Indian Med. J.* 49, 128–133, 2000.

8. Brody, T. *Nutritional Biochemistry*, 2nd ed. Academic Press, San Diego, CA, 1999, p. 94.

9. Ralston, A.W.J. and Hoerr, C.W. The solubilities of the normal saturated fatty acids. *J. Organ. Chem.* 7, 546–555, 1942.

10. USDA. Results from USDA's 1994–96 Continuing Survey of Food Intakes by Individuals. 1997.

11. Putnam, J., Allshouse, J., and Kantor, L.S. U.S. per capita food supply trends: more calories, refined carbohydrates, and fats. *U.S. Per Capita Food Review*, 25, 1–15. http://www.ers.usda.gov/publications/FoodReview/DEC2002/frvol25i3a.pdf. Accessed May 2006.

12. Henderson, L., Gregory, J., Irving, K., and Swan, G. The National Diet and Nutrition Survey: Adults Aged 19 to 64 Years Energy, Carbohydrate, Protein, Fat and Alcohol Intake. http://www.statistics.gov.uk/downloads/theme_health/NDNS_V2.pdf. Accessed October 5, 2003.

13. Westergaard, H. and Dietschy, J.M. The mechanism where by bile acid micelles increase the rate of fatty acid and cholesterol uptake into the intestinal mucosal cell. *J. Clin. Invest.* 58, 97–108, 1976.

14. Hamosh, M. Lingual and gastric lipases. *Nutrition* 6, 421–428, 1990.

15. Carriere, F., Grandval, P., Renou, C., Palomba, A., Prieri, F., Giallo, J., Henniges, F., Sander-Struckmeier, S., and Laugier, R. Quantitative study of digestive enzyme secretion and gastrointestinal lipolysis in chronic pancreatitis. *Clin. Gastroenterol. Hepatol.* 3, 28–38, 2005.

16. Fredrikzon, B., Hernell, O., and Blackberg, L. Lingual lipase. Its role in lipid digestion in infants with low birthweight and/or pancreatic insufficiency. *Acta Paediatr. Scand. Suppl.* 296, 75–80, 1982.

17. Roulet, M., Weber, A.M., Paradis, Y., Roy, C.C., Chartrand, L., Lasalle, R., and Morin, C.L. Gastric emptying and lingual lipase activity in cystic fibrosis. *Pediatr. Res.* 14, 1360–1362, 1980.

18. Faber, J., Goldstein, R., Blondheim, O., Stankiewicz, H., Darwashi, A., Bar-Maor, J.A., Gorenstein, A., Eidelman, A.I., and Freier, S. Absorption of medium chain triglycerides in the stomach of the human infant. *J. Pediatr. Gastroenterol. Nutr.* 7, 189–195, 1988.

19. Manosh, M. The role of lingual lipase in neonatal fat digestion. *Ciba. Found. Symp.* 70, 69–98, 1979.

20. DeNigris, S.J., Hamosh, M., Kasbekar, D.K., Lee, T.C., and Hamosh, P. Lingual and gastric lipases: species differences in the origin of prepancreatic digestive lipases and in the localization of gastric lipase. *Biochim. Biophys. Acta* 959, 38–45, 1988.

21. Liao, T.H., Hamosh, P., and Hamosh, M. Fat digestion by lingual lipase: mechanism of lipolysis in the stomach and upper small intestine. *Pediatr. Res.* 18, 402–409, 1984.

22. Carey, M.C., Small, D.M., and Bliss, C.M. Lipid digestion and absorption. *Ann. Rev. Physiol.* 45, 651–677, 1983.

23. Carriere, F., Grandval, P., Gregory, P.C., Renou, C., Henniges, F., Sander-Struckmeier, S., and Laugier, R. Does the pancreas really produce much more lipase than required for fat disgestion? *J. Pancreas* 6, 206–215, 2005.

24. Stipanuk, M.H. *Biochemical and Physiological Aspects of Human Nutrition.* W.B. Saunders, New York, 2000, p. 128.

25. Jandacek, R.J., Whiteside, J.A., Holcombe, B.N., Volpenhein, R.A., and Taulbee, J.D. The rapid hydrolysis and efficient absorption of triglycerides with octanoic acid in the 1 and 3 positions and long-chain fatty acid in the 2 position. *Am. J. Clin. Nutr.* 45, 940–945, 1987.

26. Hu, M. and Hoy, C.R. The digestion of dietary triacylglycerols. *Prog. Lipid Res.* 43, 105–133, 2004.

27. Shiau, Y.F. Mechanisms of intestinal absorption. *Am. J. Physiol.* 240, G1–G9, 1981.

28. Wollaeger, E.E. Role of the ileum in fat absorption. *Mayo Clin. Proc.* 48, 836–843, 1973.

29. Jeppesen, P.B. and Mortensen, P.B. The influence of a preserved colon on the absorption of medium chain fatty acids in patients with small bowel resection. *Gut* 43, 478–483, 2006.

30. Thomson, A.B.R., Keelan, M., Thiesen, A., Clandinin, M.T., Ropeleski, M., and Wild, G.E. Small bowel review normal physiology: part 1. *Dig. Dis. Sci.* 46, 2567–2587, 2001.

31. Da Costa, T.H.M. Fats: digestion, absorption, and transport. In *Encyclopedia of Human Nutrition*, 2nd ed., Vol. 2, Caballero, B., Ed., Elsevier/Academic Press, Amsterdam, 2005, pp. 2274–2276.

32. Schaffer, J.E. Fatty acid transport: the roads taken. *Am. J. Physiol. Endocrinol. Metab.* 282, E239–E246, 2002.

33. Ramirez, M., Amate, L., and Gil, A. Absorption and distribution of dietary fatty acids from different sources. *Early Hum. Dev.* 65, S95–S101, 2001.

34. Bisgaier, C. L. and Glickman, R.M. Intestinal synthesis, secretion, and transport of lipoproteins. *Ann. Rev. Physiol.* 45, 625–636, 1983.

35. Bauch, A.C., Ingenbleek, Y., and Frey, A. The usefulness of dietary medium-chain triglycerides in body weight control: fact or fancy? *J. Lipid Res.* 37, 708–725, 1996.

36. Carlier, H. and Bezard, J. Electron microscope auto radiographic study of intestinal absorption of decanoic and octanoic acids in the rat. *J. Cell Biol.* 65, 383–397, 1975.

37. Bloom, B., Chaikoff, I.L., and Reinhardt, W.O. Intestinal lymph as pathway for transport of absorbed fatty acids of different chain lengths. *Am. J. Physiol.* 166, 451–455, 1951.

38. Bloom B., Chaikoff, I.L., Reinhardt, W.O., and Dauben, W.G. Participation in lymphatic transport of absorbed fatty acids. *J. Biol. Chem.* 189, 261–267, 1951.

39. Mansbach, C.M., II, Dowell, R.F., and Pritchett D. Portal transport of absorbed lipids in rats. *Am. J. Physiol.* 261, G530–G538, 1991.

40. Chistensen, M.S., Hoy, C.E., Becker, C.C., and Redgrave, T.G. Intestinal absorption and lymphatic transport of eicosapentaenoic (EPA), docosahexaenoic (DHA), and decanoic acids: dependence on intramolecular triaclglycerol structure. *Am. J. Clin. Nutr.* 61, 56–61, 1995.

41. Bach, A.C. and Babayan, V.K. Medium-chain triglycerides: an update. *Am. J. Clin. Nutr.* 36, 950–962, 1982.

42. Sarda, P., Lepage, G., Roy, C.C., and Chessex, P. Storage of medium-chain triglycerides in adipose tissue of orally fed infants. *Am. J. Clin. Nutr.* 45, 399–405, 1987.

43. Zurier, R.B., Campbell, R.G., Hashim, S.A., and Van Itallie, T.B. Enrichment of depot fat with odd and even numbered medium chain fatty acids. *Am. J. Physiol.* 212, 291–294, 1967.

44. Verkijk, R.J., Whiteside, J.A., Holcombe, B.N., Volpenhein, R.A., and Taulbee, J.D. The rapid hydrolysis and efficient absorption of triglycerides with octanoic acid in the 1 and 3 positions and long-chain fatty acids in the 2 position. *Dig. Dis. Sci.* 45, 940–945, 1997.

45. Ledeboer, M., Masclee, A.A., Jansen, J.B., and Lamers, C.B. Effect of equimolar amounts of long-chain triglycerides and medium-chain triglycerides on small-bowel transit time in humans. *JPEN* 19, 5–8, 1995.

46. Greenberger, N.J. and Skillman, T.G. Medium-chain triglycerides: physiologic considerations and clinical implications. *NEJM* 280, 1045–1056, 1969.

47. Carnielli, V.P., Sulkers, E.J., Moretti, C., Wattimena, J.L., van Goudoever, J.B., Degenhart, H.J., Zacchello, F., and Sauer, P.J. Conversion of octanoic acid into long-chain saturated fatty acids in premature infants fed a formula containing medium-chain triglycerides. *Metabolism* 43, 1287–1292, 1994.

48. Swift, L.L., Hill, J.O., Peters, J.C., and Greene, H.L. Medium-chain fatty acids: evidence for incorporation into chylomicron triglycerides in humans. *Am. J. Clin. Nutr.* 52, 834–836, 1990.

49. Johnson, L. *Essential Medical Physiology*, 2nd ed. Lippincott-Raven, Philadelphia, PA, 1997.

50. Goldberg, I.J. Lipoprotein lipase and lipolysdis: central roles in lipoprotein metabolism and atherogenesis. *J. Lipid Res.* 37, 693–707, 1996.

51. Tso, P., Pitts, V., and Granger, D.N. Role of lymph flow in intestinal chylomicron transport. *Am. J. Physiol.* 249, G21–G28, 1985.

52. Berger, GM. Clearance defects in primary chylomicronemia: a study of tissue lipoprotein lipase activities. *Metabolism* 35, 1054–1061, 1986.

53. Gonzalez-Yanes, C. and Sanchez-Margalet, V. Signalling mechanisms regulating lipolysis. *Cell. Signalling* 18, 401–408, 2006.

54. Nebeling, L.C. and Lerner, E. Implementing a ketogenic diet based on medium-chain triglyceride oil in pediatric patients with cancer. *J. Am. Diet. Assoc.* 95, 693–697, 1995.

55. Carroll, J. and Koenigsberger, D. The ketogenic diet: a practical guide for caregivers. *J. Am. Diet. Assoc.* 98, 316–321, 1998.

56. Robinson, A.M. and Williamson, D.H. Physiological roles of ketone bodies as substrates and signals in mammalian tissues. *Physiol. Rev.* 60, 143–187, 1980.

57. Kaunitz, H. Medium chain triglycerides (MCT) in aging and atherosclerosis. *J. Environ. Pathol. Toxicol. Oncol.* 6, 115–121, 1986.

58. Reda, E., D'Iddio S., Nicolai, R., Benatti, P., and Calvani, M. The carnitine system and body composition. *Acta Diabetol.* 40, S106–S113, 2003.

59. Longo, N., di San Filippo, A., and Pasquali, M. Disorders of carnitine transport and the carnitine cycle. *Am. J. Med. Genet. C* 142, 77–85, 2006.

60. Papamandjaris, A.A., MacDougall, D.E., and Jones, P.J.H. Medium chain fatty acid metabolism and energy expenditure: obesity treatment implications. *Life Sci.* 62, 1203–1215, 1998.

61. Fats, Oils, Fatty Acids, Triglycerides: Chemical Structure. *ScientificPsychic* website. http://www.scientificpsychic.com/fitness/fattyacids1.html. Accessed May 10, 2006.

62. Fatty Acid Composition of Plant Oils Used in Pharmacy and Cosmetic. Cyberlipid Center website. http://www.cyberlipid.org/glycer/glyc0065.htm#top. Accessed May 10, 2006.

63. Gordon, M.H. Fats/occurrence. In *Encyclopedia of Human Nutrition*, 2nd ed., Vol. 2, Caballero, B., Ed. Elsevier/Academic Press, Amsterdam, 2005, pp. 2274–2276.

64. USDA/ARS Nutrient Data Laboratory website. 2004. [No longer available.]

65. Babayan, V.K. Medium chain triglycerides and structural lipids. *Lipids* 22, 417–420, 1987.

66. Misell, L.M., Lagomarcino, N.D, Schuster, V., and Kern, M. Chronic medium-chain triacylglycerol consumption and endurance performance in trained runners. *J. Sports Med. Phys. Fit.* 41, 210–215, 2001.

67. Horvath, P.J., Eagen, C.K., Fisher, N.M., Leddy, J.J., and Pendergast, D.R. The effects of varying dietary fat on performance and metabolism in trained male and female runners. *J. Am. Col. Nutr.* 19, 52–60, 2000.

68. Angus, D.J., Hargreaves, M., Dancey, J., and Febraio, M.A. Effect of carbohydrate or carbohydrate plus medium-chain triglyceride ingestion on cycling bike trial performance. *J. Appl. Physiol.* 88,113–119, 2000.

69. Horowitz, J.F., Mora-Rodriguez, R., Byerley, L.O., and Coyle, E.F. Preexercise medium-chain triglyceride ingestion does not alter muscle glycogen use during exercise. *J. Appl. Physiol.* 88, 219–225, 2000.

70. Rowland, D.S. and Hopkins, W.G. Effect of high-fat, high-carbohydrate, and high-protein meals on metabolism and performance during endurance cycling. *Int. J. Sports Nutr. Exerc. Metab.* 12, 318–335, 2002.

71. Goedecke, J.H., Elmer-English, R., Dennis, S.C., Schloss, I., Noakes, T.D., and Lambert, E.V. Effects of medium-chain triacylglycerol ingested with carbohydrate on metabolism and exercise performance. *Int. J. Sports Nutr.* 9, 35–47, 1999.

72. Hawley, J.A., Burke, L.M., Angus, D.J., Fallon, K.E., Martin, D.T., and Febbraio, M.A. Effect of altering substrate availability on metabolism and performance during intense exercise. *Br. J. Nutr.* 84, 829–838, 2000.

73. Hawley, J.A. Effect of increased fat availability on metabolism and exercise capacity. *Med. Sci. Sports Exerc.* 34, 1485–1491, 2002.

74. Hawley, J.A., Brouns, F., and Jeukendrup, A. Strategies to enhance fat utilization during exercise. *Sports Med.* 25, 241–257, 1998.

75. Jeukendrup, A.E., Thielen, J.J.H.C., Wagenmakers, A.J.M., Brouns, F., and Saris, W.H.M. Effect of medium-chain triacylglycerol and carbohydrate ingestion during exercise on substrate utilization and subsequent cycling performance. *Am. J. Clin. Nutr.* 67, 397–404,1998.

76. Satabin, P., Portero, P., Defer, G., Bricout, J., and Guezennec, C.Y. Metabolic and hormonal responses to lipid and carbohydrate diets during exercise in man. *Med. Sci. Sports Exerc.* 19, 218–223, 1987.

77. Lambert, E.V., Goedecke, J.H., van Zyl, C., Murphy, K., Hawley, J.A., Dennis, S.C., and Noakes, T.D. High-fat diet versus habitual diet prior to carbohydrate loading: effects on exercise metabolism and cycling performance. *Int. J. Sports Nutr. Exerc. Metab.* 11, 209–225, 2001.

78. Helge, J.W., Richter, E.A., and Kiens, B. Interaction of training and diet on metabolism and endurance during exercise in man. *J. Physiol.* 492, 293–306, 1996.

79. Wildman, R.E.C. and Medeiros D.M. *Advanced Human Nutrition.* CRC Press, Boca Raton, FL, 2000, pp. 297, 310–312.

80. Hill, J.O., Peters, J.C., Swith, L.L., Yang, D., Sharp, T., Abumrad, N., and Greene H.L. Changes in blood lipids during six days of overfeeding with medium or long chain triglycerides. *J. Lipid Res.* 31, 407–416, 1990.

81. Jeukendrup, A.E., Saris, W.H., Schrauwen, P., Brouns, F., and Wagenmakers, A.J. Metabolic availability of medium-chain triglycerides coingested with carbohydrates during prolonged exercise. *J. Appl. Physiol.* 79, 756–762, 1995.

82. Jeukendrup, A.E., Saris, W.H., Van Diesen, R., Brouns, F., and Wagenmakers, A.J. Effect of endogenous carbohydrate availability on oral medium-chain triglyceride oxidation during prolonged exercise. *J. Appl. Physiol.* 80, 949–954, 1996.

83. Jeukendrup, A.E., Saris, W.H.M., Brouns, F., Halliday, D., and Wagenmakers, A.J.M. Effects of carbohydrate (CHO) and fat supplementation on CHO metabolism during prolonged exercise. *Metabolism* 45, 915–921, 1996.

84. Jeukendrup, A.E., Saris, W.H.M., and Wagenmakers, A.J.M. Fat metabolism during exercise: a review. *Int. J. Sports Med.* 19, 371–379, 1998.

85. Goedecke, J.H., Clark, V.R., Noakes, T.D., and Lambert, E.V. The effects of medium-chain triacylglycerol and carbohydrate ingestion on ultra-endurance exercise performance. *Int. J. Sports Nutr. Exerc. Metab.* 14, 15–27, 2005.

86. Kern, M., Lagomarcino, N.D., Misell, L.M., and Schuster, V. The effect of medium-chain triacylglycerols on the blood lipid profile of male endurance runners. *J. Nutr. Biochem.* 11, 288–292, 2000.

87. Tholstrup, T., Ehnholm, C., Jauhiainen, M., Peterson, M., Hey C.E., Lund, P., and Sandstrom B. Effects of medium-chain fatty acids and oleic acid on blood lipids, lipoproteins, glucose, insulin, and lipid transfer protein activities. *Am. J. Clin. Nutr.* 79, 564–569, 2004.

88. Hill, J.O., Peters, J.C., Yang, D., Sharp, T., Kaler, M., Abumard, N.N., and Greene, H.L. Therogenesis in man during overfeeding with medium chain triglycerides. *Metabolism* 38, 641–648, 1989.

89. Shinohara, H., Ogawa, A., Kasai, M., and Aoyama, T. Effect of randomly interesterified triacylglycerols containing medium- and long-chain fatty acids on energy expenditure and hepatic fatty acid metabolism in rats. *Biosci. Biotechnol. Biochem.* 69, 1811–1818, 2005.

90. Cater, N.B., Heller, H.J., and Denke, M.A. Comparison of the effects of medium-chain triacylglycerols, palm oil, and high oleic acid sunflower oil on plasma triacylglycerol fatty acids and lipid and lipoprotein concentrations in humans. *Am. J. Clin. Nutr.* 65, 41–45, 1997.

91. Naohisa, N., Kasai, M., Nakamura, M., Takahashi, I., Itakura, M., Takeuchi, H., Aoyama, T., Tsuji, H., Okazaki, M., and Kondo, K. Effects of dietary medium-chain triacylglycerols on serum lipoproteins and biochemical parameters in healthy men. *Biosci. Biotechnol. Biochem.* 66, 1713–1718, 2002.

92. Calabrese, N.D., Myer, S., Munson, S., Turet, P., and Birdsall, T.C. A cross-over study of the effect of a single oral feeding of medium chain triglyceride oil vs. canola oil on post-ingestion plasma triglyceride levels in healthy men. *Altern. Med. Rev.* 4, 23–28, 1999.

93. Swift, L.L., Hill, J.O., Peters, J.C., and Greene, H.L. Plasma lipids and lipoproteins during 6 d of maintenance feeding with long-chain, medium-chain triglycerides. *Am. J. Clin. Nutr.* 56, 881–886, 1992.

94. Asakura, L., Lottenburg, A.M.P., Neves, M.Q.T.S., Nunes, V.S., Rocha, J.C., Passarelli, M., Nakandakare, E.R., and Quinttao, E.C.R. Dietary medium-chain triacylglycerol prevents the postprandial rise of plasma triacylglycerols but induces hypercholesterolemia in primary hypertriglycerdemic subjects. *Am. J. Clin. Nutr.* 71, 701–705, 2000.

95. Themme, E.H.M., Mensink, R.P., and Hornstra, G. Effects of medium chain fatty acids (MCFA), myristic acids, and oleic acid on serum lipoproteins in healthy subjects. *J. Lipid Res.* 38, 1746–1754, 1997.

96. Thomas, T.R., Horner, K.E., Langdon, M.M., Zhang, J.Q., Kurl, E.S., Sun, G.Y., and Cox, R.H. Effect of exercise and medium-chain fatty acids on postparandial lipemia. *J. Appl. Physiol.* 90, 1239–1246, 2001.

97. Stein, J. Chemically defined structured lipids: current status and future directions in gastrointestinal diseases. *Int. J. Colorect. Dis.* 14, 79–85, 1999.

98. Vistisen, B., Nybo, L., XU, X., Hey, C.E., and Kiens, B. Minor amounts of plasma medium-chain fatty acids and no improved trial performance after consuming lipids. *J. Appl. Physiol.* 95, 2434–2443, 2003.

99. Kasai, M., Nosaka, N., Maki, H., Negishi, S., Aoyama, T., Nakamura, M., Suzuki, Y., Tsuji, H., Uto, H., Okazaki, M., and Kondo, K. Effect of dietary medium- and long-chain triglycerols (MLCT) on accumulation of body fat in healthy humans. *Asia Pac. J. Clin. Nutr.* 12, 151–160, 2003.

100. Mu, H. and Hoy, C.E. Intestinal absorption of specific structured trigacylalycerols. *J. Lipid Res.* 42, 792–798, 2001.

101. Carvajal, O., Sakono, M., Sonoki, H., Nakayams, M., Kishi, T., Sato, M., Ikeda, I., Sugano, M., and Imaizumi, K. Structured triacylglycerol containing medium-chain fatty acids in sn 1(3) facilitates the absorption of dietary long-chain fatty acids in rats. *Biosci. Biotechnol. Biochem.* 64, 793–798, 2000.

102. St.-Onge, M. and Jones, P.J.H. Physiological effects of medium-chain triglycerides: potential agents in the prevention of obesity. *J. Nutr.* 132, 329–332, 2002.

103. Tsuji, H., Kasai, M., Takeuchi, H., Nakamura, M., Okazaki, M., and Kondo K. Dietary medium-chain triglycerols suppress accumulation of body fat in a double-blind, controlled trial in healthy men and women. *J. Nutr.* 131, 2853–2859, 2001.

104. Nosaka, N., Maki, H., Suzuki, Y., Haruna, H., Ohara, A., Kasai, M., Tsuji, H., Aoyama, T., Okazaki, M., Igarashi, O., and Kondo, K. Effects of margarine containing medium-chain triglycerols on body fat reduction in humans. *J. Atheroscler. Thromb.* 10, 290–298, 2003.

105. Kasai, M., Nosaka, N., Maki, H., Suzuki, Y., Takeuchi, H., Aoyama, T., Ohra, A., Harada, Y., Okazaki, M., and Kondo, K. Comparison of diet-induced thermogenesis of foods containing medium- versus long-chain triacylglcerols. *J. Nutr. Sci. Vitaminol.* 48, 536–540, 2002.

106. Noguchi, O., Takeuchi, H., Kubota, F., Tusji, H., and Aoyama T. Larger diet-induced thermogenesis and less body fat accumulation in rats fed medium-chain triacylglycerols than those fed long-chain triacylglycerols. *J. Nutr. Sci. Vitaminol.* 48, 524–529, 2002.

107. Traul, K.A., Driedger, A., Ingle, D.L., and Nakhasi, D. Review of the toxicologic properties of medium-chain triglycerides. *Food Chem. Toxicol.* 38, 79–98, 2000.

4 Omega-3 and Omega-6 Fatty Acids

Karina R. Lora and Nancy M. Lewis

CONTENTS

4.1 INTRODUCTION

The ω-3 and ω-6 fatty acids are polyunsaturated fatty acids that comprise a family of several other fatty acids that are essential for different physiological processes in humans. α-Linolenic acid and linoleic acid are the two main representative compounds of the ω-3 and ω-6 fatty acids from which arachidonic acid, eicosapentaenoic acid (EPA), and docosahexaenoic acid (DHA) are synthesized. Extensive research has been conducted to investigate the properties and effects of these polyunsaturated fatty acids in the last decades. Today there is consensus on the benefits of a diet with adequate intake and balance of ω-3 and ω-6 fatty acids to ensure nutrient adequacy, prevent nutrient deficiency, and reduce the risk of some chronic diseases. After considerable scientific information, the National Academy of Science's Institute of Medicine released the Dietary Reference Intakes for Adequate Intakes for linoleic acid and α-linolenic acid for the first time in 2002. Important information is now available about the risk of excessive ω-3 and ω-6 fatty acids intake; however, upper limit intakes have not yet been set. In that regard, although some studies have explored the effects of these polyunsaturated fatty acids on athletes, there is still not enough information to set requirements for individuals engaged in exercise, and more research is needed in that area. Research may focus on supplementation to enhance aerobic performance and to decrease exercise-induced bronchoconstriction in athletes.

This chapter provides current information on the properties, metabolism, functions, nutrient status assessment, recommended intakes, and other important characteristic of ω-3 and ω-6 fatty acids. In addition, available scientific information on the effects of ω-3 and ω-6 fatty acids supplementation on physical performance and exercise is presented.

4.2   CHEMICAL STRUCTURES AND SYNTHESIS

Fatty acids are hydrocarbon chains with a carboxyl group (–COOH) at one end and a methyl group (CH_3) at the other. Fatty acids vary in chain length, degree of unsaturation,[1] and location of double bonds[2] and can be classified as saturated (no double bonds), monounsaturated (single double bond), and polyunsaturated (several double bonds). Unsaturated fatty acids can be classified in two different ways: the delta (Δ) and the omega (ω) numbering system.[1,3] In the delta system, the carboxyl carbon is denoted as carbon 1, while in the omega system carbon 1 is the methyl carbon.[3] The number of double bonds in the fatty acid chain are counted from either the carboxyl or the methyl end. For instance, in the delta system the polyunsaturated fatty acid α-linolenic acid has the notation $18:3\Delta^{9c,12c,15c}$ or 18 carbons, and three double bonds occurring in the 9, 12, and 15 carbons. The same fatty acid in the omega system is 18:3ω3 or 18 carbons, with three double bonds and the first occurring at carbon 3.[4] Fatty acids in which the first double bond occurs three carbons from the methyl end are called omega-3 fatty acids and are symbolized as ω-3 (or n-3) fatty acids. Fatty acids in which the first double bond occurs six carbons from the methyl end are named omega-6 fatty acids with the symbol of ω-6 (or n-6) fatty acids.[2]

Mammals do not have the capacity to completely synthesize either of these two types of polyunsaturated fatty acids because they cannot desaturate the 16- or 18-carbon products of fatty acid synthesis any further than nine carbons from the carboxyl end.[3] Linoleic acid and α-linolenic acid are the two main representative compounds of the ω-6 and ω-3 fatty acids and are essential fatty acids because they prevent deficiency symptoms and cannot be synthesized by humans;[5] therefore, they need to be obtained from the diet. These two types of polyunsaturated fatty acids cannot be interconverted, have different biochemical roles,[3,5] and are precursors of other polyunsaturated fatty acids (Table 4.1). Linoleic acid is a precursor for arachidonic acid and eicosanoids. α-Linolenic acid is a precursor for DHA. Linoleic acid,

TABLE 4.1
Primary ω-3 and ω-6 Polyunsaturated Fatty Acids

ω-3 Fatty Acids		ω-6 Fatty Acids	
18:3	α-Linolenic acid	18:2	Linoleic acid
20:5	Eicosapentaenoic acid (EPA)	18:3	γ-Linolenic acid
22:5	Docosapentaenoic acid	20:3	Dihomo-γ-linolenic acid
22:6	Docosahexaenoic acid (DHA)	20:4	Arachidonic acid
		22:4	Adrenic acid
		22:5	Docosapentaenoic acid

Adapted from Institute of Medicine, *Dietary Reference Intakes for Energy, Carbohydrate, Fiber, Fat, Fatty Acids, Cholesterol, Protein, and Amino Acids,* National Academy Press, Washington, DC, 2005.

arachidonic acid, and DHA are found in cellular phospholipids.[6] The more unsaturated and longer-chain ω-3 and ω-6 fatty acids, arachidonic acid (20:4ω-6), EPA (20:5ω-3), and docosahexaenoic acid (22:6ω-3) can be synthesized from linoleic and α-linolenic acids by alternating desaturation, elongation, and partial β-oxidation process[3,7] (Figure 4.1). Nonesterified fatty acids enter cells via fatty acid transporters and are converted to fatty acyl-CoA thioesters by acyl-CoA synthetases. Fatty acyl-CoA thioesters are the substrate for reactions of elongation, desaturation, and retroconversion[8] that take place in the synthesis of ω-3 and ω-6 fatty acids in humans. The liver is the primary site for the metabolism of essential fatty acids; however, other tissues experience metabolism of these fatty acids.[9] Dietary 18:2ω-6 and 18:3ω-3 are converted to long-chain highly unsaturated fatty acids by a series of desaturation and elongation reactions that take place in the endoplasmatic reticulum, and β-oxidation, which occurs in the peroxisomes.[8]

Fatty acid desaturation is accomplished by the enzymes Δ^6-desaturase and Δ^5-desaturase.[3,5,7,8] Δ^6-Desaturase is now considered to be the rate-limiting step of the pathway.[5] Earlier it was thought that an acyl-CoA-dependent 4-desaturase was responsible for the desaturation of the ω-3 and ω-6 fatty acids; however, it was later found that the endoplasmatic reticulum does not contain this type of desaturase.[10] These two desaturases are membrane-bound enzymes that occur in the endoplasmatic reticulum of tissues in the liver, intestinal mucosa, brain, and retina.[11–16] The work of Okayasu et al.[17] showed that cytochrome b_5 and cytochrome b_5 reductase were required to desaturate 18:2ω-6 to 18:3ω-6. Later, it was accepted that the desaturase reactions require O_2, NADH, cytochrome b_5, and cytochrome b_5 reductase for the desaturation of both linoleic and α-linolenic acid.[3,7] Hormonal and dietary factors such as insulin and fatty acid-deficient diets have been observed to increase the activity of the Δ^6-desaturase, while glucose, epinephrine, and glucagon decrease desaturase activity.[18] Δ^6-Desaturase utilizes the fatty acyl chain that has a double bond at carbon 9 and inserts a new double bond at carbon 6. This desaturase converts α-linolenic acid to 18:4, and 24:5 to 24:6; and linoleic acid to 18:3, and 24:4 to 24:5. Δ^5-Desaturase operates on a fatty acyl chain that has a double bond at carbon

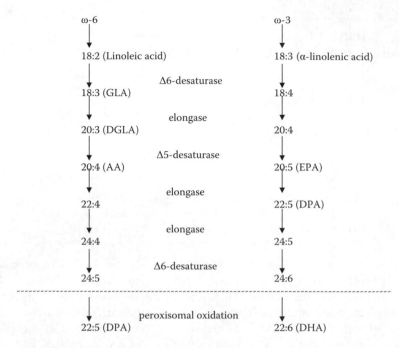

FIGURE 4.1 Pathway for the synthesis of ω-6 and ω-3 fatty acids. *Note:* GLA = γ-linolenic acid, DGLA = dihomo-γ-linolenic acid, AA = arachidonic acid, EPA = eicosapentaenoic acid, DPA = docosapentaenoic acid, DHA = docosohexanoic acid. *Source:* Adapted from Arterburn et al. (2006).[118]

8 and adds a new double bond at carbon 5. It converts 20:4 to 20:5 (EPA) and 20:3 to 20:4 (arachidonic acid).[3]

Fatty acid elongation occurs with only one type of elongase. During the elongation process, the chain is lengthened by the addition of two carbons to the carbonyl group by malonyl CoA. The carbonyl group of the fatty acyl CoA is reduced to a methylene group in reactions that need NADPH. During the elongation of the fatty acids the double bonds do not move.[3] Three elongation steps occur in the synthesis of the ω-3 and ω-6 fatty acids.

Retroconversion is the final step in the synthesis of these polyunsaturated fatty acids. The retroconversion step of peroxisomal β-oxidation is also called the Sprecher pathway.[19] The role of peroxisomes takes place when the synthesis of 22:5 and 22:6 requires intracellular communication between the endoplasmic reticulum and a site where a partial β-oxidation could occur.[10] In the retroconversion process, two carbons are removed from the carboxyl end of the fatty acid as acetyl CoA. Then the 24-carbon intermediaries are retroconverted to 22:5 and 22:6. The retroconversion process requires O_2, FAD, and NAD^+.[3]

TABLE 4.2
Selected Physical Properties of Some ω-3 and ω-6 Polyunsaturated Fatty Acids

Fatty Acid	Chemical Name	Δ Formula	ω Formula	MW	Melting Point (°C)	Solubility
Linoleic acid	All cis-9,12-octadecadienoic	$18:2\Delta^{9c,12c}$	$18:2\omega6$	280.44	−5	i.H$_2$O, ∞EtOH, eth., CHCl$_3$
γ-Linolenic acid	All cis-6,9,12-octadecatrienoic	$18:3\Delta^{6c,9c,12c}$	$18:3\omega6$	278.44		
α-Linolenic acid	All cis-9,12,15-octadecatrienoic	$18:3\Delta^{9c,12c,15c}$	$18:3\omega3$	278.44	−10	i.H$_2$O, s.EtOH, eth., CHCl$_3$
Arachidonic acid	All cis-5,8,11,14-eicosatetraenoic	$20:4\Delta^{5c,8c,11c,14c}$	$20:4\omega6$	304.50	−49.5	i.H2O, s.eth.
Eicosapentaenoic acid	All cis-5,8,11,14,17-eicosapentaenoic	$20:5\Delta^{5c,8c,11c,14c,17c}$	$20:5\omega3$	302.50		
Docosahexaenoic acid	All cis-4,7,10,13,16,19-docosahexaenoic	$22:6\Delta^{4c,7c,10c,13c,16c,19c}$	$22:6\omega3$	328.50		

Note: MW = molecular weight; i. = insoluble; ∞ = completely miscible; eth. = diethyl ether; s. = soluble.

Adapted from Small, D.M., in *Biochemical and Physiological Aspects of Human Nutrition*, Stipanuk, M.H., Ed., W.B. Saunders Company, Philadelphia, PA, 2000, pp. 43–71; and Dawson, R.C. et al., in *Data for Biochemical Research*, Dawson, R.C. et al., Eds., Oxford University Press, New York, 1986, pp. 167–189.

4.3 GENERAL PROPERTIES

Table 4.2 lists physical properties of molecular weight, melting point, and solubility of some ω-3 and ω-6 polyunsaturated fatty acids.

4.4 METABOLISM

4.4.1 DIGESTION AND ABSORPTION

The digestion and absorption of ω-3 and ω-6 fatty acids is similar to that of other long-chain fatty acids.[20] Dietary fat digestion and absorption is a complex process that further leads to the absorption of lipids by the enterocytes of the small intestine mucosa.[21] Dietary lipids undergo the action of lingual lipase in the mouth, which cleaves the sn-3 position of the triacylglycerol molecule, and its activity continues through the esophagus and into the stomach.[2] In the stomach, gastric lipase augments the activity of lingual lipase by cleaving triacylglycerols at the sn-3 position and partially digesting fats before they enter the small intestine. Gastric lipase preferentially digests triacylglycerols that contain medium-chain fatty acids rather than those that have long-chain fatty acids. The action of this lipase in the stomach releases 1,2 diacylglycerols and fatty acids that are thought to contribute to emulsification of dietary fat in the stomach.[2,21] After lipids enter the small intestine as an emulsion, they are subjected to the action of bile and pancreatic juice. Bile salts and phospholipids from bile emulsify the fat, and pancreatic lipase hydrolyzes the fat. Triacylglycerols are cleaved at the sn-1 and sn-3 positions, resulting in free fatty acids and 2-monoacylglycerides. These resulting products of digestion are absorbed into the enterocytes.

Absorption of fatty acids in the small intestine follows a complex process that varies in efficiency depending on certain qualitative characteristics of dietary fat.[22] Unsaturated fatty acids tend to be absorbed at a higher efficiency than saturated fatty acids. Fatty acids with ≤10 carbons are directly absorbed into the portal circulation, while fatty acids with ≥12 carbons are absorbed into the lymphatic system packaged as chylomicrons.[2] Fat digestion products incorporated into micelles occur largely through passive diffusion. Absorption of micellar components into intestinal mucosal cells depends on the penetration of the micelles across the unstirred water layer that separates the intestinal content from the brush border of the small intestine.[2,22]

4.4.2 TRANSPORT

Dietary fat is transported to peripheral and hepatic tissues by the exogenous transport system.[22] In the cell, lipid compounds in the cytosol of the enterocytes are transported from the apical region where they were absorbed to the endoplasmic reticulum[21] by specific fatty acid-binding protein (FABP).[23] Biosynthesis of complex lipids takes place in the endoplasmic reticulum.[21] The exogenous system starts with reorganization in the enterocytes of 2-monoacylglycerides and fatty acids in triacylglycerol via the monoacylglycerol pathway.[21,22] The formed triacylglycerols along with phospholipids, cholesterol, and glycerol form molecules called chylomicrons.[22] The main function of chylomicrons is to provide a mechanism for dietary fat and other fat-soluble compounds to be carried from the site of absorption to other parts of the body for uptake and metabolism.[24] Chylomicrons are released into the lymphatic circulation and further into the blood circulation. In the circulation, the triacylglycerol component of the chylomicrons is hydrolyzed by the enzyme lipoprotein lipase (LPL). LPL is synthesized in the adipose tissue and skeletal muscle.[2] The hydrolysis of triglycerides by LPL ensures the peripheral tissues a delivery of dietary fat for diverse metabolic processes such as oxidation, metabolism, and storage.[2,22] Chylomicrons are released from peripheral tissues as chylomicron remnants and further used by the liver.

Humans are unable to insert a double bond at the n-3 position of a fatty acid of 18 carbons in length or a cis double bond at the n-6 position of a fatty acid chain; therefore, ω-3 and ω-6 fatty acids are essential nutrients.[20] α-Linolenic and linoleic acids are the precursors of other polyunsaturated fatty acids of the ω-3 and ω-6 fatty acids family. The liver is the primary site for the metabolism of essential fatty acids and where the synthesis of arachidonic acid (20:4ω-6) from linoleic acid and EPA (20:5ω-3) and DHA (22:6ω-3) from α-linolenic acid takes place. However, other tissues experience metabolism of these fatty acids.[9] For instance, the desaturase enzymes occur in the endoplasmatic reticulum tissues of the intestinal mucosa, brain, and retina.[11–16] The metabolism of ω-6 fatty acids involves the synthesis of arachidonic acid and eicosanoid precursors from linoleic acid, which is accomplished by reactions as elongation, desaturation, and retroconversion,[8] explained previously. EPA is the precursor for series-3 eicosanoids and series-5 leukotrienes. DHA is a component of membrane structural lipids that are enriched in phospholipids found in nervous tissue, retina, and spermatozoa.[20] Arachidonic acid is found primarily in membrane phospholipids and is a precursor for eicosanoids that are involved in platelet aggregation, hemodynamics, and coronary vascular tone.[25]

4.4.3 BODY RESERVES

DHA is the most abundant ω-3 fatty acid in most tissues,[8] is in higher concentrations in the myocardium, retina, brain, and spermatozoa, and is essential for proper functioning of these tissues and growth.[26] In the nervous system, the tissue most highly enriched in DHA is the photoreceptor outer segment.[27] Different classes of lipids in the body contain ω-3 fatty acids. For instance, α-linolenic acid is found in triglycerides, cholesterol esters, and, in small concentrations, phospholipids. EPA is found in cholesterol esters, triglycerides, and phospholipids, while DHA is found mostly in phospholipids.[28]

4.4.4 EXCRETION

Polyunsaturated ω-3 and ω-6 fatty acids are almost completely absorbed. Small amounts of these two fatty acids are lost during sloughing of skin and other epithelial cells.[20]

4.5 FUNCTIONS AND PROBABLE FUNCTIONS

Polyunsaturated fatty acids are recognized to be essential for humans and animals for two reasons: synthesis of lipid mediators and production of membranes that have the optimum lipid bilayer structure and functional properties. The main function of ω-3 fatty acids is related to membrane structure, and DHA plays a role. The polyunsaturated ω-6 fatty acids have a role in formation of lipid mediators, which includes the eicosanoids and the inositol phosphoglycerides. Arachidonic acid is the main fatty acid of the ω-6 family involved in this process; however, EPA also can play a role in the formation of eicosanoids.[3]

The ω-3 fatty acids are major structural components of membrane phospholipids of tissues and influence membrane fluidity and ion transports. These polyunsaturated fatty acids are rich in the brain, myocardium, and retina, are essential for proper functioning and growth, and modulate many physiological processes.[26] Along with arachidonic acid, DHA is the major polyunsaturated fatty acid found in the brain and is recognized to be important for brain development and function.[29] These two types of fatty acids have an effect on the neuronal membrane fluidity index, and it appears that the relative amounts of ω-3 and ω-6 fatty acids in the cell membranes are responsible for affecting cellular function.[30] Reported effects of polyunsaturated fatty acids on brain functions are modifications of membrane fluidity, the activity of membrane-bound enzymes, the number and affinity of receptors, the function of ion channels, and the production and activity of neurotransmitters and signal transduction.[31]

Omega-3 fatty acids have been recognized to lower the risk of coronary heart disease (CHD) and protect against sudden cardiac death through antiarrhythmic, antiatherogenic, antithrombotic, and vasoprotective mechanisms. Omega-3 fatty effects on inhibition of platelet aggregation and serum lipids (triglycerides and high-density lipoprotein [HDL]) may prevent CHD. However, the antiarrhythmic rather than the antiatherothrombotic effect seems to be the major function of ω-3 fatty acids in preventing CHD.[26]

The ω-3 fatty acid DHA is also essential for proper development of the retina, particularly at the synapse and the outer segment of photoreceptors,[32] by influencing membrane fluidity in the temporal response of the G-protein-coupled signaling system in the retinal rod outer segment (ROS).[8,29]

One of the most characterized physiological functions of these polyunsaturated fatty acids is the role of eicosanoids. Eicosanoids work as autocrine/paracrine hormones and mediate a variety of functions, such as immune response, blood pressure regulation, blood coagulation,[33] movement of calcium and other substances into and out of cells, relaxation and contraction of muscles, and cell division and growth.[34] The eicosanoids include substances such as prostaglandins and leukotrienes. Arachidonic acid is the precursor for a group of eicosanoids that include series-2 prostaglandins and series-4 leukotrienes, while EPA is the precursor for a group of eicosanoids that include series-3 prostaglandins and series-5 leukotrienes.[28] Eicosanoids derived from ω-6 fatty acids are pro-inflammatory and pro-aggregatory agonists, while those derived from ω-3 fatty acids tend to inhibit platelet aggregation and be anti-inflammatory.[35,36] Adequate production of the series-3 prostaglandins is thought to have protective effects against heart attacks.[28]

The effects of ω-3 and ω-6 fatty acids in inflammation and autoimmune diseases have been linked to the concentration of the type of prostaglandins and leukotrienes present in the cells. EPA-derived eicosanoids are less potent inducers of inflammation than the arachidonic acid-derived eicosanoids,[5] and competition between ω-3 and ω-6 fatty acids occurs in the prostaglandins' formation.[36] For instance, an increased level of interleukin (IL) 1, a pro-inflamatory cytokine, is present in CHD, depression, aging, and cancer. Similarly, high levels of IL1 and series-4 leukotrienes produced by ω-6 fatty acids are present in arthritis and other autoimmune diseases.

Other probable effects of ω-3 fatty acids are membrane-mediated processes, such as insulin transduction signals; activity of lipases, which are affected by alteration of the fatty acid composition of the membrane phospholipids; and regulation of genes involved in lipid and glucose metabolism, and adipogenesis.[37]

A newly discovered metabolite (10,17S-docosatriene) synthesized in the brain has been indicated to have a response to an ischemic insult and to have opposite anti-inflammatory effects.[29]

4.6 DIETARY AND SUPPLEMENTAL SOURCES

The predominant food sources of ω-3 fatty acids in the diet are vegetable oils and fish. Fish is the major source of EPA and DHA, and vegetable oils (canola, soybean, flaxseed/linseed, olive) are the major source of α-linolenic acid. Other sources include nuts and seeds, vegetables and some fruit, egg yolk, poultry, and meat.[38,39] Enrichment of diets with fish oil,[40,41] extracts of algae oils,[42,43] and mixtures of fish oil and linseed, and canola and sunflower oil[44] have been fed to hens to produce enriched eggs as a source of ω-3 fatty acids for humans. Vitamin E is usually added to the hens' diet to avoid lipid peroxidation and extend shelf life.[45,46] A trial has reported feeding subjects with a variety of ω-3-enriched foods, including bread, milk, spread, eggs, biscuits, cereals, soups, pancake mix, muffin mix, salad dressing, dips, snacks, and chocolates, to test the feasibility of enriched products to consumers.[47] Food sources of ω-6 polyunsaturated fatty acids include nuts, seeds, certain vegetables, and vegetable oils such as soybean, safflower, and corn oil.[20] Blackcurrant seed oil and evening primrose oil have high contents of γ-linolenic acid. Arachidonic acid is formed only in animal cells from linoleic acid and is present in small quantities in meat, poultry, and eggs[20] (Table 4.3).

Dietary fish oil supplements are available on the market and vary in the amounts and ratios of EPA and DHA. Common amounts of ω-3 fatty acids in fish oil capsules are 180 mg of EPA and 120 mg of DHA.[38,39] Cod liver oil supplement capsules usually contain 173 mg of EPA and 120 mg of DHA. Fish oil supplements need to be consumed with caution due to their high content of vitamins A and D.[39] Because vitamin E deficiency may occur when fish oil supplements are taken for several months, manufacturers add vitamin E to many commercial fish oil products.[38] A DHA source from algae that provides 100 mg/capsule is available on the market.[39]

4.7 NUTRIENT STATUS ASSESSMENT

The measurements of the total amount of various essential fatty acids as ω-3 fatty acids in plasma, serum, or erythrocyte membrane phospholipids have been indicated as useful markers of essential polyunsaturated fatty acids.[5,26] Essential fatty acid deficiency is a clinical condition that derives from inadequate status of ω-3 and ω-6 fatty acids; however, the symptoms are nonspecific and may not present prior to marginal essential fatty acid status.[48] Widely used biomarkers for biochemical essential fatty acid deficiency are mead acid and the triene/tetraene ratio.[49–51] However, the total plasma triene/tetraene ratio has been considered the gold standard for essential fatty acid deficiency.[48,52] Mead acid, or 5,8,11-eicosatrienoic acid (5,8,11–20:3 ω-9)[5,52] is synthesized from endogenous oleic acid and is increased when there is insufficient concentrations of linoleic and α-linolenic acid to meet the needs of polyunsaturated fatty acids.[5,52] Under normal conditions only trace amounts of mead acid are found in plasma.[52] EPA and DHA inhibit mead acid synthesis.[5] Mead acid measurement is an indicator of essential fatty acid deficiency state, while essential fatty acid depletion is associated with a decrease in plasma linoleate and arachidonate percentages.[52] Assessment of long-term essential fatty acid intake is measured in adipose tissue, and it is considered the best indicator because of its slow turnover.[53–55] Cutoff values for the assessment of essential fatty acids and ω-3 fatty acid status in erythrocytes have been reported.[48] Proposed cutoff values for children older than 0.2 years are 0.46 mol% 20:3 ω-9 (mead acid) for early suspicion of essential fatty acid deficiency, 0.068 mol/mol docosapentaenoic/arachidonic acid

TABLE 4.3
Polyunsaturated (ω-3 and ω-6) Fatty Acid Composition of Food Commodities

	ω-3 Fatty Acids			ω-6 Fatty Acids	
	LNA	EPA	DHA	LA	AA
Commodities	mg/100 g			mg/100 g	
Poultry meats	73	5	25	1443	98
Chicken, with skin[a]	140	10	30	2880	80
Chicken, without skin[a]	20	10	30	550	80
Turkey, with skin[a]	110	0	20	1700	110
Turkey, without skin[a]	20	0	20	640	120
Pig meats	53	3	2	831	68
Pork loin, without fat	12	3	2	262	53
Pork loin, without fat[a]	20	NA	NA	440	60
Pork, with fat[a]	90	NA	NA	1310	80
Eggs	31	0	44	1272	156
Bovine meats	105	5	4	277	24
Beef rib eye	10	5	2	178	46
Beef rib eye[a]	10	NA	NA	240	20
Beef sirloin	20	5	10	94	9
Beef Swiss steak	61	9	8	182	18
Nelore *longissimus dorsi*	15	3	2	115	11
Canchim *longissimus dorsi*	13	4	2	101	9
Beefalo *longissimus dorsi*	16	3	2	98	9
Beef, with fat[a]	190	NA	NA	410	30
Goat and mutton	178	5	21	460	64
Lamb loin chop	54	5	10	369	84
Lamb steak leg	126	14	84	202	12
Lamb, raw feet	27	0	9	198	66
Lamb, Australian[a]	202	NA	NA	422	69
Lamb, New Zealand[a]	420	NA	NA	550	10
Lamb, domestic[a]	330	NA	NA	1090	70
Goat shoulder	44	9	5	337	109
Goat leg	49	0	9	262	65
Goat[a]	20	NA	NA	100	60
Freshwater fish	93	245	461	295	104
Trout, rainbow[a]	58	260	668	710	25
Bass, freshwater[a]	111	238	357	87	144
Demersal fish	37	82	199	19	89
Flatfish, flounder and sole[a]	8	93	106	8	38
Halibut[a]	65	71	292	30	139
Pelagic fish	74	185	619	60	90
Tuna, bluefin[a]	0	283	890	53	43
Salmon, Atlantic[a]	295	321	1115	172	267
Cod, Atlantic[a]	1	64	120	5	22
Pollock, Atlantic[a]	0	71	350	9	26

TABLE 4.3 (CONTINUED)
Polyunsaturated (ω-3 and ω-6) Fatty Acid Composition
of Food Commodities

	ω-3 Fatty Acids			ω-6 Fatty Acids	
	LNA	EPA	DHA	LA	AA
Commodities	mg/100 g			mg/100 g	
Crustacean, shrimp[a]	14	258	222	28	87
Mollusks, mussel[a]	20	188	253	18	70
Marine fish, other	36	178	323	31	84
Coconut vegetable oil[a]	0	0	0	1800	0
Cottonseed vegetable oil[a]	200	0	0	51,500	100
Groundnut oil	0	0	0	32,000	0
Maize germ oil	700	0	0	58,000	0
Olive oil	600	0	0	7900	0
Palm kernel vegetable oil[a]	0	0	0	1600	0
Palm vegetable oil[a]	200	0	0	9100	0
Canola oil[a]	9300	0	0	20,300	0
Rice bran vegetable oil[a]	1600	0	0	33,400	0
Sesame oil[a]	300	0	0	41,300	0
Soybean oil[a]	6800	0	0	51,000	0
Sunflower vegetable oil[a]	0	0	0	65,700	0

Note: LNA = α-linolenic acid; EPA = eicosapentaenoic acid; DHA = docoso-hexanoic acid; LA = linoleic acid; AA = arachidonic acid; NA = not available.

[a] Information retrieved from the U.S. Department of Agriculture National Nutrient Database for Standard Reference, Release 17.

Adapted from Hibbeln, J.R. et al., *Am. J. Clin. Nutr.*, 83, 1483S–1493S, 2006.

for ω-3 fatty acid deficiency, 0.22 mol/mol docosapentaenoic/docosahexaenoic acid for ω-3 fatty acid/docosahexaenoic acid marginality, and 0.48 mol/mol docosapen-taenoic/docosahexaenoic acid for ω-3 fatty acid/docosahexaenoic acid deficiency.[48] Recently, fasting whole blood has been proposed as a biomarker of essential fatty acid intake.[56]

The triene/tetraene ratio (20:3 ω-9/20:4 ω-6) more commonly indicative of essential fatty acid deficiency is greater than 0.4,[57,58] although ratios of 0.2 have been used.[59,60] Currently, there is no accepted cutoff value of plasma or tissue DHA concentrations for indicating impaired health.[20] The triene/tetraene ratio is considered a sensitive diagnostic index of essential fatty acid deficiencies associated with total parenteral nutrition.[57] Food frequency questionnaires and 24-hour recalls to assess ω-3 fatty acid intake in cardiac patients,[61] pregnant women,[62] physically active adults,[63] and hypercholestolemic subjects[64] have been used.

4.8 INTERACTIONS WITH OTHER NUTRIENTS AND DRUGS

The synergistic effects of ω-3 and ω-6 fatty acids and drugs used in the treatment of Crohn's disease have been reported.[65,66] Amino-salicylic acid (5-ASA) therapy with ω-3 fatty acids supplementation in the treatment of pediatric patients with Crohn's disease delayed the relapse of episodes. The synergistic effect of the drug and supplement were observed by 5-ASA inhibition of factors of the inflammatory cascade [cyclooxygenase, thromboxane-synthetase, and platelet activating factor (PAF) synthetase], production of IL-1 and free radicals, antioxidant activity, and ω-3 fatty acid inhibition of the PAF synthetase.[65] Omega-3 but not ω-6 fatty acids have shown immunomodulatory properties and an increase in pro-inflamatory cytokines in patients receiving enteral ω-3 and ω-6 fatty acids used as adjuvant therapy to corticosteroid medication for the treatment of Crohn's disease.[66] Omega-3 fatty acids have been shown to decrease the nephrotoxicity caused by cyclosporine therapy used to prevent rejection in organ transplantation.[67,68] Female rats fed with a mixture of ω-3 and ω-6 fatty acids and receiving intraperitoneal cyclosporine treatment showed that the metabolites of arachidonic acid increased the levels of thromboxane A, which plays a role in cyclosporine nephrotoxicity. Additionally, the polyunsaturated fatty acid mixture improved prostaglandin synthesis, which plays a beneficial role in the prevention of renal dysfunction.[67] It has also been reported that the interaction of ω-3 fatty acids supplementation to patients early after kidney graft as an adjunctive treatment to immunosuppressive regimen with cyclosporine reduces the nephrotoxic effects of this drug.[68]

Omega-3 fatty acids may increase the risk of bleeding when taken with drugs that increase the risk of bleeding, including aspirin, anticoagulants such as warfarin or heparin, antiplatelet drugs such as clopidogrel, and nonsteroidal anti-inflammatory drugs such as ibuprofen or naproxen.[38] A reported case of 1000 to 2000 mg/day intake of fish oil with warfarin medication indicated increased anticoagulation, and the ω-3 fatty acid in the oil may have affected platelet aggregation or vitamin K-dependent coagulation factors, and lowered thromboxane and decreased factor VII concentrations.[69] In contrast, there was no effect on vitamin K-dependent coagulation factors, but lowered platelet integrin activation and plasma levels of fibrinogen factor V have been reported with an intake of 3 g of ω-3 fatty acids daily for 4 weeks.

Omega-3 fatty acids supplementation may lower blood pressure by their anti-hypertensive and hypotriglyceridemic effects, and add to the effects of drugs that may also affect blood pressure, such as beta-blockers or diuretics.[38,70]

Omega-3 fatty acids lower triglyceride concentrations and may have a synergistc effect with the triglyceride-lowering effects of agents such as niacin, fibrates such as gemfibrozil, or resins such as cholestyramine. However, ω-3 fatty acids may work against the low-density lipoprotein (LDL) cholesterol-lowering properties of statin drugs.[49]

Modulation of interleukins by ω-3 fatty acid and intakes of 500 IU of vitamin E in the diet have been reported. These two nutrients may modulate the levels of IL-6, IL-10, IL-12, and tumor necrosis factor-α (TNF-α) in mice.[71] Omega-3 fatty acids have been reported to increase the risk of bleeding with the use of Ginkgo biloba, garlic, and saw palmetto; add to the effects of agents that may also affect blood pressure, such as eucalyptol, eucalyptus oil, flaxseed/flaxseed oil, garlic, ginger, and ginkgo, among others; and enhance lower blood sugar properties of aloe vera, American ginseng, bilberry, bitter melon, maitake mushroom, marshmallow, milk thistle, Panax ginseng, rosemary, shark cartilage, and Siberian ginseng, among others.[38] Omega-3 fatty acids can increase LDL cholesterol concentrations and may work against the potential LDL-lowering properties of agents like barley, garlic, guggul, psyllium, soy, or sweet almond.[38]

4.9   CLINICAL EFFECTS OF INADEQUATE INTAKES

Inadequate status of ω-3 and ω-6 fatty acid families presents a clinical condition of essential fatty acid deficiency.[48] Dietary deficiencies of α-linolenic and linoleic acids during development result in lower levels of arachidonic and docosahexaenoic acids in the central nervous system, resulting in altered learning behavior and visual function.[52] Deficiency of the ω-3 fatty acids family leads to neuronal-specific defects, including reduced learning, impaired vision, numbness, leg pain, and abnormal electroretinogram.[72,73] A normal electroretinogram is observed when α-linolenic acid is included in the diet again. Reduction in visual function is accompanied by decreased brain and retina DHA and an increase in docosapentaenoic acid. Changes in learning behavior have been reported in animals fed low α-linolenic diets containing less than 1%, and high content of linoleic acid.[20] Deficiency of ω-6 fatty acids in humans, although rare,[48] has been linked to several nonneuronal abnormalities, reduced growth, reproductive failure, skin lesions such as scaly skin rash, fatty liver and polydipsia, increased transepidermal water loss, and elevation of the plasma triene/tetraene ratio of eicosatrienoic acid/arachidonic acid to values greater than 0.4.[20,72,73] Inadequate essential fatty acid intake or impaired absorption leads to a decrease in tissue concentration of arachidonic acid, reduction in the inhibition of the desaturation of oleic acid, and increased synthesis of eicosatrienoic acid from oleic acid.[20] Protein-energy malnutrition is associated with deficiency in linoleic and arachidonic acid in infants, children, and malnourished elderly patients, and cutaneous hypersensitivity presented in these groups may be attributed to essential fatty acid deficiency.[52]

4.10   TOXICITY

According to the 2005 edition of the Dietary Reference Intakes (DRIs), there is insufficient evidence to set an upper limit (UL) for ω-3 and ω-6 fatty acids. However, an Acceptable Macronutrient Distribution Range (AMDR) has been estimated for linoleic and α-linolenic acids.[20] An AMDR of 5 to 10% of energy is estimated for ω-6 fatty acids (linoleic acid), and an AMDR of 0.6 to 1.2% of energy is given for α-linolenic acid. Approximately 10% of the AMDR for α-linolenic acid can be consumed as EPA and DHA (0.06 to 0.12% of energy).[20] High ω-6-fatty-acid diets may increase the risk for inflammatory disorders, such as increased plasma arachidonic acid concentrations after dietary supplementation of γ-linolenic acid, leading to platelet aggregation problems,[74] LDL oxidation,[75,76] and risk of nutrient excess by inhibition of the synthesis of ω-3 fatty acids.[20] An increase in the risk of cancer was reported when ω-6 fatty acids were fed as 15% of energy;[77] however, a more recent review of literature concluded that high intakes of linoleic acid were unlikely to increase the risk of several types of cancer.[78] Adverse effects of EPA and DHS have been reported because they are more potent than their precursor, α-linolenic acid.[20] High intakes of EPA and DHA may have adverse effects on immune function and increase the risk of bleeding and hemorrhagic stroke. High intakes of α-linolenic acid can affect the biosynthesis of ω-6 fatty acids important for prostaglandins and eicosanoid synthesis.[20] Several studies *in vitro* or *ex vivo* have shown suppression of different aspects of human immune function in individuals fed ω-3 fatty acid supplements or experimental diets. Doses of EPA from 0.9 to 9.4 g/day and DHA from 0.6 to 6.0 g/day are reported to cause some type of immunosuppression.[20] Oxidative damage of erythrocytes, liver and kidney membranes, and bone marrow DNA with high consumption of DHA have been reported.[79–81] It has been reported that high intake of dietary α-linolenic acid (40% of total fatty acids) in male hamsters adversely affected the hepatobiliary metabolism of sterols.[82] The high intake of α-linolenic acid decreased the ratio of cholic to chenodeoxicholic acid, probably by an inhibition of sterol 12-hydroxylase via SREBP1, and affected the bile acid transformation in the colon.[82] The combination of the drug prevastatin plus fish oil, although reported to reduce total plasma cholesterol and plasma triglycerides, was documented to develop nausea in one subject.[83]

Omega-3 fatty acid supplements should be used with caution in diabetic patients due to potential increases in blood sugar concentrations, in patients at risk for bleeding, and in individuals with high levels of LDL.[38] Other reported side effects of the use of fish oil are gastrointestinal symptoms such as gastrointestinal upset, nausea,[84,85] diarrhea and potentially severe diarrhea at very high doses,[85] burping,[86] acid reflux indigestion,[87] bloating,[88] and abdominal pain.[89] Small reductions in blood pressure with intake of ω-3 fatty acids have been reported and are dose–responsive.[90–93] Increase in LDL cholesterol levels by 5 to 10% with ω-3 fatty acid intakes of 1 g/day or greater,[38] mild elevation in alanine aminotransferase enzyme,[94] and rare reports of neurologic and psychiatric effects have also been reported.[38]

4.11 EFFECTS ON PHYSICAL PERFORMANCE

Physical activity is recognized as one factor that affects polyunsaturated fatty acid status.[5] Physical activity per se induces changes in the phospholipid fatty acid composition of muscle membranes.[5,95] The effects of an aerobic exercise program (55% VO$_2$ peak) on phospholipid fatty acid composition of ω-3 and ω-6 fatty acids in the skeletal muscle have been examined in sedentary subjects.[95] Six weeks of physical training showed changes in the levels of ω-3 (EPA, DHA, and docosapentaenoic acid) fatty acids, decreased the proportion of ω-6 (linoleic acid, dihomo-γ-linolenic acid, and arachidonic acid) fatty acids in muscle phospholipids, and reduced the ω-6 to ω-3 ratio.[96] Similar results were reported by Helge et al.[95] when investigating the effect of endurance training of the knee extensor of one leg for 4 weeks on the muscle membrane phospholipid fatty acid composition. After 4 weeks of training, the phospholipid fatty acid contents of oleic acid and DHA were higher in the trained than the untrained leg, and the ratio of ω-6 to ω-3 was lower in the trained than in the untrained leg.[95] The beneficial effect of exercise on lipoproteins and subfractions has been reported previously. The ω-3 fatty acid role in physiological metabolism includes an amelioration of lipid profiles, specifically triglycerides and cholesterol fractions, and increased fluidity in membranes, of which similar effects have been attributed to regular aerobic exercise.[97] It has been indicated that a single session of aerobic exercise has shown effects on triglyceride concentrations similar to those shown by ω-3 supplementation.[98]

Brilla and Landerholm[97] assessed the effect of aerobic exercise for 1 hour three times a week (mean range VO_2 max post-exercise: 35.6 to 49.5 ml kg^{-1} min^{-1}), and fish oil supplementation (4 g/day of ω-3 fatty acids) on serum lipids and aerobic fitness on healthy sedentary males for 10 weeks. Subjects in the exercise only and fish oil plus exercise groups had significantly higher VO_2 max. Subjects in the fish only, exercise only, and fish oil plus exercise groups had significantly higher ventilatory anaerobic thresholds (VATs) than controls; however, there were no differences in blood lipid values among all groups.[97] The improvement in aerobic indicators may be explained by incorporation of ω-3 fatty acids into membranes and their effect on the increase of the deformability of red blood cells, enhancing oxygen transport, and probably improving exercise performance.[97,99] Contrasting results on plasma lipoproteins were reported on recreationally active males who completed an aerobic exercise session of 60 min on the treadmill (60% VO_2 max) and were supplemented with 4 g/day of ω-3 fatty acids (600 mg of EPA and 400 mg of DHA/g) for 4 weeks. Supplementation increased plasma EPA and DHA, supplementation or exercise each affected HDL and subfractions (HDL_2 for supplementation and HDL_3 for exercise), exercise increased LDL, and the combined treatments affected HDL_3 and LDL_1.[100] The lowering effect of ω-3 fatty acids in the form of fish oil on triglycerides is thought to involve the suppression on enzymes engaged in the triglyceride synthesis and stimulation of β-oxidation in the liver.[101,102] Chronic supplementation with fish oil of 4 g/day (600 mg of EPA and 400 mg of DHA/g) rather than an acute high dose of 16 to 22 g/day (600 mg of EPA and 400 mg of DHA/g) has been reported to increase fat oxidation during 60 min of aerobic exercise (60% VO_2 max) in recreationally active males.[103] The effect on fat oxidation may be linked to the activation of skeletal muscle peroxisomal poliferator-activated receptor-α (PPAR-α) by EPA and DHA, resulting in decreased accumulation of triglycerides in myotubes.[103]

Contrary to studies that reported improvement in ventilatory indicators, Raastad et al.[104] showed that the effect of ω-3 fatty acids supplementation on cardiac output and peripheral blood flow on increasing aerobic performance did not show positive results. Well-trained soccer players supplemented with 5.2 g/day of fish oil (1.60 g/day EPA and 1.04 g/day DHA) for 10 weeks did not demonstrate an improvement in maximal aerobic power, anaerobic threshold, and running performance. However, supplemented subjects had significantly reduced plasma triglycerides and elevated plasma concentrations of EPA and DHA.

Omega-3 fatty acid supplementation has been utilized for muscle inflammation and soreness, and its use is based on the anti-inflammatory response that these polyunsaturated fatty acids have shown through modulation of the eicosanoid pathways.[28] Intakes of ω-3 fatty acids to reduce joint tenderness in patients with rheumatoid arthritis[28,105] and myalgic pain[106] have been reported, and intake of cod liver oil to mitigate musculoskeletal pain has been examined in a cross-sectional study that included nonathletic males and females older than 18 years.[107] However, supplementation of ω-3 fatty acids (1.8 g/day) for 30 days before and during iso-kinetic eccentric elbow flexion exercise was not effective in decreasing the physical parameters linked with delayed-onset muscle soreness (DOMS).[108]

The effect of ω-3 fatty acids, specifically EPA and DHA, has been tested on cytokine production during strenuous exercise due to their modulation on the production of pro-inflamatory and immunoregulatory cytokines.[109] Strenuous exercise induces an acute-phase response with increased plasma concentration of IL-6,[110] IL-1 receptor antagonist,[111] and TNF-α.[112] It is also thought that the anti-inflammatory cytokine, and transforming growth factor (TGF)-β_1, is increased in physiological states similar to strenuous exercise.[109] Therefore, the effect of 6.0 g/day of fish oil supplementation containing 3.6 g of ω-3 fatty acids (approximately 1.9 g of EPA and 1.1 g of DHA), and tocopherol for 6 weeks on male runners before participating in a marathon was examined.[109] The study aimed to investigate whether fish oil supplementation could modulate the acute-phase response to strenuous exercise. Subjects supplemented with fish oil showed incorporation of ω-3 fatty acids and less arachidonic acid in blood mononuclear cells than the nonsupplemented group, and although cytokine concentrations increased as a result of exercise, the cytokine concentrations of the supplemented and nonsupplemented groups did not differ.[109]

Omega-3 fatty acids supplementation on the effect of exercise-induced bronchoconstriction (EIB) in athletes has gained attention lately.[113–116] Fish oil supplementation in doses of 3.2 g/day of EPA and 2.0 to 2.2 g/day of DHA for 3 weeks has been reported to reduce the severity of EIB in athletes challenged to aerobic exercise (treadmill) until exhaustion, as seen by decreases in the forced expiratory volume (FEV_1) pre- and post-exercise of 64 to 80% at 15 min after exercise.[114,116] Inflammatory mediators of urinary LTE_4 and 9α, 11β-PGF_2, blood LTB_4, TNF-α, and IL-1β,[114] and sputum LTC_4-LTE_4, PGD_2, IL-1β, and TNF-α[116] were decreased in subjects on the ω-3 fatty acid diet compared to placebo and after exercise,[114] and before and following exercise in the fish oil group compared to placebo.[116]

Supplementation intakes of ω-3 fatty acids have ranged from 1.8 to 6 g/day, and one study reported using an acute high dose of up to 22 g/day. To our knowledge, there are no existing studies that have addressed the effect of inadequate or toxic intakes on physical performance or reported the use and effects of ω-6 fatty acids supplementation on athletes.

4.12 RECOMMENDED INTAKES

Because a Recommended Dietary Allowance (RDA) cannot be determined, an Adequate Intake (AI) has been estimated for ω-3 (α-linolenic acid) and ω-6 (linoleic acid) fatty acids. The AIs for α-linolenic acid for men and women older than 19 years are 1.6 and 1.1 g/day, respectively, and the AIs for linoleic acid for men and women 19 to 50 years are 17 and 12 g/day, respectively; for men and women older than 51 years, they are 14 and 11 g/day, respectively.[20] AI recommendations differ by age and gender groups and for special conditions, such as pregnancy and lactation. It has been recommended that an optimal dietary intake of α-linolenic acid should be 2 g/day, or 0.6 to 1% of total energy intake.[26] The Food and Drug Administration classifies intake of up to 3 g/day of ω-3 fatty acids from fish as GRAS (Generally Regarded As Safe).[38] A statement of the American Heart Association declared that people who have elevated triglycerides may need 2 to 4 g of EPA and DHA per day provided as a supplement, but it cautions patients taking more than 3 g of supplemental ω-3 fatty acids because it could cause excessive bleeding.[117] An AMDR, defined as a range of intakes for a particular energy source that is associated with reduced risk of chronic diseases while providing adequate intakes of essential nutrients, has been set for linoleic and α-linolenic acid.[20] An AMDR of 5 to 10% of energy is estimated for ω-6 fatty acids (linoleic acid), and an AMDR of 0.6 to 1.2% of energy is given for α-linolenic acid, and approximately 10% of the AMDR for α-linolenic acid can be consumed as EPA and DHA (0.06 to 0.12% of energy).[20]

4.13 FUTURE RESEARCH NEEDS

Future research needs to focus on long-term epidemiologic studies on the effects of diets supplemented with EPA, DHA, and α-linolenic acid, compared to ω-6 fatty acids diets, and their outcome in autoimmune and chronic diseases. It is suggested that future research in the area of ω-3 and ω-6 fatty acids and physical performance should focus on large long-term controlled intervention studies to assess the effects and probably benefits of long-term supplementation in athletes. It is also suggested that studies of the effects of supplemental doses on physical performance need to be evaluated with caution, as adverse effects have been reported for these polyunsaturated fatty acids. Recently, adequate intakes for α-linolenic and linoleic acids have been set for a healthy population, as there is not enough evidence to set an RDA; therefore, the need for well-designed studies in the field of exercise and physical performance is critical to further assess the effect of inadequate or toxic intakes on athletes. It is recommended that older and female athletes be included to examine the effect of age and gender, as most of the studies have included only young males.

4.14 SUMMARY

Omega-3 and ω-6 fatty acids are essential for life. Research has shown either beneficial effects of supplementation or detrimental results of nutritional deprivation or lower intake on metabolism. DHA and EPA in the form of dietary fish or fish oil supplements have been shown to lower triglycerides and reduce the risk of heart attack and strokes in people with known cardiovascular disease. α-Linolenic acid seems to have similar benefits, although they seem to be less considerable. Omega-3 and ω-6 fatty acids play a crucial role in brain function as well as normal growth and development. High intakes of ω-3 and ω-6 fatty acids need to be approached with caution, as side effects and interaction with drugs have been reported. Some studies have reported ω-3 fatty acids supplementation to have an effect on aerobic capacity, probably by its incorporation into membranes and its effect in the increase of the deformability of red blood cells, enhancing oxygen transport and then improving exercise performance. However, other studies have shown contrasting results. Therefore, enhanced aerobic exercise performance has not been clearly demonstrated, and more research is needed to elucidate the effect of supplementation. Based on available information, ω-3 fatty acids supplementation seems to reduce the severity of EIB in athletes by reduction of several inflammatory mediators. Additional research is needed in this area, as the research on supplementation of ω-3 fatty acids on nonathlete individuals does not show enough evidence to form a clear conclusion.

ACKNOWLEDGMENT

The authors thank Paula Ritter-Gooder, M.S., for reading the chapter and providing feedback.

REFERENCES

1. Stryer, L., Fatty acid metabolism, in *Biochemistry*, Stryer, L., Ed., W.H. Freeman and Company, New York, 1995, pp. 603-627.
2. Lichtenstein, A.H. and Jones P.J.H., Lipids: absorption and transport, in *Present Knowledge in Nutrition*, Bowman, B.A. and Rusell, R.M., Eds., ILSI Press, Washington, DC, 2001, pp. 92–103.
3. Spector, A.A., Lipid metabolism: essential fatty acids, in *Biochemical and Physiological Aspects of Human Nutrition*, Stipanuk, M.H., Ed., W.B. Saunders Company, Philadelphia, PA, 2000, pp. 365–383.
4. Small, D.M., Structure and properties of lipids, in *Biochemical and Physiological Aspects of Human Nutrition*, Stipanuk, M.H., Ed., W.B. Saunders Company, Philadelphia, PA, 2000, pp. 43–71.
5. Benatti, P., Peluso, G., Nicolai, R., and Calvani, M., Polyunsaturated fatty acids: biochemical, nutritional and epigenetic properties, *J. Am. Coll. Nutr.*, 23, 281–302, 2004.
6. Salem, N., Litman, B., Kim, H.Y., and Gawrisch. K., Mechanisms of action of docosahexaenoic acid in the nervous system, *Lipids*, 36, 945–359, 2001.
7. Innis, S.M., Essential dietary lipids, in *Present Knowledge in Nutrition*, Ziegler, E.E. and Filer, L.J., Eds., ILSI Press, Washington, DC, 1996, pp. 58–66.
8. Jump, D.B., The biochemistry of n-3 polyunsaturated fatty acids, *J. Biol. Chem.*, 277, 8755–8758, 2002.
9. Hughes, C.L. and Dhima, T.R., Dietary compounds in relation to dietary diversity and human health, *J. Med. Food*, 5, 51–68, 2002.
10. Sprecher, H., Luthria, D.L., Mohammed, B.S., and Baykousheva, S.P., Reevaluation of the pathways for the biosynthesis of polyunsaturated fatty acids, *J. Lipid Res.*, 36, 2471–2477, 1995.
11. Innis, S.M., Essential fatty acids in growth and development, *Prog. Lipid Res.*, 30, 39–103, 1991.

12. Sprecher, H., Interconversions between 20- and 22-carbon ω-3 and ω-6 fatty acids via 4-desaturase independent pathways, in *Essential Fatty Acids and Eicosanoids*, Sinclair, A. and Gibson, R., Eds., American Oil Chemists' Society, Champaign, IL, 1992, pp. 18–22.

13. Moore, S.A., Yoder, E., and Spector, A.A., Role of the blood-brain barrier in the formation of long-chain omega-3 and omega-6 fatty acids from essential fatty acid precursors, *J. Neurochem.*, 55, 391–402, 1990.

14. Moore, S.A., Yoder, E., Murphy, S., Dutton, G.R., and Spector, A.A., Astrocytes, not neurons, produce docosahexaenoic acid (22:6 omega-3) and arachidonic acid (20:4 omega-6), *J. Neurochem.*, 56, 518–524, 1991.

15. Wang, N. and Anderson, R.E., Synthesis of docosahexaenoic acid by retina and retinal pigment epithelium, *Biochemistry*, 32, 13703–13709, 1993.

16. Wetzel, M.G., Li, J., Alvarez, R.A., Anderson, R.E., and O'Brien, P.J., Metabolism of linolenic acid and docosahexaenoic acid in rat retinas and rod outer segments, *Exp. Eye Res.*, 53, 437–446, 1991.

17. Okayasu, T., Nagao, M., Ishibashi, T., and Imai, Y., Purification and partial characterization of linoleoyl-CoA desaturase from rat liver microsomes, *Arch. Biochem. Biophys.*, 206, 21–28, 1981.

18. Brenner, R.R., Nutritional and hormonal factors influencing desaturation of essential fatty acids, *Prog. Lipid Res.*, 20, 41–47, 1981.

19. Sprecher, H., Chen, Q., and Yin, F.Q., Regulation of the biosynthesis of 22:5n-6 and 22:6n-3: a complex intracellular process, *Lipids*, 34, S153–S156, 1999.

20. Food and Nutrition Board, Institute of Medicine, *Dietary Reference Intakes for Energy, Carbohydrate, Fiber, Fat, Fatty Acids, Cholesterol, Protein, and Amino Acids*, National Academy Press, Washington, DC, 2005, pp. 422–541.

21. Tso, P. and Crissinger, K., Digestion and absorption of lipids, in *Biochemical and Physiological Aspects of Human Nutrition*, Stipanuk, M.H., Ed., W.B. Saunders Company, Philadelphia, PA, 2000, pp. 125–141.

22. Jones, P.J. and Kubow, S., Lipids, sterols, and their metabolites, in *Modern Nutrition in Health and Disease*, Shils, M.E., Oson, J.A., Shike, M., and Ross, A.C., Eds., Lippincott Williams & Wilkins, Baltimore, MD, 1999, pp. 67–94.

23. Ockner, R.K. and Manning, J.A., Fatty acid binding protein in small intestine. Identification, isolation and evidence for its role in cellular fatty acid transport, *J. Clin. Invest.*, 54, 326–338, 1974.

24. Hussain, M.M., A proposed model for the assembly of chylomicrons, *Atherosclerosis*, 148, 1–15, 2000.

25. Kinsella, J.E., Lokesh, B., and Stone, R.A., Dietary polyunsaturated fatty acids and amelioration of cardiovascular disease: possible mechanisms, *Am. J. Clin. Nutr.*, 52, 1–28, 1990.

26. Lee, K.W. and Lip, G.Y.H., The role of omega-3 fatty acids in the secondary prevention of cardiovascular disease, *Q. J. Med.*, 96, 465–480, 2003.

27. Fliesler, S.J. and Anderson, R.E., Chemistry and metabolism of lipids in the vertebrate retina, *Prog. Lipid Res.*, 22, 79–131, 1983.

28. Simopoulos, A.P., Omega-3 fatty acids in health and disease and in growth and development, *Am. J. Clin. Nutr.*, 54, 438–463, 1991.

29. Maclean, C.H., Newberry, S.J., Mojica, W.A., Issa, A., Khanna, P., Lim, Y.W., Morton, S.C., Suttorp, M., Tu, W., Hilton, L.G., Garland, R.H., Traina, S.B., and Shekelle, P.G., Effects of omega-3 fatty acids on cancer, *Evid. Rep. Technol. Assess.*, 113, 1–4, 2005.

30. Yehuda, S., Rabinovitz, S., and Mostofsky, D.I., Essential fatty acids and the brain: from infancy to aging, *Neurobiol. Aging*, 1, 98S–102S, 2005.

31. Robinson, D.R., Urakaze, M., Huang, R., Taki, H., Sugiyama, E., Knoell, C.T., Xu, L., Yeh, E.T., and Auron, P.E., Dietary marine lipids suppress continuous expression of interleukin-1 beta gene transcription, *Lipids*, 31, 23S–31S, 1996.

32. Marszalek, J.R. and Lodish, H.F., Docosahexaenoic acid, fatty acid-interacting proteins, and neuronal function: breastmilk and fish are good for you, *Annu. Rev. Cell Dev. Biol.*, 21, 633–657, 2005.

33. Samuelsson, B., From studies of biochemical mechanism to novel biological mediators: prostaglandin endoperoxides, thromboxanes, and leukotrienes, *Biosci. Rep.*, 3, 791–813, 1983.

34. Luo, M., Flamand, N., and Brock, T.G., Metabolism of arachidonic acid to eicosanoids within the nucleus, *Biochim. Biophys. Acta*, 1716, 618–625, 2006.

35. Simopoulos, A.P., Essential fatty acids in health and chronic disease, *Am. J. Clin. Nutr.*, 70, 560S–569S, 1999.

36. Simopoulos, A.P., Omega-3 fatty acids in inflammation and autoimmune diseases, *J. Am. Coll. Nutr.*, 21, 495–505, 2002.

37. Lombardo, Y.B. and Chicco, A.G., Effects of dietary polyunsaturated n-3 fatty acids on dyslipidemia and insulin resistance in rodents and humans. A review, *J. Nutr. Biochem.*, 17, 1–13, 2006.

38. Omega-3 Fatty Acids, Fish Oil, Alpha-Linolenic Acid, Medline Plus website, http://www.nlm.nih.gov/medlineplus/druginfo/natural/patient-fishoil.html. Accessed June 9, 2006.

39. Kris-Etherton, P.M., Taylor, D.S., Yu-Poth, S., Huth, P., Moriarty, K., Fishell, V., Hargrove, R.L., Zhao, G., and Etherton, T.D., Polyunsaturated fatty acids in the food chain in the United States, *Am. J. Clin. Nutr.*, 71, 179S–188S, 2000.

40. Lewis, N.M., Seburg, S., and Flanagan, N.L., Enriched eggs as a source of n-3 polyunsaturated fatty acids for humans, *Poult. Sci.*, 79, 971–974, 2000.

41. Baucells, M.D., Crespo, N., Barroeta, A.C., Lopez-Ferrer, S., and Grashorn, M.A., Incorporation of different polyunsaturated fatty acids into eggs, *Poult. Sci.*, 79, 51–59, 2000.

42. Bourre, J.M., Where to find omega-3 fatty acids and how feeding animals with diet enriched in omega-3 fatty acids to increase nutritional value of derived products for human: what is actually useful? *J. Nutr. Health Aging*, 9, 232–242, 2005.

43. Nitsan, Z., Mokady, S., and Sukenik, A., Enrichment of poultry products with omega-3 fatty acids by dietary supplementation with the alga *Nannochloropsis* and mantur oil, *J. Agric. Food Chem.*, 47, 5127–5132, 1999.

44. Farrell, D.J., Enrichment of hen eggs with n-3 long-chain fatty acids and evaluation of enriched eggs in humans, *Am. J. Clin. Nutr.*, 68, 538–544, 1998.

45. Grune, T., Kramer, K., Hoppe, P.P., and Siems, W., Enrichment of eggs with n-3 polyunsaturated fatty acids: effects of vitamin E supplementation, *Lipids*, 36, 833–838, 2001.

46. Meluzzi, A., Sirri, F., Manfreda, G., Tallarico, N., and Franchini, A., Effects of dietary vitamin E on the quality of table eggs enriched with n-3 long-chain fatty acids, *Poult. Sci.*, 79, 539–545, 2000.

47. Murphy, K.J., Mansour, J., Patch, C.S., Weldon, G., Ross, D., Mori, T.A., Tapsell, L.C., Meyer, B.J., Noakes, M., Clifton, P.A., Puddey, I.B., and Howe, P.R., Development and evaluation of foods enriched with omega-3 fatty acids (Omega3) from fish oil, *Asia Pac. J. Clin. Nutr.*, 12, S35, 2003.

48. Fokkema, M.R., Smit, E.N., Martini, I.A., Woltil, H.A., Boersma, E.R., and Muskiet, F.A., Assessment of essential fatty acid and omega3-fatty acid status by measurement of erythrocyte 20:3omega9 (mead acid), 22:5omega6/20:4omega6 and 22:5omega6/22:6omega3, *Prostaglandins Leukot. Essent. Fatty Acids*, 67, 345–356, 2002.
49. Innis, S.M., Essential fatty acids in growth and development, *Prog. Lipid Res.*, 30, 39–103, 1991.
50. Holman, R.T., The ratio of trienoic:tetranoic acids in tissue lipids as a measure of essential fatty acid requirement, *J. Nutr.*, 70, 405–410, 1960.
51. Lundberg, W.O., The significance of cis, cis, cis 5,8,11 eicosatrienoic acid in essential fatty acid deficiency, *Nutr. Rev.*, 38, 233–235, 1980.
52. Sauberlich, H.E., Essential fatty acids deficiencies, in *Assessment of Nutritional Status*, Sauberlich, H.E., Ed., CRC Press, Boca Raton, FL, 1999, pp. 471–477.
53. Hirsch, J., Farquhar, J.W., Ahrens, E.H., Peterson, M.L., and Stoffel, W., Studies of adipose tissue in man. A microtechnic for sampling and analysis, *Am. J. Clin. Nutr.*, 8, 499–511, 1960.
54. Godley, P.A., Campbell, M.K., Miller, C., Gallagher, P., Martinson, F.E., Mohler, J.L., and Sandler, R.S., Correlation between biomarkers of omega-3 fatty acid consumption and questionnaire data in African American and Caucasian United States males with and without prostatic carcinoma, *Cancer Epidemiol. Biomarkers Prev.*, 5, 115–119, 1996.
55. vanStaveren, W.A., Deurenberg, P., Katan, M.B., Burema, J., de Groot, L.C., and Hoffmans, M.D., Validity of the fatty acid composition of subcutaneous fat tissue microbiopsies as an estimate of the long-term average fatty acid composition of the diet of separate individuals, *Am. J. Epidemiol.*, 123, 455–463, 1986.
56. Baylin, A., Kim, M.K., Donovan-Palmer, A., Siles, X., Dougherty, L., Tocco, P., and Campos, H., Fasting whole blood as a biomarker of essential fatty acid intake in epidemiologic studies: comparison with adipose tissue and plasma, *Am. J. Epidemiol.*, 162, 373–381, 2005.
57. Goodgame, J.T., Lowry, S.F., and Brennan, M.F., Essential fatty acid deficiency in total parenteral nutrition: time course of development and suggestions for therapy, *Surgery*, 84, 271–277, 1978.
58. O'Neill, J.A., Caldwell, M.D., and Meng, H.C., Essential fatty acid deficiency in surgical patients, *Ann. Surg.*, 185, 535–542, 1977.
59. Holman, R.T., Johnson, S.B., and Ogburn, P.L., Deficiency of essential fatty acids and membrane fluidity during pregnancy and lactation, *Proc. Natl. Acad. Sci. U.S.A.*, 1991, 4835–4839, 1991.
60. Jeppesen, P.B., Hoy, C.E., and Mortensen, P.B., Essential fatty acid deficiency in patients receiving home parenteral nutrition, *Am. J. Clin. Nutr.*, 68, 126–133, 1998.
61. Ritter-Gooder, P., Lewis, N., Heidal, K.B., and Eskridge, K.M., Validity and reliability of quantitative food frequency questionnaire measuring n-3 fatty acid intakes in cardiac patients in the Midwest: a validation pilot study, *J. Am. Diet. Assoc.*, 106, 1251–1255, 2006.
62. Lewis, N.M., Widga, A.C., Buck, J.S., and Frederick, A.M., Survey of omega-3 fatty acids in diets of Midwest low-income pregnant women, *J. Agromed.*, 2, 49–57, 1994.
63. Sindelar, C., Scheerger, S., Plugge, S., Eskridge, K., Wander, R.C., and Lewis, N.M., Serum lipids of physically active adults consuming omega-3 fatty acid-enriched eggs or conventional eggs, *Nutr. Res.*, 24, 731–739, 2004.

64. Lewis, N.M., Schalch, K., and Scheideler, S.E., Serum lipid response to n-3 fatty acid enriched eggs in persons with hypercholesterolemia, *J. Am. Diet. Assoc.*, 100, 365–367, 2000.
65. Romano, C., Cucchiara, S., Barabino, A., Annese, V., and Sferlazzas, C., Usefulness of omega-3 fatty acid supplementation in addition to mesalazine in maintaining remission in pediatric Crohn's disease: a double-blind, randomized, placebo-controlled study, *World J. Gastroenterol.*, 11, 7118–7121, 2005.
66. Nielsen, A.A., Jorgensen, L.G., Nielsen, J.N., Eivindson, M., Gronbaek, H., Vind, I., Hougaard, D.M., Skogstrand, K., Jensen, S., Munkholm, P., Brandslund, I., and Hey, H., Omega-3 fatty acids inhibit an increase of proinflammatory cytokines in patients with active Crohn's disease compared with omega-6 fatty acids, *Aliment. Pharmacol. Ther.*, 22, 1121–1128, 2005.
67. Tsipas, G. and Morphake, P., Beneficial effects of a diet rich in a mixture of n-6/n-3 essential fatty acids and of their metabolites on cyclosporine: nephrotoxicity, *J. Nutr. Biochem.*, 14, 626–632, 2003.
68. Busnach, G., Stragliotto, E., Minetti, E., Perego, A., Brando, B., Broggi, M.L., and Civati, G., Effect of n-3 polyunsaturated fatty acids on cyclosporine pharmacokinetics in kidney graft recipients: a randomized placebo-controlled study, *J. Nephrol.*, 11, 87–93 1998.
69. Buckley, M.S., Goff, A.D., and Knapp, W.E., Fish oil interaction with warfarin, *Ann. Pharmacother.*, 38, 50–53, 2004.
70. Lungershausen, Y.K., Abbey, M., Nestel, P.J., and Howe, P.R., Reduction of blood pressure and plasma triglycerides by omega-3 fatty acids in treated hypertensives, *J. Hypertens.*, 12, 1041–1045, 1994.
71. Venkatraman, J.T. and Chu, W.C., Effects of dietary omega-3 and omega-6 lipids and vitamin E on serum cytokines, lipid mediators and anti-DNA antibodies in a mouse model for rheumatoid arthritis, *J. Am. Coll. Nutr.*, 18, 602–613, 1999.
72. Connor, W.E., Neuringer, M., and Reisbick, S., Essential fatty acids: the importance of n-3 fatty acids in the retina and brain, *Nutr. Rev.*, 50, 21–29, 1992.
73. Holman, R.T., Johnson, S.B., and Hatch, T.F., A case of human linolenic acid deficiency involving neurological abnormalities, *Am. J. Clin. Nutr.*, 35, 617–623, 1982.
74. Rodier, M., Colette, C., Crastes de Paulet, P., Crastes de Paulet, A., and Monnier, L., Relationships between serum lipids, platelet membrane fatty acid composition and platelet aggregation in type 2 diabetes mellitus, *Diabetes Metab.*, 19, 560–565, 1993.
75. Abbey, M., Belling, G.B., Noakes, M., Hirata, F., and Nestel, P.J. Oxidation of low-density lipoproteins: intraindividual variability and the effect of dietary linoleate supplementation, *Am. J. Clin. Nutr.*, 57, 391–398, 1993.
76. Berry, E.M., Eisenberg, S., Haratz, D., Friedlander, Y., Norman, Y., Kaufmann, N.A., and Stein, Y. Effects of diets rich in monounsaturated fatty acids on plasma lipoproteins: the Jerusalem Nutrition Study: high MUFAs vs. high PUFAs, *Am. J. Clin. Nutr.*, 53, 899–907, 1991.
77. Pearce, M.L. and Dayton, S., Incidence of cancer in men on a diet high in polyunsaturated fat, *Lancet*, 1, 464–467, 1971.
78. Zock, P.L. and Katan, M.B., Hydrogenation alternatives: effects of trans fatty acids and stearic acid versus linoleic acid on serum lipids and lipoproteins in humans, *J. Lipid Res.*, 33, 399–410, 1992.
79. Ando, K., Nagata, K., Beppu, M., Kikugawa, K., Kawabata, T., Hasegawa, K., and Suzuki, M., Effect of n-3 fatty acid supplementation on lipid peroxidation and protein aggregation in rat erythrocyte membranes, *Lipids*, 33, 505–512, 1998.

80. Song, J.H. and Miyazawa, T., Enhanced level of n-3 fatty acid in membrane phospholipids induces lipid peroxidation in rats fed dietary docosahexaenoic acid oil, *Atherosclerosis*, 155, 9–18, 2001.
81. Umegaki, K., Hashimoto, M., Yamasaki, H., Fujii, Y., Yoshimura, M., Sugisawa, A., and Shinozuka, K., Docosahexaenoic acid supplementation-increased oxidative damage in bone marrow DNA in aged rats and its relation to antioxidant vitamins, *Free Radic. Res.*, 34, 427–435, 2001.
82. Morise, A., Mourot, J., Riottot, M., Weill, P., Fenart, E., and Hermier, D., Dose effect of alpha-linolenic acid on lipid metabolism in the hamster. *Reprod. Nutr. Dev.*, 45, 405–418, 2005.
83. Contacos, C., Barter, P.J., and Sullivan, D.R., Effect of pravastatin and omega-3 fatty acids on plasma lipids and lipoproteins in patients with combined hyperlipidemia, *Arterioscler. Thromb.*, 13, 1755–1762, 1993.
84. Anonymus, Dietary supplementation with n-3 polyunsaturated fatty acids and vitamin E after myocardial infarction: results of the GISSI-Prevenzione trial. Gruppo Italiano per lo Studio della Sopravvivenza nell'Infarto miocardico, *Lancet*, 354, 447–455, 1999.
85. Glaum, M., Metzelthin, E., Junker, S., Luley, C., and Klor, H.U., Comparative effect of oral fat loads with saturated, omega-6 and omega-3 fatty acids before and after fish oil capsule therapy in healthy probands. *Klin. Wochenschr.*, 68, 103–105, 1990.
86. Deutch, B., Jorgensen, E.B., and Hansen, J.C., Menstrual discomfort in Danish women reduced by dietary supplements of omega-3 PUFA and B_{12} (fish oil or seal oil capsules), *Nutr. Res.*, 20, 621–631, 2000.
87. Cobiac, L., Nestel, P.J., Wing, L.M., and Howe, P.R., A low-sodium diet supplemented with fish oil lowers blood pressure in the elderly, *J. Hypertens.*, 10, 87–92, 1992.
88. Salomon, P., Kornbluth, A.A., and Janowitz, H.D., Treatment of ulcerative colitis with fish oil n-3-omega-fatty acid: an open trial, *J. Clin. Gastroenterol.*, 12, 157–161, 1990.
89. Maresta, A., Balduccelli, M., Varani, E., Marzilli, M., Galli, C., Heiman, F., Lavezzari, M., Stragliotto, E., and De Caterina, R., Prevention of postcoronary angioplasty restenosis by omega-3 fatty acids: main results of the Esapent for Prevention of Restenosis Italian Study (ESPRIT), *Am. Heart J.*, 143, E5, 2002.
90. Morris, M.C., Sacks, F., and Rosner, B., Does fish oil lower blood pressure? A meta-analysis of controlled trials, *Circulation*, 88, 523–533, 1993.
91. Morris, M.C., Taylor, J.O., Stampfer, M.J., Rosner, B., and Sacks, F.M., The effect of fish oil on blood pressure in mild hypertensive subjects: a randomized crossover trial, *Am. J. Clin. Nutr.*, 57, 59–64, 1993.
92. Appel, L.J., Miller, E.R., Seidler, A.J., and Whelton, P.K., Does supplementation of diet with 'fish oil' reduce blood pressure? A meta-analysis of controlled clinical trials, *Arch. Intern. Med.*, 153, 1429–1438, 1993.
93. Mori, T.A., Bao, D.Q., Burke, V., Puddey, I.B., and Beilin, L.J., Docosahexaenoic acid but not eicosapentaenoic acid lowers ambulatory blood pressure and heart rate in humans, *Hypertension*, 34, 253–260, 1999.
94. Henderson, W.R., Astley, S.J., and Ramsey, B.W., Liver function in patients with cystic fibrosis ingesting fish oil, *J. Pediatr.*, 125, 504–505, 1994.
95. Helge, J.W., Wu, B.J., Willer, M., Daugaard, J.R., Storlien, L.H., and Kiens, B., Training affects muscle phospholipid fatty acid composition in humans, *J. Appl. Physiol.*, 90, 670–677, 2001.

96. Andersson, A., Sjodin, A., Olsson, R., and Vessby, B., Effects of physical exercise on phospholipid fatty acid composition in skeletal muscle, *Am. J. Physiol.*, 274, E432–E438, 1998.
97. Brilla, L.R. and Landerholm, T.E., Effect of fish oil supplementation and exercise on serum lipids and aerobic fitness, *J. Sports Med. Phys. Fitness*, 30, 173–180, 1990.
98. Borsheim, E., Knardahl, S., and Hostmark, A.T., Short-term effects of exercise on plasma very low density lipoproteins (VLDL) and fatty acids, *Med. Sci. Sports Exerc.*, 31, 522–530, 1991.
99. Carr, T.P. and Cowles, R.L., Lipid supplements in exercise and sports, in *Energy-Yielding Macronutrients and Energy Metabolism in Sport Nutrition*, Driskell, J.A. and Wolinsky, I., Eds., CRC Press, Boca Raton, FL, 2000, pp. 183–189.
100. Thomas, T.R., Smith, B.K., Donahue, O.M., Altena, T.S., James-Kracke, M., and Sun, G.Y., Effects of omega-3 fatty acid supplementation and exercise on low-density lipoprotein and high-density lipoprotein subfractions, *Metabolism*, 53, 749–754, 2004.
101. Connor, W.E., Importance of n-3 fatty acids in health and disease, *Am. J. Clin. Nutr.*, 71, 171S–175S, 2000.
102. Harris, W.S., Connor, W.E., Alam, N., and Illingworth, D.R., Reduction of postprandial triglyceridemia in humans by dietary n-3 fatty acids, *J. Lipid Res.*, 29, 1451–1460, 1988.
103. Huffman, D.M., Michaelson, J.L., and Thomas, T.R., Chronic supplementation with fish oil increases fat oxidation during exercise in young men, *JEP*, 7, 48–56, 2004 (online).
104. Raastad, T., Hostmark, A.T., and Stromme, S.B., Omega-3 fatty acids supplementation does not improve maximal aerobic power, anaerobic threshold and running performance in well trained soccer players, *Scand. J. Med. Sci. Sports*, 7, 25–31, 1997.
105. Kremmer, J.M., Fish-oil supplementation in active rheumatoid arthritis, *Ann. Intern. Med.*, 106, 497–503, 1987.
106. Behan, P.O., Behan, W.M., and Horrobin, D., Effect of high doses of essential fatty acids on the postviral fatigue syndrome, *Acta Neurol. Scand.*, 82, 209–216, 1990.
107. Eriksen, W., Sandvik, L., and Bruusgaard, D., Does dietary supplementation of cod liver oil mitigate musculoskeletal pain? *Eur. J. Clin. Nutr.*, 50, 689–693, 1996.
108. Lenn, J., Uhl, T., Mattacola, C., Boissonneault, G., Yates, J., Ibrahim, W., and Bruckner, G., The effects of fish oil and isoflavones on delayed onset muscle soreness, *Med. Sci. Sports Exerc.*, 34, 1605–1613, 2002.
109. Toft, A.D., Thorn, M., Ostrowski, K., Asp, S., Møller, K., Iversen, S., Hermann, C., Søndergaard, S.R., and Pedersen, B.K., N-3 polyunsaturated fatty acids do not affect cytokine response to strenuous exercise, *J. Appl. Physiol.*, 89, 2401–2406, 2000.
110. Northoff, H. and Berg, A., Immunologic mediators as parameters of the reaction to strenuous exercise, *Int. J. Sports Med.*, 12, S9–S15, 1991.
111. Ostrowski, K., Rohde, T., Zacho, M., Asp, S., and Pedersen, B.K., Evidence that interleukin-6 is produced in human skeletal muscle during prolonged running, *J. Physiol.*, 508, 949–953, 1998.
112. Espersen, G.T., Elbaek, A., Ernst, E., Toft, E., Kaalund, S., Jersild, C., and Grunnet, N., Effect of physical exercise on cytokines and lymphocyte subpopulations in human peripheral blood, *APMIS*, 98, 395–400, 1990.
113. Arm, J.P., Horton, C.E., Mencia-Huerta, J.M., House, F., Eiser, N.M., Clark, T.J., Spur, B.W., and Lee, T.H., Effect of dietary supplementation with fish oil lipids on mild asthma, *Thorax*, 43, 84–92, 1988.

114. Mickleborough, T.D., Murray, R.L., Ionescu, A.A., and Lindley, M.R., Fish oil supplementation reduces severity of exercise-induced bronchoconstriction in elite athletes, *Am. J. Respir. Crit. Care Med.*, 168, 1181–1189, 2003.

115. Mickleborough, T.D. and Rundell, K.W., Dietary polyunsaturated fatty acids in asthma- and exercise-induced bronchoconstriction, *Eur. J. Clin. Nutr.*, 59, 1335–1346, 2005.

116. Mickleborough, T.D., Lindley, M.R., Ionescu, A.A., and Fly, A.D., Protective effect of fish oil supplementation on exercise-induced bronchoconstriction in asthma, *Chest*, 129, 39–49, 2006.

117. Kris-Etherton, P.M., Harris, W.S., and Appel, L.J., American Heart Association Scientific Statement. Fish consumption, fish oil, omega-3 fatty acids, and cardiovascular disease, *Circulation*, 106, 2747–2757, 2002.

118. Arterburn, L.M., Hall, E.H., and Oken, H., Distribution, interconversion, and dose response of n-3 fatty acids in humans, *Am. J. Clin. Nutr*, 83, 1467S–1476S, 2006.

119. Dawson, R.C., Elliot, D.C., Elliot, W.H., and Jones, K.M., Lipids and long chain fatty acids, in *Data for Biochemical Research*, Dawson, R.C., Elliot, D.C., Elliot, W.H., and Jones, K.M., Eds., Oxford University Press, New York, 1986, pp. 167–189.

120. Hibbeln, J.R., Nieminen, L.R.G., Blasbalg, T.L., Riggs, J.A., and Lands, W.E.M., Healthy intakes of n-3 and n-6 fatty acids: estimations considering worldwide diversity, *Am. J. Clin. Nutr.*, 83, 1483S–1493S, 2006.

5 Conjugated Linoleic Acid

Celeste G. Koster and Martha A. Belury

CONTENTS

5.1 INTRODUCTION

Conjugated linoleic acid (CLA) refers to a group of stereo and positional isomers of octadecadienoate (18:2) (Figure 5.1).[1] This group of polyunsaturated fatty acids is formed by partial biohydrogenation in the rumen of cattle and lamb, and is therefore found in the meat and milk products from these ruminant sources (Table 5.1).[2–4] Levels of CLA and individual isomers in meat and milk result from differences in diet and farming management of cows.[5] CLA can also be prepared synthetically by heating linoleic acid in the presence of alkali or by partial dehydrogenation of linoleic acid; however, synthetic preparation of CLA from precursors such as linoleic acid results in an alteration of the isomeric composition (Table 5.2).[6] In foods, c9t11 CLA, also called rumenic acid,[7] is the most predominant isomer,[4,8] followed by t7c9 CLA, c11t13 CLA, c8t10 CLA, and t10c12 CLA.[8] In synthetic preparations of CLA, c9t11 CLA and t10c12 CLA are the dominant isomeric forms, followed by t7c9 CLA, c8t10 CLA, and c11t13 CLA. Importantly, most research on CLA in health has utilized the synthetic form of CLA oil containing the altered ratio of c9t11 CLA:t10c12 CLA of 0.95.

5.2 HEALTH PROPERTIES OF CONJUGATED LINOLEIC ACID

Several animal and human studies have found CLA to have various health properties, including action as an anticarcinogen[9] and anti-atherosclerotic agent,[10,11] as well as an antidiabetic agent.[12] CLA also reduces body mass in growing animals[13–16] and

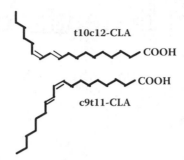

FIGURE 5.1 Structures of t10c12-conjugated linoleic acid and c9t11-conjugated linoleic acid.

adult humans[17,18] when provided as a synthetic mixture of CLA isomers. The t10c12 isomer appears to have a greater effect on adiposity than the c9t11 isomer in mice.[18,19] Because of favorable effects of CLA on adiposity and lean mass in experimental animals, CLA has received some attention as an ergogenic aid for resistance-trained athletes and bodybuilders. This review will summarize the effects of CLA on energy expenditure, body composition, and muscle mass with and without resistance training. We will review and present the current state of knowledge surrounding proposed mechanisms of action, and finally, we will speculate about the possibility of CLA to act as an ergogenic aid in people.

5.3   EFFECTS OF CONJUGATED LINOLEIC ACID ON MUSCLE MASS AND STRENGTH

Along with reducing adiposity in several animal models of obesity, CLA may have positive effects on muscle mass (Table 5.3). A relationship between CLA supplementation and muscle size and strength was first reported in 1997.[20] In a placebo-controlled study, 24 male novice bodybuilders were supplemented with 7.2 g/day of CLA or a vegetable oil placebo while completing 6 weeks of bodybuilding exercises. Arm circumference and skin-fold measurements were used to determine body mass. Arm girth increased from 7175 ± 978 to 7562 ± 1000 mm^2 in the CLA group compared with the placebo (from 7777 ± 1532 to 7819 ± 1516 mm^2). The greater increase in arm girth in the CLA group suggests that more muscle was built in the CLA group than in the placebo group. Body mass in the CLA group increased from 77.6 ± 11.8 to 79.0 ± 12 kg, while the control group remained relatively even at 77.8 ± 11.9 kg to 77.8 ± 11.8 kg. As a measure of strength, leg press increased from 263.6 ± 63.0 to 335 ± 75 kg in the CLA group, while there was a smaller increase in the placebo group: 271.5 ± 62.9 kg to 306.8 ± 70.2 kg. Skin-fold measurements, total body fat, and total body water measured by bioelectrical impedance analysis (BIA) of both whole body and upper limb were similar between groups.

In a randomized, placebo-controlled study with similar design by Ferreira et al.,[21] experienced resistance-trained men were supplemented with CLA or an olive oil placebo for 28 days.[21] In men supplemented with CLA, performance on the 1-RM (repetition maximum) bench press and leg press was slightly improved; however,

TABLE 5.1
Content of Conjugated Linoleic Acid in Selected Foods

Food	Total CLA (mg/g fat)	c9t11 Isomer (%)
Dairy Products		
Homogenized milk	5.5	92
Butter	4.7	88
Sour cream	4.6	90
Plain yogurt	4.8	84
Nonfat yogurt	1.7	83
Ice cream	3.6	86
Sharp cheddar cheese	3.6	93
Mozzarella cheese	4.9	95
Colby cheese	6.1	92
Cottage cheese	4.5	83
American processed cheese	5.0	93
Meat (Uncooked)		
Fresh ground beef	4.3	85
Beef round	2.9	79
Veal	2.7	84
Lamb	5.6	92
Pork	0.6	82
Poultry (Uncooked)		
Chicken	0.9	84
Fresh ground turkey	2.5	76
Seafood (Uncooked)		
Salmon	0.3	
Lake trout	0.5	
Shrimp	0.6	
Processed Foods		
Beef frank	3.3	83
Turkey frank	1.6	70
Peanut butter	0.2	
Canned Foods		
Spam™	1.3	71
Baked beans	0.7	56
Corned beef	6.6	85
Vegetable Oils		
Safflower	0.7	44
Sunflower	0.4	38
Canola	0.5	44

Reprinted from *J. Food Compos. Anal.*, Vol. 5, Chin, S.F. et al., Dietary sources of conjugated dienoic isomers of linoleic acid, a newly recognized class of anti-carcinogens, 185. Copyright 1992, with permission from Elsevier.

TABLE 5.2
Approximate Isomeric Content (%CLA) of Conjugated Linoleic Acid: Selected Foods vs. Synthetic Mixture

	c9t11 CLA	c7t9 CLA, c8t10 CLA	t10c12 CLA, Others	c9t11 CLA:t10c12 CLA Ratio
Beef	74.8	15.8	9.0	8.31
Cheese	82.6	8.3	9.0	9.18
CLA mix	48.7		51.3	0.95

TABLE 5.3
Summary of the Role of Conjugated Linoleic Acid to Alter Muscle Mass in Humans

Source	Action with CLA
Lowery et al., 1998[20]	↑ Arm girth in novice bodybuilders ↑ Body mass ↑ Leg press
Ferreira et al., 1997[21]	↑ Bench press in experienced resistance-trained men ↑ Leg press
Kreider et al., 1998[22]	↑ Bone mineral content in experienced resistance-trained athletes ↓ Neutrophil/lymphocyte levels
Kreider et al., 2002[23]	↔ No change in experienced resistance-trained athletes

the improvement was not statistically different from the control group. In addition, blood urea nitrogen levels were lower in men supplemented with CLA, suggesting an anabolic effect. Total body masses measured by dual x-ray absorptiometry (DEXA), fat-free mass, fat mass, and percent body fat were similar between groups.

In a separate study of CLA in relation to bone mineral content, bone mineral density, and immune stress, 23 experienced resistance-trained males were supplemented with 6.0 g/day of CLA, 3.2 g/day of CLA, or an olive oil placebo for 28 days.[22] Bone mineral content increased and the neutrophil/lymphocyte ratio decreased in the CLA-supplemented groups, suggesting less immune stress. In a subsequent study, supplementation with 3.0 g/day of CLA had no effect for 23 experienced resistance-trained males on total body mass, fat-free mass, fat mass, percent body fat, bone mass, strength, serum substrates, general markers of catabolism, and immunity during training during a 28-day study.[23] Perhaps the relatively higher doses of 6 g/day of CLA are more effective than a 3 g/day supplement.

Notably, all studies on the role of CLA as an ergogenic aid to enhance strength have involved humans. Unfortunately, the results are mixed, with some studies finding a correlation between supplementation of CLA and strength via leg press[20,21] and others finding no relationship.[22,23] More attention to the prospective relationship between strength and CLA is needed, including using women in addition to men, since it is very possible that the different sexes metabolize and utilize CLA differently.

5.4 EFFECTS OF CONJUGATED LINOLEIC ACID ON BODY COMPOSITION

CLA has been shown to have an inverse relationship with adiposity. A reduction in body fat mass has been found in growing animals such as mice, rats, pigs, and cattle as well as adult humans. In fact, when 6-week-old male ICR mice were supplemented with 0.5% CLA plus 5% corn oil to their diet for 32 days, a 57% reduction in body fat and a 5% increase in lean body mass was observed compared with their respective controls.[13] In the same study, 6-week-old females were fed a 0.5% CLA plus 5% corn oil-supplemented diet for 28 days and showed a 60% reduction in body fat and a 14% increase in lean body mass compared with their respective controls. The control male and female mice were fed a diet with 5.5% corn oil. It is interesting to note the similarity of body fat reduction, but there was a nearly threefold difference in lean body mass between the male and female mice; perhaps male and female mice metabolize and incorporate CLA differently. In a separate study, a 50% reduction in adipose tissue mass was observed when 8-week-old female ICR mice were fed a diet containing 0.5% of a CLA mixture for 4 weeks.[14] The adipose tissue reduction was sustained after the CLA was removed from the diet. When AKR/J mice were fed a semipurified diet supplemented with 2.46 mg/kcal of CLA mixture for 6 weeks, a significant reduction in adipose tissue deposition (43 to 88%) independent of the high-fat (45 kcal%) and low-fat (15 kcal%) diet composition was observed.[15]

To determine whether a metabolite of CLA could explain the reducing effect of CLA on body weight and adiposity, the effect of CLA and conjugated linolenic acid (CLNA) on body fat in male Sprague-Dawley rats was determined.[16] CLNA is a highly unsaturated conjugated fatty acid and is expected to affect lipid metabolism. The 4-week-old male rats were fed a purified diet with either 1% CLA or CLNA for 4 weeks. Peri-renal and epididymal adipose tissue weight was reduced in both the CLA and CLNA groups; however, the effects were heightened within the CLNA group. These results suggest that CLNA and CLA may work differently in reducing adipose tissue weight.

In studies involving human subjects, research findings have been mixed. A study supplementing varying amounts of CLA from 1.7 to 6.8 g/day to overweight and obese humans for 12 weeks showed a reduction in body fat mass, measured by DEXA, for the CLA group.[17] In people with type 2 diabetes mellitus, supplementation with CLA (mixture of c9t11 CLA and t10c12 CLA isomers) or placebo was provided at 8.0 g/day. Supplementing for 8 weeks with the CLA mixture resulted in reduced body weight.[18] Further, it was noted that the t10c12 CLA isomer was more significantly associated with the decreased body weight than the c9t11 CLA isomer, suggesting that t10c12 CLA may be the bioactive isomer responsible for weight loss. Another study, involving weanling ICR rats, also found that the t10c12 CLA isomer was associated with reduced body fat, enhanced body water, enhanced body protein, and enhanced body ash, whereas the c9t11 and t9t11 CLA isomers did not affect these parameters.[19]

In addition to reducing adipose tissue mass, the t10c12 CLA isomer has been linked to increased insulin resistance in men who have symptoms of the metabolic syndrome.[26,27] A CLA mixture also appeared to cause hyperinsulinemia in C57BL/6J mice[24] that was accompanied by severe adipose tissue ablation and decreased leptin levels. The effects of the CLA mixture on adipose tissue depletion were reversed by continuous leptin infusion. In a follow-up study, decreasing the amount of a CLA mixture from 1 to 0.1 g/100 g diet, while increasing the amount of total fat in the diet from 4 to 34 g/100 g diet, did not lead to lipodystrophy, while fat mass was modestly reduced.[25] Insulin resistance was present in the group fed the 1 g CLA/100 g diet, but not present in the 0.1 g CLA/100 g diet group.

In men who were supplemented with 3.4 g/day of a CLA mixture, purified t10c12 CLA isomer, or olive oil placebo, the t10c12 CLA isomer exerted an increase in insulin resistance that correlated with increased urinary isoprostane levels, suggesting an increase in oxidative stress in these same individuals. Previously, in a study from the same group, 60 abdominally obese men supplemented with 3.4 g/day of the t10c12 CLA isomer, a CLA mixture, or equal amounts of olive oil became more insulin resistant when supplemented with t10c12 CLA than did people supplemented with the CLA mix or olive oil control.[27] These results are significant in the clinical usages of various isomers of CLA as a dietary supplement.

In contrast to the above studies, women supplemented with 3 g/day of CLA had no significant difference in body composition compared with the placebo.[28] Seventeen women were supplemented with either a 3 g/day capsule of a CLA mixture or a sunflower oil placebo while being confined to a metabolic suite for 94 days. Their diet and activity were held constant. It is possible that 3 g/day is not enough to elucidate a change in body composition in women.

In 1994, it was proposed that CLA acted as an *in utero* anabolic stimulus for rats, since it appeared to enhance weight gain in rats.[29] Eight-week-old female Fisher rats were fed a nonpurified diet and allowed to mate with a male counterpart. Immediately after mating, the females were separated and fed a mixture of either 0.5 g CLA/100 g or 0.25 g CLA/100 g or corn oil mixed with a semipurified diet. Diets with CLA did not affect the weight of dams but increased the weight of the pups in the CLA-fed groups. Conversely, Poulos et al. later performed a similar study in which pregnant Sprague-Dawley rats were provided diets with 6.5 g/100 g soybean oil and 0.5 g/100 g CLA or 7 g/100 g soybean oil.[30] The maternal treatment continued until day 21 of lactation, at which time the pups were weaned. The pups were assigned control or CLA diets until 11 weeks of age. No difference was found in the number of pups per litter, weights of whole litters, litter weight gain, litter efficiency, or food intake of the dams fed. Parametrial fat pad weight and retroperitoneal pad weight were less in dams fed CLA, and pups from dams fed CLA were significantly heavier at weaning than the pups from the control dams. Heavier gastrocnemius and soleus muscles and longer tail lengths, which are markers of skeletal growth, were found at 11 weeks of age in male pups than in dams fed CLA. These results suggest that CLA treatment in relation to body composition may be dependent on the sex and age of the animal as well as the duration of feeding.

TABLE 5.4
Summary of the Role of Conjugated Linoleic Acid in Energy Expenditure and Food Intake

Source	Action with CLA
Animal Models	
West et al., 1998[15]	↓ Energy intake in AKR/J mice
West et al., 2000[32]	↔ No change in energy intake in AKR/J mice
	↑ Energy expenditure
Bouthegard et al., 2002[31]	↔ No change in energy expenditure in Syrian hamsters
Human Models	
Zambell et al., 2000[28]	↔ No change in energy expenditure or intake in women

5.5 EFFECTS OF CONJUGATED LINOLEIC ACID ON ENERGY INTAKE AND EXPENDITURE

The inverse association of CLA with body mass and adiposity prompted research to elucidate the role of CLA to modulate energy intake and expenditure (Table 5.4). Seventeen healthy, nonobese women between the ages of 20 and 41 were supplemented with 3 g/day CLA or a sunflower oil placebo for 64 days.[28] Energy expenditure measured by respiratory gas exchange, energy intake, or body composition was associated with CLA provided as a low dose and in a short-duration protocol. Similarly, no effect of CLA on energy expenditure was found in adult male Syrian hamsters fed diets with the c9t11 CLA isomer to equate 1.6% of energy or a CLA mixture of 3.2% of energy for 6 to 8 weeks.[31] In contrast, male AKR/J mice supplemented with CLA reduced energy intake and growth rate.[15] The group fed a diet with 1.2% CLA mixture in a high-fat diet and 1.0% CLA mixture in a low-fat diet also had an increased metabolic rate and a decreased nighttime respiratory quotient compared with the controls fed without CLA. In a separate study, West et al. also found no reduction in energy intake when AKR/J mice were fed diets with 1% CLA mixture for 5 weeks.[32] However, energy expenditure was increased and appeared to account for lower body fat stores in the CLA group.

5.6 SUMMARY

The effects of CLA as a modulator of muscle mass have been given little attention. While there is evidence that CLA may help to increase muscle mass, there is also some evidence that CLA has no effect as an ergogenic aid. In the studies that presented evidence that CLA did increase muscle mass, the increase was slight and only 20 to 30 subjects were tested. A larger subject base along with longer supplementation time could possibly provide more significantly impressive data.

CLA has been found to lower adipose tissue, body fat mass, and body weight in animal and human models. While lowering adipose tissue in mice, it was also found to increase hyperinsulinemia, which was later found to be lowered with a lower concentration of CLA supplementation. More clinical research varying the amount of CLA and the duration of supplementation is necessary because the data with human subjects are not conclusive.

The research regarding CLA's effect on energy intake and expenditure is also variant between research groups. In animal models, CLA has been shown to increase or demonstrate no effect on energy intake. Energy expenditure was shown to decrease and stay at baseline with CLA supplementation. No effect was found in humans. There is good evidence to support that CLA does in fact modulate energy intake and expenditure; however, the mechanisms of this action remain unclear.

Based on ambiguous but suggestive findings, more research examining the effects of CLA on energy expenditure and metabolism is warranted. These studies are clearly required for a better understanding and for making recommendations to the public regarding the practice of using CLA as an ergogenic or performance-enhancing aid (Figure 5.2).

ACKNOWLEDGMENTS

The authors are grateful to Dr. J. Buell, A. Purushotham, and A. Wendel for their helpful feedback regarding this manuscript.

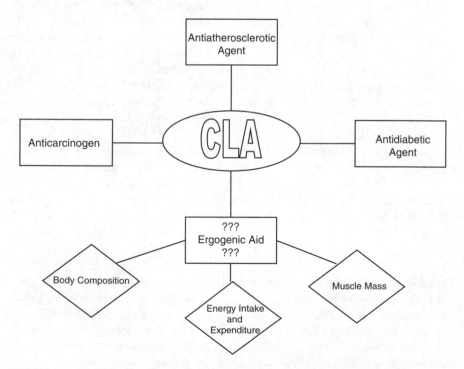

FIGURE 5.2 Health properties that may be responsive to conjugated linoleic acid.

REFERENCES

1. Pariza MW, Park Y, and Cook ME. 2000. Mechanisms of action of conjugated linoleic acid: evidence and speculation. *Exp. Bio. Med.*, 223, 8.
2. Chin SF, Liu W, Storkson JM, Ha YL, and Pariza MW. 1992. Dietary sources of conjugated dienoic isomers of linoleic acid, a newly recognized class of anti-carcinogens. *J. Food Compos. Anal.*, 5, 185.
3. Griinari JM, Cori BA, Lacy SH, Chouinard PY, Nurmela KVV, and Bauman DE. 2000. Conjugated linoleic acid is synthesized endogenously in lactating dairy cows by delta(9)-desaturase. *J. Nutr.*, 130, 2285.
4. Ma D, Wierzbicki A, Field C, and Clandinin MT. 1999. Conjugated linoleic acid in Canadian dairy and beef products. *J. Agric. Food Chem.*, 47, 1956.
5. Parodi PW. 2002. Conjugated linoleic acid. *Food Aust.*, 54, 96.
6. Banni S. 2002. Conjugated linoleic acid metabolism. *Curr. Opin. Lipidol.*, 13, 261.
7. Kramer JKG, Parodi PW, Jensen RG, Mossoba MM, Yurawecz MP, and Adlof RO. 1998. Rumenic acid: a proposed common name for the major conjugated linoleic acid isomer found in natural products. *Lipids*, 33, 83.
8. Fritsche J, Rickert R, and Steinhart H. 1999. Formation, contents and estimation of daily intake of conjugated linoleic acid isomers and trans-fatty acids in foods. In *Advances in Conjugated Linoleic Acid Research*, Yurawecz MP, Mossaba MM, Kramer JKG, Pariza MW, Nelson, GJ, Eds., Vol. 1. AOCS Press, Champaign, IL, p. 378.
9. Belury MA. 2002. Inhibition of carcinogenesis by conjugated linoleic acid: potential mechanisms of action. *J. Nutr.* 132, 2995.
10. Lee KN, Kritchevsky D, and Pariza MW. 1994. Conjugated linoleic acid and atherosclerosis. *Atherosclerosis*, 108, 19.
11. Wilson KL, Nicolosi RJ, Chrysam M, and Kritchevsky D. 2000. Conjugated linoleic acid reduces early aortic atherosclerosis greater than linoleic acid in hypercholesterolemic hamsters. *Nutr. Res.*, 20, 1795.
12. Houseknect KL, Vanden Heuvel JP, Moya-Camarena SY, Portocarrero CP, Peck LW, Nickel KP, and Belury MA. 1998. Dietary conjugated linoleic acid normalizes impaired glucose tolerance in the zucker diabetic fatty rat. *Biochem. Biophys. Res. Commun.*, 244, 678.
13. Park Y, Albright KJ, Liu W, Storkson JM, Cook ME, and Pariza MW. 1997. Effect of conjugated linoleic acid on body composition in mice. *Lipids*, 32, 853.
14. Park Y, Albright KJ, Storkson JM, Liu W, Cook ME, and Pariza MW. 1999. Changes in body composition in mice during feeding and withdrawal of conjugated linoleic acid. *Lipids*, 34, 243.
15. West DB, Delany JP, Camet PM, Blohm F, Truett AA, and Scimeca J. 1998. Effects of conjugated linoleic acid on body fat and energy metabolism in the mouse. *Am. J. Physiol.*, 275, R667.
16. Koba K, Akahoshi A, Masao Y, Tanaka K, Yamada K, Iwata T, Kamegai T, Tsutsumi K, and Sugano M. 2002. Dietary conjugated linolenic acid in relation to CLA differently modifies body fat mass and serum lipid levels in rats. *Lipids*, 37, 243.
17. Blankson H, Stakkestad JA, Fagertun H, Thom E, Wadstein J, and Gudmundsen O. 2000. Conjugated linoleic acid reduces body fat mass in overweight and obese humans. *J. Nutr.*, 130, 2943.
18. Belury MA, Mahon A, and Banni S. 2003. The conjugated linoleic acid (CLA) isomer, t10c12-CLA, is inversely associated with changes in body weight and serum leptin in subjects with type 2 diabetes mellitus. *J. Nutr.*, 133, 257S.

19. Park Y, Storkson JM, Albright KJ, Liu W, and Pariza MW. 1999. Evidence that the trans-10, cis-12 isomer of conjugated linoleic acid induces body composition changes in mice. *Lipids*, 34, 235.

20. Lowery LM, Appicelli PA, and Lemon PWR. 1998. Conjugated linoleic acid enhances muscle size and strength gains in novice bodybuilders. *Med. Sci. Sports Exerc.*, 30, S182.

21. Ferreira M, Kreider R, Wilson M, and Almada A. 1997. Effects of conjugated linoleic acid supplementation during resistance training on body composition and strength. *J. Strength Cond. Res.*, 11, 280.

22. Kreider R, Ferreira M, Wilson M, and Almada A. 1998. Effects of conjugated linoleic acid (CLA) supplementation during resistance-training on bone mineral content, bone mineral density and markers of immune stress. *FASEB J.*, 12, A244.

23. Kreider R, Ferreira M, Greenwood M, Wilson M, and Almada A. 2002. Effects of conjugated linoleic acid supplementation during resistance training on body composition, bone density, strength and selected hematological markers. *J. Strength Cond. Res.*, 16, 325.

24. Tsuboyama-Kasoka N, Takahashi M, Tanemura K, Kim HJ, Tange T, Okuyama H, Kasai M, Ikemoto S, and Ezaki O. 2000. Conjugated linoleic acid supplementation reduced adipose tissue by apoptosis and develops lipodystrophy in mice. *Diabetes*, 49, 1534.

25. Tsuboyama-Kasaoka N, Miyazaki H, Kasaoka S, and Ezaki O. 2003. Increasing the amount of fat in a conjugated linoleic acid-supplemented diet reduces lipodystrophy in mice. *J. Nutr.*, 133, 1793.

26. Riserus U, Arner P, Brismar K, and Vessby B. 2002. Treatment with dietary trans 10 cis 12 conjugated linoleic acid causes isomer-specific insulin reistance in obese men with the metabolic syndrome. *Diabetes Care*, 25, 1516.

27. Riserus U, Basu S, Jovinge S, Fredrikson GN, Arnlov J, and Vessby B. 2002. Supplementation with conjugated linoleic acid causes isomer-dependent oxidative stress and elevated C-reaction protein. *Circulation*, 106, 1925.

28. Zambell KL, Keim NL, Van Loan MD, Gale B, Benito P, Kelley DS, and Nelson GJ. 2000. Conjugated linoleic acid supplementation in humans: effects on body composition and energy expenditure. *Lipids*, 35, 777.

29. Chin SF, Storkson JM, Albright KJ, Cook ME, and Pariza MW. 1994. Conjugated linoleic acid is a growth factor for rats as shown by enhanced weight gain and improved feed efficiency. *J. Nutr.*, 124, 2344.

30. Poulos SP, Sisk M, Hausman DB, Azain MJ, and Hausmann GJ. 2001. Pre- and postnatal dietary conjugated linoleic acid alters adipose development, body weight gain and body composition in Sprague-Dawley rats. *J. Nutr.*, 131, 2722.

31. Bouthegourd JC, Even PC, Gripois D, Tiffon B, Blouquit MF, Roseau S, Lutton C, Tome D, and Martin JC. 2002. A CLA mixture prevents body triglyceride accumulation without affecting energy expenditure in Syrian hamsters. *J. Nutr.*, 132, 2682.

32. West DB, Blohm FY, Truett AA, and DeLany JP. 2000. Conjugated linoleic acid persistently increases total energy expenditure in AKR/J mice without increasing uncoupling protein gene expression. *J. Nutr.*, 130, 2471.

6 Octacosanol and Wheat Germ Oil

Susan H. Mitmesser

CONTENTS

6.1 INTRODUCTION

Over the past few years, nutraceuticals have become increasingly popular among the general public.[1] Octacosanol is one such supplement that has been the subject of many research studies. As with other types of supplementation, the benefits must outweigh the risks.

Octacosanol is the main active component of policosanol and wheat germ oil. Octacosanol is a long carbon chain: $CH_3(CH_2)_{26}CH_2O_{14}$. It has a natural mixture of high molecular weight alcohols and is primarily isolated from sugar cane (*Saccharum officinarum* L) wax. Small quantities of octacosanol are available in the human diet through plants (mainly as a wax in the superficial layers of fruits), leaves, skins of common plants, and whole seeds. Most studies have used wheat germ oil extract or policosanol to elicit an octacosanol response.

Early work by Thomas Cureton examined the physiological effects of wheat germ oil on humans during exercise. He discovered that extracts from wheat germ oil had beneficial effects on the physical performance of athletes.[2,3] Based on Cureton's work, other researchers began to take notice of the benefits of wheat germ oil. Soon its components were isolated and examined separately. Octacosanol appeared to be the primary active compound in wheat germ oil. With the help of Gonzalez-Bravo et al., the analytical procedure for determining octacosanol in plasma was refined.[4] This procedure allowed for higher recovery (94.5 to 98.7%) and precision (1.8 to 5.8%) than was ever before permitted.

6.2 MECHANISM OF ACTION

While only small amounts of octacosanol are ingested in the diet, many health benefits have surfaced, in part due to researchers developing octacosanol in a supplement form. Most studies to date have used a wheat germ oil extract or policosanol, a natural mixture of primary alcohols isolated from sugar cane wax, of which octacosanol is the primary component. Octacosanol has the potential to benefit human health in many areas, in particular exercise performance, platelet aggregation, and plasma cholesterol levels. Of the potential health benefits associated with octacosanol, its ergogenic properties and cholesterol-lowering effects have been the most studied.

6.2.1 EXERCISE PERFORMANCE

Ergogenic aids, substances that enhance athletic performance and increase stamina and capability to exercise, are believed to improve performance by either renewing or increasing energy stores in the body, which facilitates biochemical reactions contributing to fatigue, or by maintaining optimal body weight.[5] Because the U.S. Food and Drug Administration does not require nutritional supplements to be proven safe or effective, many athletes take such supplements without realizing potential side effects. Likewise, nutritional supplements are not covered by the U.K. Medicines Act, and therefore no regulations for manufacture, quality, or usage exist, making them subject to abuse.[6] Additionally, it is often difficult to fully determine whether an improvement in performance or muscle size is due to a nutritional supplement or to other factors, such as improved training techniques or diet.

Octacosanol is one such ergogenic supplement proposed to enhance performance and delay fatigue. Thomas Cureton was the first to report that wheat germ oil had ergogenic effects. During his career, Cureton performed approximately 42 studies that addressed the ergogenic potential of wheat germ oil.[2] In 1963, Cureton published a study involving 30 trainees in the U.S. Navy. The subjects received either 3.7 ml (10 capsules containing 0.37 ml each) of octacosanol in cottonseed oil, cottonseed oil (used as the placebo), or whole-wheat germ oil daily for 6 weeks. While the octacosanol-supplemented group had higher mean exercise performance, they did not differ significantly from that of the placebo group.[2]

In 1986, Saint-John and McNaughton investigated human subjects taking octacosanol supplements in relationship to chest strength, stamina, grip, cardiovascular function, and reaction time. Specifically, 1000 µg of octacosanol was administered to healthy human subjects daily. Grip strength and reaction time significantly improved in response to a visual stimulus. The researchers concluded octacosanol was an "active energy releasing factor" and improved performance when compared with the placebo.[7] This research led others to hypothesize that octacosanol might exhibit properties affecting the nervous system because reaction time was able to change according to nerve impulses throughout the body. A study was conducted in 1998 on a group of patients with coronary heart disease taking a policosanol supplement that improved their response to exercise angina and significantly increased maximum oxygen uptake.[8] Animal studies have also exhibited ergogenic properties of octacosanol. Exercised-trained octacosanol-supplemented Sprague-Dawley rats ran 46% longer and had significantly higher plasma ammonia and lactate concentrations than control rats. While the exercised-trained octacosanol-supplemented rats ran significantly longer until exhausted, their plasma glucose level and gastronecmius muscle gycogen concentrations were not different from those of the control rats. These results suggest that octacosanol supplementation allows for muscle glycogen sparing and an increase in the oxidative capacity of the muscle.[9] On the other hand, Bucci reported a failure of other researchers to significantly substantiate the ergogenic benefit of octacosanol.[10]

If octacosanol truly does possess ergogenic properties, the mechanism of action is not fully understood at this point. Kabir and Kimura attempted to address this phenomenon using rats. The researchers set out to investigate the biodistribution of radioactive (^{14}C) octacosanol in response to exercise.[11] They found the amount of voluntary exercise to be significantly higher in octacosanol-fed rats than in control rats. Additionally, the amount of radioactive octacosanol in the muscle of exercised animals was significantly higher. The muscle seemed to be able to store a considerable amount of octacosanol in response to exercise. While the exact mechanism behind this increase in physical activity caused by octacosanol is unclear, it is quite possible that octacosanol has the ability to increase the mobilization of free fatty acids from fat cells within the muscle. The results from this study indicate that octacosanol possesses an adipolinetic activity that could potentially affect lipolysis in muscle.[11]

All in all, the studies assessing octacosanol as an ergogenic aid are nonspecific. The trials up to this point appear to have many confounding factors. It is essential in clinical trials, especially when athletic performance is measured, to eliminate the placebo effect as much as possible. Many of the studies presented here, which are considered the most reliable to date, lack consistency. This lack of congruency makes it difficult to compare studies. Furthermore, completely randomized, double-blinded studies comparing athletes participating in similar exercise regimens are warranted.

6.2.2 ANTIAGGREGATORY PROPERTIES

Platelet aggregation occurs when blood is converted from a thin consistency to a thicker form or even a clot, which can cause a deep-vein thrombosis or stroke. Exogenous factors such as arachidonic acid, collagen, and adenosine diphosphate can cause aggregation. Platelet aggregation is an important factor in coronary artery disease and vascular arterial disease. Patients at risk for one of these diseases have an increased risk for the other.[12] Arruzazabala and colleagues found that 5 to 20 mg/kg of policosanol given to rats resulted in antiaggregatory effects.[8] These researchers suggested the action was due to the inhibition of arachidonic acid metabolism. The same group of researchers found that when 50 to 200 mg/kg of policosanol was administered, a significant inhibition of platelet aggregation was observed.[12] This study emphasized the need for a large dose to allow policosanol to exhibit antiaggregatory effects.

In 1997, the same research group investigated the effects of policosanol and aspirin on platelet aggregation.[13] Aspirin is commonly used to prevent thrombosis and cerebral ischemia, but can cause gastric irritation. Policosanol works by inhibiting thromboxane A_2 (TxA_2) synthesis instead of prostaglandin synthesis; therefore, fewer side effects such as gastric irritation occur. A daily dose of 20 mg of policosanol caused a significant reduction in platelet aggregation, establishing that policosanol was just as effective as 100 mg/day of aspirin.

6.2.3 CHOLESTEROL-LOWERING EFFECTS

Researchers noticed that during exercise endurance experiments on mice, octacosanol had the ability to alter hepatic and serum lipid concentrations.[14] This led them to begin focusing on octacosanol as a cholesterol-lowering agent. In 1992, Hernandez et al. investigated the effects on healthy individuals with normal cholesterol levels given 10 or 20 mg of policosanol or a placebo.[15] The policosanol-supplemented group had a significant decrease in serum cholesterol levels. The group taking 20 mg of policosanol also demonstrated an increase in high-density lipoprotein (HDL) levels. Aside from the cholesterol-lowering effect, this study revealed a good tolerance in all subjects taking the policosanol supplement.

Kato and colleagues set out to test the effect of octacosanol on lipid metabolism through rats fed a high-fat diet supplemented with octacosanol.[16] The addition of 10 g octacosanol/kg to a high-fat diet led to a significant reduction in the perirenal adipose tissue weight without causing a decrease in cell number. This suggests that octacosanol may suppress lipid accumulation in this tissue. Furthermore, octacosanol supplementation decreased the serum triacylglycerol concentration, most likely through the inhibition of hepatic phosphatidate phosphohydrolase. High amounts of lipoprotein lipase in the perirenal adipose tissue and an increase in the total oxidation rate of fatty acid in the muscle were also observed. Lipid absorption, however, was unaffected by octacosanol supplementation. This study suggests that the dietary incorporation of octacosanol affects some aspects of lipid metabolism. The action of octacosanol may depend on specific dietary conditions, such as fat content, as suggested by this study.

While statin drugs (drugs currently used to reduce blood cholesterol levels) inhibit 3-hydroxy-3-methylglutaryl coenzyme A reductase in the cholesterol synthesis pathway, policosanol inhibits the same pathway but a step earlier. Policosanol could, therefore, prove to be a useful alternative to statin drugs.

In 1999, a study examined just that — the effects of policosanol and pravastatin (a statin drug) on the lipid profile of hypercholesterolemic patients.[17] The researchers demonstrated that policosanol was more effective than pravastatin in lowering low-density lipoprotein (LDL), as well as improving the ratios of LDL to HDL and total cholesterol to HDL. As seen in previous studies, policosanol also increased HDL.[15,16] It is important to note that both drugs in this study were well tolerated with little or no side effects reported.

A similar study examined the effects of policosanol and fluvastatin, another commonly used statin drug, on hypercholesterolemic patients.[18] Policosanol exhibited LDL-lowering and HDL-raising effects. Again, policosanol was well tolerated by the hypercholesterolemic patients. As in the studies discussed here, many others have also investigated the effects of policosanol on hypercholesterolemia, and in all cases the results were similar: LDL cholesterol decreased and HDL cholesterol increased.[17–21]

From these studies we can conclude that octacosanol/policosanol appears to be a promising lipid-lowering agent that is well tolerated with fewer reported side effects than its statin counterpart. Additionally, the cost of octacosanol/policosanol supplementation is only a fraction of statin drugs, which would make it more available to lower-income hypercholesterolemic patients. It is important to note that most of the studies examined here are considered short term (<1 year long). Larger trials extending over longer periods of time are needed to assess the longer-term effects of octacosanol.

6.3   BIODISTRIBUTION

To evaluate some of the health claims regarding octacosanol, researchers began to focus on the distribution of orally administered octacosanol throughout the body. Kabir and Kimura set out to further understand the mechanism of increased physical exercise and motor endurance by octacosanol.[22] ^{14}C-labeled octacosanol administered to rats was found to primarily accumulate in adipose tissue, especially brown adipose tissue. Additionally, they found excretion through the feces to be very low, but present in measurable quantities in the urine and expired as $^{14}CO_2$. This study suggests that a portion of ^{14}C-octacosanol might be converted into fatty acids, which in turn supplies $^{14}CO_2$ and energy through the process of β-oxidation. There is, however, the possibility that all the free acid produced from octacosanol does not undergo direct oxidation and part of it is stored in the fat pool of the adipose tissue. Neptune et al. reported similar findings; the conversion of long-chain fatty acids to $^{14}CO_2$ constituted only a small fraction of the total CO_2 in the rat diaphragm.[23]

Kabir and Kimura further investigated the tissue distribution of ^{14}C-octacosanol in liver and muscle of rats after a series of administrations.[24] They found the highest amount of radioactivity in the liver (9.5% of administered dose), followed by the digestive tract (8.2% of administered dose) and the muscle (3.5% of administered dose). Interestingly enough, the radioactivity in the liver disappeared rapidly, while the muscle seemed to be able to store a considerable amount in response to the dose administered. More recently, Menendez et al. demonstrated that octacosanoic acid, as well as short-chain saturated and unsaturated fatty acids, are formed after an oral dosing of policosanol in rats and monkeys. These results reinforce the idea that octacosanol metabolism is linked to fatty acid metabolism via β-oxidation.[25]

6.4   SUMMARY

Octacosanol has many potential uses for various health concerns. The most widely studied to date are its cholesterol-lowering properties and exercise performance effects. The studies presented thus far have supported the potential octacosanol has in benefiting human health with regard to cholesterol lowering and platelet antiaggregation. Additionally, it has the potential to treat these health conditions without the major side effects often associated with currently marketed drugs. Thus, octacosanol is an important drug of the future in view of the ever-increasing prevalence of obesity and coronary heart disease in the U.S. However, the ability to pinpoint optimal doses for the aforementioned health benefits is lacking in the current literature. Likewise, toxicity of octacosanol has not been observed and remains unknown at this point. More studies are needed to address the long-term effectiveness of octacosanol as well as long-term problems that may arise with supplementation such as this. Furthermore, trials need to be consistent to optimize a comparison of studies that reflect true human function. For example, studies assessing octacosanol as an ergogenic aid need to be completely randomized and double blinded (to eliminate placebo effect), comparing athletes participating in similar exercise regimens. A study containing all of these aspects has not yet been reported. Future research must begin to focus on defining guidelines for octacosanol supplementation, which need to be specific for each health claim. This is especially important because supplementation of this sort does not fall under the U.S. Food and Drug Administration's jurisdiction.

REFERENCES

1. Wildman, R., in *Handbook of Nutraceuticals and Functional Foods*, R. Wildman, Ed. CRC Press, Boca Raton, FL, 2001, pp. 198–206.
2. Cureton, T., Improvements in physical fitness associated with a course of U.S. Navy underwater trainees, with and without dietary supplements. *Res Q*, 34: 440, 1963.
3. Cureton, T., *The Physiological Effects of Wheat Germ Oil on Humans in Exercise*. Charles C. Thomas Publisher, Springfield, IL, 1972.
4. Gonzalez-Bravo, L. et al., Analytical procedure for the determination of l-octacosanol ion plasma by solvent extraction and capillary gas chromatography. *J Chromat B*, 682: 359, 1996.
5. Beltz, S. and P. Doering, Efficacy of nutritional supplements used by athletes. *Clin Pharm*, 12: 900, 1993.
6. Cockerill, D. and L. Bucci, Increases in muscle girth and decreases in body fat associated with a nutritional supplement program. *Chiroprac Sports Med*, 1: 73, 1987.
7. Saint-John, M. and L. McNaughton, Octacosanol ingestion and its effects on metabolic responses to submaximal cycle ergometry, reaction time and chest and grip strength. *Int Clin Nutr Rev*, 6: 81, 1986.
8. Arruzazabala, M., R. Mas, and V. Molina, Effects of policosanol on platelet aggregation in type II hypercholesterolaemic patients. *Tissue React*, 20: 119, 1998.
9. Kim, H. et al., Octacosanol supplementation increases running endurance time and improves biochemical parameters after exhaustion in trained rats. *J Med Food*, 6: 345, 2003.
10. Bucci, L., Nutritional ergoenic aids, in *Nutrition in Exercise and Sport*, I. Wolinsky and J. Hickson, Eds. CRC Press, Boca Raton, FL, 1989, pp. 107–184.
11. Kabir, Y. and S. Kimura, Distribution of radioactive octacosanol in response to exercise in rats. *Nahrung*, 38: 373, 1994.
12. Arruzazabala, M., D. Carbajal, and R. Mas, Effects of policosanol on platelet aggregation in rats. *Throm Res*, 69: 321, 1993.

13. Arruzazabala, M., S. Valdes, and R. Mas, Comparative study of policosanol, aspirin and the combination therapy policosanol-aspirin on platelet aggregation in healthy volunteers. *Pharmacol Res*, 36: 106, 1997.

14. Shimura, S., T. Hasegawa, and S. Takano, Studies on the effect of octacosanol on motor endurance in mice. *Nutr Rep Int*, 36: 1029, 1987.

15. Hernandez, F., J. Illait, and R. Mas, Effect of policosanol on serum lipids and lipoproteins in healthy volunteers. *Curr Ther Res*, 51: 568, 1992.

16. Kato, S. et al., Octacosanol affects lipid metabolism in rats fed on a high-fat diet. *Br J Nutr*, 73: 433, 1995.

17. Pons, P., M. Rodriguez, and R. Mas, One-year efficacy and safety of policosanol in patients with type II hypercholesterolaemia. *Curr Ther Res*, 55: 1084, 1994.

18. Aneiros, E., R. Mas, and B. Calderon, Effect of policosanol in lowering cholesterol levels in patients with type II hypercholesterolaemia. *Curr Ther Res*, 56: 176, 1995.

19. Castano, G., L. Tula, and M. Canetti, Effects of policosanol in hypertensive patients with type II hypercholesterolaemia. *Curr Ther Res*, 57: 691, 1996.

20. Mas, R., G. Castano, and J. Illnait, Effects of policosanol inpatients with type II hypercholesterolaemia and additional coronary risk factors. *Clin Pharmacol Ther*, 65: 439, 1999.

21. Stusser, R. et al., Long-term therapy with policosanol improves treadmill exercise-ECG testing performance of coronary heart disease patients. *Int J Clin Pharmacol Ther*, 36: 469, 1998.

22. Kabir, Y. and S. Kimura, Biodistribution and metabolism of orally administered octacosanol in rats. *Ann Nutr Metab*, 37: 33, 1993.

23. Neptune, E. et al., Phospholipid and triglyceride metabolism of exercised rat diaphragm and the role of these lipids in fatty acid uptake and oxidation. *J Lipid Res*, 1: 229, 1960.

24. Kabir, Y. and S. Kimura, Tissue distribution of (8-14C)-octacosanol in liver and muscle of rats after serial administration. *Ann Nutr Metab*, 39: 279, 1995.

25. Menendez, R. et al., *In vitro* and *in vivo* study of octacosanol metabolism. *Arch Med Res*, 36: 113, 2005.

Section III

Proteins

7 Protein: Quantity and Quality

Mark A. Tarnopolsky and Brian W. Timmons

CONTENTS

7.1 INTRODUCTION

The *quantity* of protein intake for athletic populations has been a matter of controversy for several years. Interest in protein intake can even be traced to ancient Greece, where records from the Olympics indicated that athletes consumed huge amounts of meat to try to maximize strength performance.[1] By the 18th century, muscle contraction was believed to be fueled by the oxidation of muscle protein.[2] As the importance of lipid and carbohydrate (CHO) oxidation in muscle metabolism became clear, a central role for protein oxidation in the supply of energy during muscle contraction waned.[3] In contrast, the *quality* of protein intake for athletic populations has received much less scientific attention. Only recently have researchers attempted to distinguish the potential benefits of varying compositions of amino acids and protein type (e.g., whey vs. casein). The question as to whether physical activity of any type alters the dietary requirement for protein remains open for debate.[4-6]

In this chapter, the pathways of protein metabolism in skeletal muscle with emphasis on the effects of exercise on metabolic and anabolic regulation will be reviewed, including the factors that modify these responses. We will then review studies that have attempted to determine whether athletes require dietary protein intakes higher than those for sedentary individuals and whether protein quality influences metabolic and anabolic regulation. Throughout the chapter, exercise will be broadly classified as either endurance or resistance to highlight the two major classifications of exercise at opposite ends of the metabolic demand spectrum. Endurance activities can be broadly defined as those that utilize predominantly oxidative phosphorylation as the primary energy source; resistance activities lead to increases in strength, power, and muscle mass as outcomes.

7.2 PROTEIN METABOLISM

Proteins are important molecules comprised of amino acids — compounds containing an amino group ($-NH_2$), a carboxylic acid group ($-COOH$), and a radical group (different for each of the amino acids). Structural proteins include cytoskeletal proteins such as dystrophin, vimentin, and desmin, and connective tissue proteins such as collagen; regulatory proteins include enzymes such as lactate dehydrogenase, citrate synthase, or cytochrome c oxidase. There are 20 amino acids that are found as constituents of proteins or present as free amino acids. Nine amino acids are considered essential or indispensable (histidine, isoleucine, leucine, lysine, methionine, phenylalanine, threonine, tryptophan, valine),[7] and arginine is sometimes considered to be conditionally essential. The essential amino acids must come from the diet or from endogenous protein breakdown. Since proteins serve such critical roles in the survival of the organism, it is not surprising that their metabolism is complex, tightly regulated, and in a constant state of flux with simultaneous synthesis and degradation.

7.2.1 Protein Synthesis

Protein synthesis is initiated when a signal (e.g., nutrient, hormone, mechanical) to the cell is communicated to the DNA to induce gene expression (transcription),[8] resulting in formation of messenger RNA (mRNA). The mRNA is translated into a protein through the process of translation by the ribosomes, which are free in the cytosol or bound to rough endoplasmic reticulum. The process of translation requires a second form of RNA, called transfer RNA, and three distinct steps: initiation, elongation, and termination. Following translation, the nascent protein can be further modified through processes such as glycosylation or degradation (posttranslational modification).

When the entire process of muscle protein synthesis is considered, there is ample evidence that this increases in a similar manner after both endurance[9,10] and resistance[11–14] exercise. Factors such as the intensity and duration of exercise also have profound effects on gene expression.[15] The sites of regulation and how this generalized protein synthetic response is fine-tuned to allow for phenotypical divergence are just becoming unravelled. We have used microarray technology and found that over 200 mRNA species are differentially expressed by only 3 h after endurance exercise,[16] and only a minority of these same species are expressed in a similar fashion following resistance exercise.[17] Others have found that phosphorylation of proteins such as p70S6k, 4E-BP1, eIF-2B, and AMPK is altered in response to different contraction patterns in skeletal muscle.[18,19] Collectively, the data show that there are changes at multiple levels (e.g., transcription and translation) within the protein synthetic pathway that simultaneously respond to exercise. It is also likely that the state of training will have a major role in determining the absolute and relative importance of transcriptional and translational control of certain proteins and how this relates to protein synthesis,[8,20,21] ultimately modulating the phenotypic response to a given pattern of muscle contraction. Innovative approaches have revealed that muscle conserves the ability to acutely and directionally respond to divergent stimulii, even if its training history is at the opposite end of the metabolic demand spectrum.[22]

The relationship between exercise and nutrition and the fundamental aspects of gene expression and translation are only now being explored.[23–26] For example, low muscle glycogen content causes an induction of IL-6 mRNA content in skeletal muscle,[24] which may function as a homeostatic sensor to increase hepatic glucose production.[27] During exercise, glucose supplementation, compared with water intake, can attenuate increases in the expression of PDF-4 and UCP-3 — genes involved in metabolic regulation.[28] Insulin and amino acids also influence the assembly of the initiation complex required for protein translation.[29] Recent evidence suggests that diet and exercise may influence different components of the synthetic pathway, for amino acids altered p70 S6 kinase and eukaryotic initiation factor 4E-binding protein-1 phosphorylation status, while resistance exercise had no effect at the same time point.[30] Consequently, nutrition and exercise may alter protein metabolism through independent and possibly complementary pathways. If and how these changes will impact upon protein and amino acid requirements at various phases of the training continuum is not clear. It is theoretically possible that endurance exercise training could impact upon amino acid requirements through increased synthesis of enzymes, capillaries, hemoglobin, and myoglobin (in addition to oxidation). The amino acids for these processes may be derived from an increase in dietary protein intake or an increase in the efficiency of amino acid reutilization.

7.2.2 Protein Breakdown

Protein degradation is the process of breaking down proteins into their constituent amino acids. These amino acids contribute to the intracellular free amino acid pool, which may be exported into the plasma, directly oxidized, or reincorporated back into tissue protein (synthesis). Although most athletes think only of maximizing protein synthesis, it is equally logical to try to attenuate degradation, for net protein balance is a function of synthesis minus degradation. A bodybuilder, for example, could achieve net protein retention by decreasing degradation even without a change in synthesis.

The three main pathways for protein degradation in human skeletal muscle include the lysosomal (cathepsin) and nonlysosomal (calpain and ubiquitin) pathways. The lysosomal pathway degrades endocytosed proteins, some cytosolic proteins, hormones, and immune modulators.[31] This pathway is not a major contributor to human skeletal muscle protein degradation,[32] except when there is significant muscle damage and inflammation.[33] The two major nonlysosomal pathways in human skeletal muscle are the (ATP)-dependent ubiquitin pathway[31] and the calcium-activated neutral protease or calpain pathway.[34–36] The calpain pathway is felt to play a role in skeletal muscle proteolysis during exercise.[34] The ubiquitin pathway is activated after the targeting of proteins for degradation (e.g., oxidative modification). Following targeting, ubiquitin molecules are linked to lysine residues through a series of pathways catalyzed by three enzymes, termed E1, E2, and E3, and are then degraded by the 26S proteosome into peptides.[31] This pathway is activated during starvation and muscle atrophy.[37] Evidence suggests that activation of apoptotic pathways, particularily caspase 3, is a prerequisite for initiation of ubiquitin-proteosome-mediated proteolysis of acto-myosin.[38] It is not currently known whether endurance exercise training has an effect on the activation or content of any of the specific protein breakdown pathways.

In addition to dietary protein intake, protein degradation is the only other source of amino acid contribution to the intracellular free amino acid pool. In human skeletal muscle, at least eight amino acids (alanine, asparagine, aspartate, glutamate, isoleucine, leucine, lysine, and valine) can be oxidized.[39] During exercise, however, the branched-chain amino acids (BCAAs; isoleucine, leucine, and valine) are preferentially oxidized.[39–42] The BCAAs are transaminated to their ketoacids via branched-chain aminotransferase (BCAAT), with subsequent oxidation occurring via branched-chain oxo-acid dehydrogenase enzyme (BCOAD).[43,44] In the cytosol, the amino-N group is usually transaminated with α-ketoglutarate to form glutamate, which is in turn transaminated with pyruvate to form alanine[45] or aminated via glutamine synthase to form glutamine. Some of the amino-N may end up as free ammonia released from muscle; however, during high-intensity contractions most of the ammonia comes from the myoadenylate deaminase pathway.[46–48] The BCOAD enzyme is rate limiting in BCAA oxidation, with about 5 to 8% active (dephosphorylated) at rest and 20 to 25% active during exercise.[40,43] BCOAD activation is related to a decrease in the ATP/ADP ratio, a decrease in pH, and a depletion of muscle glycogen.[48–51] The inverse correlation between BCOAD activation and muscle glycogen concentration[48,49] provides theoretical support for strategies to ensure

CHO availability during exercise to attenuate BCOAD-mediated amino acid oxidation. Somewhat surprisingly, glucose supplementation during exercise does not appear to significantly attenuate BCOAD activation even though leucine oxidation was attenuated at higher protein intakes (1.8 g/kg/day).[52]

7.2.3 MODELS AND MEASUREMENT OF PROTEIN METABOLISM

There are several measurements of protein turnover at the whole-body and tissue level. At the most basic level, the balance between all protein intake and excretion would provide a net balance measurement. This protein balance can be measured using nitrogen balance (NBAL) methods. With the NBAL method, measurements are made of all sources of nitrogen intake (diet and intravenous) and output (urine, feces, sweat, and miscellaneous) and a balance is calculated. If the balance is positive, the person is in a state of net retention, and if it is negative, the person is in a state of net depletion. The measurement of nitrogen is based upon the fact that proteins are about 16% nitrogen by weight.

If an essential amino acid such as leucine is used to study protein turnover, the only sources are from dietary intake (I) or protein breakdown (B). Amino acids like leucine can be removed from the plasma, either for protein synthesis (S), oxidation (O), or incorporation into other metabolic pathways after transamination/deamination. In the case of leucine, this amino acid can also be completely oxidized in the human body to CO_2, allowing for the measurement of O as well. A simple model in the measurement of protein turnover/flux therefore takes into consideration the above factors so that flux (Q) is equal to I + B, which is in turn equal to S + O (i.e., $Q = I + B = S + O$). Isotope studies are used to derive these variables of protein turnover, since amino acid tracers can be used to measure Q and O, and if intake equals zero, then Q = B, and by subtraction, S = Q – O.[53] Isotopes are molecules that share the same atomic number (protons), yet have different numbers of neutrons (atomic mass). Stable isotopes occur naturally and do not emit ionizing radiation, whereas radioactive isotopes undergo spontaneous decay. For these reasons, stable isotopes have become very popular in exercise research.[10,40,41,53–56] Although useful, this model is very simplistic in that there are multiple amino acid pools turning over at very different rates.

Using arteriovenous catheters, one can also measure the amino acid balance across a limb, and measurements of amino acid transport, muscle protein synthesis, and breakdown can be made by simultaneously using stable isotopes.[12,54,57] Another method to measure protein synthesis is the fractional synthetic rate (FSR) method. This requires the infusion of an isotope and the measurement of the incremental increase in isotopic enrichment within a tissue or specific protein over time. We, and others, have used muscle biopsies to look at mixed-skeletal muscle FSR after exercise using this method.[10,11,13,25] Myofibrillar and mitochondrial FSR can also be determined using stable isotopic tracer incorporation in combination with a gel separation of the component proteins.[58] A recent development has been the measurement of collagen synthesis in both muscle and tendons using the FSR method.[14] With this method it has been shown that acute resistance exercise results in a rapid increase in the rate of collagen protein synthesis, possibly to remodel the extracellular matrix.[59]

A significant limitation to our understanding of protein turnover has been the lack of an adequate method to measure muscle protein breakdown. Initially, there was much enthusiasm for the use of 3-methylhistidine (3-MH), which is a posttranslational modification of histidine residues in the actin and myosin of skeletal muscle.[60,61] This method requires accurate urinary collections and assumes that most of the 3-MH arises from skeletal myofibrillar proteolysis and that the proportional contribution from other sources relative to muscle remains constant under varying physiological situations.[60] These limitations are not as much of an issue in crossover studies where the subject is his or her own control, yet the collection issues are still an issue. A method for the determination of mixed-muscle fractional breakdown rate (FBR) using a stable isotopic decay kinetic method has been developed in the laboratory of Wolfe;[13] we have used this method to show that FBR is not altered following resistance training in the fed state.[62]

7.3 ACUTE EXERCISE EFFECTS ON PROTEIN METABOLISM

7.3.1 ENDURANCE EXERCISE

The majority of the energy for endurance exercise is derived from the oxidation of lipid and CHO. As mentioned above, skeletal muscle has the metabolic capacity to oxidize certain amino acids for energy. While it may seem counterproductive to oxidize proteins during exercise since they serve either a structural or functional role, amino acid oxidation may also be required for exchange reactions in the tricarboxylic acid cycle, and this may increase their net utilization.[63]

Early studies evaluated urea excretion as an indicator of protein oxidation (urea is a breakdown product formed in the liver following amino acid oxidation) and found that urinary urea excretion was higher following endurance exercise than at rest.[4,64] This increase is missed if sweat is not collected because urea and other nitrogen compounds are contained in sweat.[65,66] For example, a person exercising

---

TABLE 7.1
Energy Requirements during a 1-h Run at 65 to 75% of VO_{2max}

	Energy (kcal/h)	% Fat	% Protein	% CHO
Males[a]	816 (122)	24 (19)	5 (3)	71 (24)
Females	603 (45)	38 (17)	2 (2)	60 (18)

[a] Males are different from females for all variables ($p < 0.01$). Values are mean (SD) from 41 females and 40 males using pooled data.[40,41,55,64,74,75]

---

in high ambient temperatures or humidity with a sweat rate of up to 2 l/h would be expected to have a high urea sweat loss that may contribute to a more negative nitrogen balance. Since urea excretion represents the full extent of amino acid oxidation, this method provides only indirect evidence for amino acid oxidation and, in some cases, does not correlate well with direct measures of amino acid oxidation.[45]

By far, the amino acid leucine has been most often used to trace the effects of exercise on amino acid oxidation, and many studies have shown that endurance exercise increases leucine oxidation.[40–42,66–69] An increase in lysine oxidation has also been observed during endurance exercise.[67] During endurance exercise, leucine oxidation demonstrates a positive correlation with exercise intensity.[70] Leucine oxidation[40,41] and plasma urea content[71] also increase with exercise duration. Finally, leucine oxidation increases with glycogen depletion, which may partially explain the increase in leucine oxidation with exercise duration.[48] Following endurance exercise, there is a prompt return toward baseline leucine oxidation levels,[41] although there appears to be a slight increase in leucine oxidation following eccentric exercise that may persist for up to 10 days.[72] This may partially explain why nitrogen balance is negative at the onset of unaccustomed endurance exercise, yet becomes more positive as the person adapts to the stress.[73] The increase in amino acid oxidation during endurance exercise may account for 1 to 6% of the total energy cost for an endurance exercise session at about 65% VO_{2peak} (Table 7.1). If only a few of the nonessential amino acids are oxidized during endurance exercise, then the predicted effect on protein requirements may be minimal. Conversely, an increase in essential amino acid oxidation (e.g., leucine and lysine) may affect protein requirements since they can only come from dietary intake or protein breakdown.

7.3.2 RESISTANCE EXERCISE

In contrast to endurance exercise, acute whole-body resistance exercise does not alter leucine oxidation.[56] In this same study we also did not find an effect of acute resistance exercise on whole-body protein synthesis, either during exercise or for up to 2 h post-exercise.[56] We hypothesized that since muscle protein synthesis (MPS) accounted for only 25% of whole-body synthesis,[76] changes in MPS either may be not measurable or would be negated by a reciprocal change in the synthesis of another protein, such as one in the gastrointestinal tract.

To measure the acute effect of resistance exercise on muscle-specific protein synthesis, several groups have used the FSR tracer incorporation method described above. We demonstrated that mixed-muscle FSR was elevated for up to 36 h following a single bout of resistance exercise.[11,77] Other groups have also shown the increase in muscle protein synthesis after an acute bout of resistance exercise using FSR[13,14,59] and arteriovenous balance[12] methods. Phillips and colleagues[13] demonstrated that FSR was elevated for up to 48 h after a single bout of resistance exercise in relatively untrained men and women, and increases in FSR in older adults have also been found following an acute bout of resistance exercise.[78,79] The acute increase in FSR following a bout of resistance exercise is attenuated after a period of training in young men, yet the basal FSR rate is elevated.[62]

Muscle protein breakdown after resistance exercise can also be studied using the intracellular tracer dilution[13] and the arteriovenous balance or tracer[12] methods. In parallel with muscle FSR, Phillips and colleagues[13] demonstrated that fractional protein breakdown (FBR) was increased after resistance exercise, yet the magnitude of the increase was less than for FSR (i.e., the muscle was in a more positive balance). Furthermore, they showed that FBR returned to baseline values before FSR.[13] Biolo and co-workers[12] found that muscle synthesis and breakdown were increased following an acute bout of resistance exercise. The net balance (synthesis minus degradation) was negative prior to exercise and was more positive (but still net negative) after exercise, for the subjects were in the fasted state. Taken together, these data indicate that muscle FSR and FBR are increased in the post-exercise period following resistance exercise. In the fasted state, net protein balance is negative, and resistance exercise renders the muscle in a less negative balance. Therefore, the post-exercise period is an important time for the delivery of nutrients, as discussed below.

7.3.3 FACTORS AFFECTING PROTEIN METABOLISM

7.3.3.1 Energy Intake

Energy is a classical determinant of protein metabolism, with suboptimal energy intake leading to a relative increase in protein oxidation.[80,81] For example, in starvation there is a clear net negative protein balance that results in cachexia. Conversely, an increase in total energy intake was associated with an improvement in protein balance in young women who performed endurance exercise on a daily basis.[82] Most men and women consume enough energy and protein to accommodate any possible increase in protein requirements; however, the goal of the sport nutritionist is to identify and work with athletes who have unique and special needs. Over the years, our group and others have expressed concern that a varying number of female athletes appear to report very low energy intakes.[41,64,65,74,83–88] Unfortunately, energy restriction is on a continuum from dieting to severe cases of anorexia, and these disordered eating patterns are not uncommon among various types of female athletes.[89] It is this minority of athletes that require most attention with regard to energy and protein balance. Fortunately, strategies such as changing the timing of nutritional delivery (see below) can have beneficial effects on protein balance and performance, without altering total energy intake.[82]

7.3.3.2 Carbohydrate (CHO) Intake

It has been known for many years that CHO intake has a significant sparing effect upon amino acid oxidation and protein balance.[81,90] The dietary interaction between protein and CHO may have implications for those athletes who habitually consume fad diets that stress a very low CHO intake. Given that CHO is the predominant fuel utilized during endurance exercise,[40,41] and that this substrate can become depleted during prolonged endurance exercise,[40] it is important for amino acid metabolism to be considered in light of CHO intake and storage (i.e., glycogen) status of the athlete. CHO loading has been shown to attenuate plasma and sweat urea excretion following endurance exercise.[91] Furthermore, CHO supplementation increases whole-body protein synthesis[92] and attenuates proteolysis.[93] We have reported that both men and women show attenuated total amino acid oxidation (serial urinary urea excretion) during endurance exercise when CHO supplements are consumed during exercise.[55] These findings have been confirmed in well-trained cyclists.[94] These latter two studies[55,94] emphasize the fact that CHO consumption during exercise is an effective strategy to attenuate potential exercise-induced increases in amino acid oxidation. Furthermore, we have also found that urea excretion in urine was lower during a period of intensive endurance exercise training when women consumed a post-exercise supplement containing CHO with a small amount of protein, compared to consuming the same supplement at a time separated from the exercise bout by more than 4 h.[8] This finding was replicated in men performing resistance exercise,[95] where a post-exercise CHO supplement resulted in a more positive nitrogen balance and an attenuation of 3-MH excretion (myofibrillar proteolysis).[95] It is important to note that these post-exercise nutritional strategies net positive effects on nitrogen balance over a 24-h period and not just in the immediate post-exercise period.[82,95] Finally, glucose consumption during endurance exercise appears to reduce leucine oxidation ($\sim$20%), but only when dietary protein intakes are rather high (1.8 g/kg/day) and not when they are low (0.7 g/kg/day — below any Recommended Dietary Allowance [RDA] for any country).[52] The positive effects of CHO on net protein balance are probably due to an insulin-mediated stimulation of protein synthesis and an attenuation of protein breakdown (see below). The convenience and relative inexpense of CHO supplementation makes this an attractive strategy to favorably alter net protein balance in resistance sports.

7.3.3.3 Dietary Protein Intake

The level of dietary protein intake influences protein metabolism in response to exercise. During and after endurance exercise, the provision of extra protein (beyond requirement) resulted in an increase in leucine oxidation[68,96,97] and in one study appeared to attenuate muscle FSR.[10] The latter study measured mixed-muscle FSR in response to three different protein intakes (0.8, 1.8, 3.6 g/kg/day) in endurance-trained athletes and found that FSR was lowest at the highest protein intake level,[10] yet whole-body leucine oxidation was greatest (a nutrient excess).[97] Our group has shown that the provision of dietary protein at levels above requirement (e.g., 2.8 vs. 1.8 g/kg/day) resulted in an exponential increase in amino acid oxidation with no further increase in protein synthesis in male strength athletes.[53] In addition, the provision of dietary protein at 2.6 g/kg/day during resistance exercise training in young males doing weight training did not confer any strength or mass benefits compared to a diet supplying 1.35 g/kg/day.[98] Taken together, these data indicate that protein consumed in excess of need is oxidized as energy and does not have a net anabolic effect per se. However, there is a lower limit of protein intake where a further reduction in protein intake will have a negative impact on protein synthesis. It is the determination of these inflection/plateau points that ultimately will determine the optimal protein intake for a given type of exercise (exponential increase in oxidation and plateau in synthesis).

7.3.3.4 Amino Acids

In addition to CHO, there has been interest in whether amino acids per se stimulate net protein balance (e.g., increase synthesis or decrease degradation). There appears to be a potentiation of amino acid transport into muscle after an acute bout of training,[99,100] and there is good evidence that an intravenous amino acid infusion has a stimulatory effect on muscle protein synthesis[99,101–104] independent of the insulin effect.[102] Leucine appears to have a particularly potent effect on stimulating muscle protein synthesis, with its addition showing a marked stimulatory effect on FSR following endurance exercise.[105] Furthermore, the essential and branched-chain amino acids seem to increase the sensitivity of the muscle to the protein stimulatory effects of insulin.[101] Net balance, however, only becomes positive with feeding, and several studies have found that it is the essential amino acids that are critical to this response.[54,106] In contrast, amino acids appear to have equivocal effects on protein degradation;[102–104] however, the addition of carbohydrate to protein appears to attenuate the breakdown process following resistance exercise.[107] The problem with this body of literature is that it does not directly answer the question about protein requirements, for it is impossible to determine whether the amino acids acted to stimulate protein synthesis during a state of deficiency, compared to a situation of adequate protein status.

7.3.3.5 Interaction of Nutrients

Complete proteins that contain high biological value (quality) amino acids (whey and casein) stimulate post-resistance exercise net protein anabolism without a difference between the two sources.[108] CHO has an interactive effect with amino acids in that amino acids appear to increase protein synthesis, whereas CHO reduces protein breakdown.[107,109] A combination of high-quality protein, amino acids, and carbohydrate clearly results in a more positive net protein balance following acute resistance exercise than does isoenergetic carbohydrate alone.[110] One study found that the provision of CHO and essential amino acids *before* a bout of resistance exercise increased amino acid (phenylalanine) uptake to a greater extent than when provided immediately after, and that this was due to a greater delivery of amino acids.[111] In a similar fashion, there is some evidence that the consumption of milk following resistance exercise may also increase the utilization of available amino acids for protein synthesis.[112] This latter observation is of interest because it reflects the potentially beneficial role of a whole food product, as opposed to dietary supplements, in optimizing exercise adaptation. Other investigations of nutrient interactions have measured muscle FSR and whole-body protein turnover after resistance exercise in response. Compared with trials of CHO only, CHO + protein, and CHO + protein + free leucine, the CHO + protein + leucine trial resulted in the most positive protein balance through a reduction in breakdown and an increase in FSR.[105] This latter study is the first to our knowledge supporting that the addition of an amino acid to a complete protein confers advantage in terms of post-exercise protein balance.

7.3.3.6 Timing of Nutrient Delivery

There has been an interest in the timing of nutrient delivery and the effects on glycogen synthesis in the recovery from endurance exercise.[113,114] Studies have demonstrated that glycogen resynthesis is more rapid if the glucose is provided in the immediate post-exercise period vs. a 2-h delay,[114] and that there may be a synergistic effect from the addition of protein to glucose drinks.[113] However, in a recent study our group did not find evidence for a synergistic increase in post-endurance exercise glycogen recovery with isoenergetic protein–glucose supplements vs. glucose alone.[75] At higher levels of energy intake some have found that the addition of protein to carbohydrate may enhance the rate of post-exercise glycogen resynthesis compared with an isoenergetic carbohydrate only drink,[115] while others have not,[116] even with nonisoenergetic diets.[117] Following resistance exercise, we found that isoenergetic glucose–protein supplements were similar in terms of glycogen resynthesis compared to glucose supplements alone.[118] We also demonstrated that whole-body protein synthesis was greater for post-resistance exercise protein–glucose and glucose supplements than for placebo.[119] Our group[82] also found that the provision of a CHO + PRO + FAT defined formula diet given immediately post-endurance exercise in female athletes during a period of increased training volume enhanced performance, maintained weight, and tended ($p = 0.06$) to enhance nitrogen balance, compared to consumption of the same diet at a different time of the day. A series of studies by Burke and colleagues demonstrated that muscle glycogen content 24 h after endurance exercise was similarly restored whether subjects ate four large meals or many small snacks[120] and whether protein and fat were consumed with the meals.[121] These results suggest that the timing of post-exercise CHO intake may not be critical if the next performance is not until 24 h later. However, if a sport requires several workouts or performances per day (e.g., a tournament), then a more rapid glycogen resynthesis may enhance performance. This phenomenon has also been shown for resistance exercise, where a CHO vs. placebo supplement given after one bout of exercise resulted in performance enhancement in a subsequent bout 4 h later.[122]

Taken together, the aforementioned observations suggest that the immediate post-exercise period, or at the onset or during exercise,[111] is an important time to consume protein and CHO, particularly for the resistance athlete. This may have an impact on protein requirements and permit optimal muscle strength gains with any given protein intake. For the endurance athlete, the immediate provision of CHO is not as critical to glycogen resynthesis over the ensuing 24 h, provided that the daily CHO intake is high (~10 g/kg/day). Notwithstanding our current understanding, we still need to more fully examine the impact of immediate post-exercise intake of protein and CHO on 24-h whole-body protein retention. However, the acute response of protein turnover to exercise and amino acid consumption appears to reflect the balance over the ensuing 24 h.[123] Together the findings in the aforementioned several paragraphs would predict that the timing (early post-exercise) and composition (protein + amino acids + carbohydrate) of the diet would positively influence (i.e., attenuate any possible increase) protein requirements.

7.3.3.7   Hormones

Although there are many hormones that directly and indirectly affect protein turnover (e.g., insulin, cortisol, testosterone, growth hormone, and insulin-like growth factor), only testosterone and insulin will be discussed here. Testosterone is of interest because of the significant controversy surrounding its unethical use in sporting events and its potent effects on protein metabolism. For many years testosterone was assumed to possess stimulatory effects on net protein synthesis, based on observations of male/female differences in lean mass as well as the increases noted for those who supplemented with pharmacological doses. Consequently, proper investigations into the metabolism and efficacy of testosterone administration followed.[57,124–127] Even without resistance exercise, testosterone administration can increase lean body mass,[124,126,127] and a resistance exercise training program can magnify these effects.[127] At the muscle level, testosterone acts by increasing protein synthesis and intracellular amino acid reutilization and not degradation.[57] Given the fact that acute resistance exercise also increases plasma testosterone concentration,[128,129] it will be important to conduct properly designed studies to compare the efficacy of an optimal nutritional intervention to that of exogenous testosterone supplementation. Another interesting finding with potential relevance to an athlete's enthusiasm for very high protein intakes is the apparent negative correlation between protein intake and plasma testosterone concentration.[128]

Another key hormone important in protein metabolism and a major factor in the efficacy of CHO–protein nutrition is insulin. Insulin has a net stimulatory effect upon muscle protein synthesis,[130] primarily through a reduction in muscle proteolysis.[102,103,107,131–133] The effect of insulin on protein synthesis appears to depend on whether there is an abundance of amino acids.[130] Several studies have failed to find a stimulation of insulin on muscle protein synthesis,[102,103,132,134] which is likely due to the hypoaminoacidemia induced by insulin.[130] When amino acids are provided simultaneously with insulin (to prevent hypoaminoacidemia), there appears to be a stimulation of protein synthesis.[102,103,131–133] Other studies have found that hyperinsulinemia stimulates both muscle FSR and amino acid transport.[12] Finally, the effects of insulin on protein metabolism are different before and after resistance exercise.[130] In the resting state, insulin induces a more positive protein balance by increasing synthesis and increasing amino acid transport; after exercise, there was no effect on synthesis, yet there was a significant reduction in degradation and a threefold increase in amino acid transport.[130] These findings provide the theoretical basis for the provision of protein and CHO in the early post-exercise period in athletes performing resistance-type exercise, a finding recently confirmed.[109]

7.3.3.8   Hydration Status

There is no question that dehydration can significantly alter exercise performance and ultimately lead to more severe medical disorders such as heat stress and heat stroke.[135,136] Hydration status is also a determinant of amino acid oxidation, with cellular dehydration inducing an increase in leucine oxidation and cellular hyperhydration showing the opposite in resting young men.[137] Although dehydration during exercise should undoubtedly increase amino acid oxidation, no study has yet been completed during endurance exercise in men or women to explore this concept. Although most athletes strive to attain optimal hydration, there are a number of factors that can limit oral intake of fluids during exercise, and every athlete in the world has undoubtedly experienced some degree of dehydration during training or competition. Consequently, the varying and episodic dehydration that all athletes experience could have some impact on protein requirements.

7.3.3.9 Gender/Sex

A number of studies have examined the influence of gender/sex on metabolic fuel selection during endurance activity.[40,41,64,67,74,75,138–140] Overall, women appear to oxidize proportionately more lipid and less CHO than men during endurance exercise.[40,41,64,67,74,75,138–140] The lower contribution from CHO in exercising females would imply that amino acid oxidation should also be lower than in men. In an earlier study using 24-h urinary urea excretion as a marker of total amino acid oxidation, we found that men, but not women, showed elevated 24-h urinary urea during a day in which they completed a 15.5-km treadmill run as compared to a rest day.[64] Using leucine as a stable isotope tracer, our group[41] and others[67,141] found that women oxidized proportionately less leucine than men during endurance cycling. The reduced leucine oxidation observed for women during endurance exercise is apparent prior to and following 31 days of endurance exercise training.[40] In the latter study we did not find that the gender difference could be explained based upon either the total or active proportion of skeletal muscle BCOAD.[40] This finding suggests that the locus of the gender difference in amino acid oxidation cannot be explained at the skeletal muscle level, and may be at the hepatic level. To further uncover the mechanisms involved in gender-related differences in protein metabolism during exercise, we supplemented healthy men with the sex hormone estrogen. Following 8 days of supplementation, the men demonstrated a reduced dependence on amino acids and CHO and an increased reliance on lipids as a fuel source during endurance exercise.[142] A summary of the effects of exercise on protein metabolism in men and women is found in Table 7.1.

7.4 CHRONIC EXERCISE EFFECTS ON PROTEIN METABOLISM

7.4.1 Endurance Training

Since proteins serve either a structural or functional role within the cell, chronic endurance exercise training would be expected to achieve adaptations that would attenuate the oxidation of protein for energy. This would also be predicted based on the sparing of muscle glycogen that accompanies chronic endurance training, which would tend to attenuate BCOAD activation. Early work by Gontzea et al.[73] showed that untrained persons who started endurance training were in a negative nitrogen balance, but as they continued to train, the nitrogen balance became less negative.

To date, human data have not yielded consistent findings on the effects of chronic exercise training on protein metabolism. Following endurance exercise training, whole-body protein synthesis at rest is increased.[69,143] There is also a greater proportion of leucine flux at rest diverted toward oxidation in the untrained vs. trained athlete.[69] However, differences in leucine turnover between trained and untrained subjects disappeared when the data were expressed relative to lean mass.[42] These findings are not consistent with the hypothesis that endurance exercise training attenuates glycogen use and spares protein oxidation. For this reason we designed an experiment to train sedentary individuals for 38 days and to measure their leucine oxidation and BCOAD activation during exercise, before and after the training.[40] We found that leucine oxidation during exercise was lower after training, as was BCOAD activation.[40] However, consequent to the increase in total mitochondrial content, the absolute capacity of BCOAD enzyme activity was higher in the trained state.[40] Our findings were confirmed in a recent study that showed that resting amino acid oxidation was lower after endurance exercise training.[144] Taken together, data from the latter two studies confirm that chronic endurance training results in a sparing of amino acid oxidation. With the greater total amount of BCOAD activity after endurance exercise training,[40] the *maximal capacity* for amino acid oxidation would be higher in the trained state. However, it is likely that only top sport athletes training for long hours and at a high relative intensity or during periods of nutritional stress (i.e., low energy or CHO intake) could ever strain metabolic capacity such that the daily amount of amino acid oxidation would exceed that in the untrained or moderately trained individual.

7.4.2 RESISTANCE TRAINING

Although there are fewer training studies concerning resistance exercise, it is logical that protein requirements/synthesis would be greater in the early stages of adaptation when the initial hypertrophy is achieved than in a long-term maintenance phase (assuming no compensatory changes in reutilization). We demonstrated that whole-body protein synthesis and degradation were greater in resistance-trained athletes than in sedentary controls;[53] furthermore, others have found that basal FSR was higher after a period of resistance exercise training.[20,62] In addition, there is an attenuation of the acute exercise-induced increase in mixed-muscle FSR following a period of resistance exercise training.[20,62] This latter finding would predict that a trained weight lifter could have either a lower (reduced post-exercise pulse) or a higher (elevated basal FSR) protein requirement. The elevation in basal mixed FSR after training is consistent with the finding of a higher whole-body protein synthesis in well-trained resistance athletes than in sedentary controls.[53] However, protein requirements[65] appear to be lower for well-trained resistance-trained athletes[65] than for those starting a training program,[98] but still marginally elevated as compared with sedentary individuals.[65] A study of resistance training in older adults suggested that protein efficiency was enhanced following a resistance training program.[145]

7.5   ASSESSMENT OF DIETARY PROTEIN
   REQUIREMENTS

Overall, dietary protein requirements represent the amount of protein that is required to support net protein synthesis (growth, repair of damaged tissues, lactation, pregnancy, muscle hypertrophy, enzyme synthesis), amino acid oxidation, and the inefficiency inherent in the amino acid recycling process. The two methods of determining protein requirements are the NBAL method and those using isotope tracers.

7.5.1   NITROGEN BALANCE

As defined above, NBAL is the method whereby the investigator determines all of the protein that enters a person (diet, intravenous, etc.) and all of the nitrogen that is excreted.[7,146] Since the body excretes nitrogenous compounds rather than whole proteins and since proteins are ~16% nitrogen by weight, the technique involves measurement of the total nitrogen intake and the total nitrogen excretion (urine, feces, sweat, and miscellaneous, e.g., menstrual loss, hair, semen, and skin). If the person is in a state of net anabolism, then there is a positive NBAL, whereas if the person is losing protein, then there is a negative NBAL. The protein intake requirement for a given physiological state (e.g., exercise, pregnancy, and lactation) is determined by feeding the person varying protein intakes and determining the NBAL at each level of intake. From this, one can calculate a regression equation from which a zero NBAL can be interpolated. In order to account for interindividual variability in the development of general guidelines, two standard deviations are added to the zero estimate. In this way, the safe protein intake level is estimated to cover 97% of the given population. It is important to note that the NBAL experiment must indicate the biological value of the dietary protein used in the study. For example, a protein requirement of 1.0 g/kg/day, based on egg white and milk protein, would have to be higher for a diet based on lower biological value proteins, such as grains. Most countries in the world base their dietary protein intake recommendations relative to a biological value estimated to be the mean for the population.[7]

One of the problems with the NBAL method is that the protein requirement estimates may underestimate what is required for optimal functioning. This concern comes from the fact that as protein intake decreases there is an increase in the efficiency of amino acid reutilization and a lower overall amino acid flux.[7,53,147,148] Therefore, NBAL may be achieved with a compromise in some physiologically relevant processes. For example, an endurance athlete may slow the induction of aerobic enzyme activity or a resistance athlete may not achieve the same degree of skeletal muscle hypertrophy over a period of training. Therefore, the ultimate method to determine the dietary requirements for athletes would be to provide a large group of sedentary individuals with a variety of graded protein intakes over a prolonged period of training and determine which was the optimal intake to achieve maximal improvements in several physiological outcome variables (e.g., VO_{2max}, muscle strength, muscle mass). Furthermore, one would also want to determine that the optimal protein intake resulted in optimal function in other critical areas, such as resistance to infections. Unfortunately, this approach would be prohibitively expensive and time-consuming and as such is not likely to ever be completed.

7.5.2 TRACER METHODS

Because of the limitations in the NBAL method, Young and Bier have been instrumental in devising a conceptual framework from which to determine optimal protein intakes using stable isotopic tracers. They have coined the terms nutrient deficiency, accommodation, adaptation, and nutrient excess.[147,148] In a state of protein deficiency, there would be a maximal reduction in amino acid oxidation and a reduction in protein synthesis to all but the essential organs (e.g., brain) that ultimately would result in muscle wasting (negative NBAL). The state of accommodation would be the state where NBAL is achieved with a decrease in a physiologically relevant process. The state of adaptation would be the dietary intake that provided for optimal rates of protein synthesis for growth, interorgan amino acid exchange, and immune function. Finally, the state of protein excess would be defined as that intake where amino acids are oxidized for energy or used in fat storage, and protein synthesis is not further simulated by an increase in intake. These four states can be determined using amino acid tracers during studies at varied protein intakes. The optimal protein intake would be that where amino acid oxidation starts to increase exponentially and protein synthesis starts to plateau. There have only been a few of these studies performed in athletes.[10,53,96,97]

7.6   HABITUAL PROTEIN INTAKES OF ATHLETES

Athletes are a group of individuals who are constantly striving for optimal performance. Because of this, many of them fall victim to false or unsubstantiated claims concerning diet and nutrient supplements. For example, the protein and amino acid supplement market in the U.S. is a multi-million-dollar industry sustained by a motive to sell product rather than to encourage optimal nutrition through food. It is common to observe individuals consuming protein and amino acid intakes that would clearly be considered a gross nutrient excess. This is particularly true for resistance-trained athletes, in whom there are anecdotes of extreme protein intakes — a football player who consumed 80 egg whites + 4 l of milk + 250 g of protein powder per day. Although some athletes believe that "more is better," there is a limit to how much dietary protein that can be incorporated into muscle mass, and anything above this level is used as energy.

The problem with excessive protein intakes is that they are quite expensive, the high protein may displace other food sources such as CHO (many of which contain fiber, vitamins, and minerals), many protein sources also contain fat, and prolonged very high protein intakes may be associated with adverse health consequences in certain people (i.e., high protein intakes can increase calcium excretion, and in people with mild renal impairment, there is a more rapid progression of renal dysfunction).[149,150] On average, athletes consume about twice the RDA for protein. However, there may be a role for limited supplement/prepackaged defined formula use, such as when an athlete is traveling to a foreign country and the availability of familiar foods may be limited. In addition, there may be cases where an individual is on a weight-restrictive diet and protein intake may not be adequate to meet the needs of a rigorous training program. Included in this group is the bodybuilder who is getting ready for a competition and the combative athlete who is trying to "make weight." Even under such instances it should be possible to take advantage of factors such as timing of nutrient intake (see previous text) to optimize protein balance. For the most part, however, the problem of protein excess is predominantly one affecting resistance athletes and not endurance athletes. In general, resistance training athletes, who are not energy restricting, consume protein that is already in excess of their protein requirement (see Table 7.2).

In contrast, some individuals may suffer from protein deficiency where chronically low intakes may lead to a compromise of function and ultimately to a loss of body protein (atrophy). There are four groups of athletes who appear to be at highest risk from protein and energy deficiency, including amenorrheic female runners,[85,151] male wrestlers,[152,153] male and female gymnasts,[152,154] and female dancers.[152,154] Table 7.3 provides mean intakes for groups of endurance athletes. It is important to remember that these nutritional surveys reflect average intakes for a group and the range can be wide within a group. For example, in one study, the mean energy and protein intakes reported by male gymnasts were 2080 kcal and 1.1 g/kg/day, respectively; however, some athletes reported intakes as low as 568 kcal and 0.16 g/kg/day.[154] Similarly, in a study of female runners, Deuster and colleagues[86] found that the mean reported energy and protein intakes were 2397 kcal and 1.56 g/kg/day, respectively, yet the lowest reported intakes were 1067 kcal and 0.53 g/kg/day.

TABLE 7.2
Habitual Protein Intakes of Resistance Athletes

Reference	Participants	Protein (g/kg/day)	(% EIN)
Roy et al., 1998[118]	N = 10 males (trained)	1.6	18
Tarnopolsky et al., 1992[53]	N = 7 males (footballers)	1.8	16
Lemon et al., 1992[98]	N = 12 males (bodybuilders)	1.4	14
Chesley et al., 1992[11]	N = 12 males (bodybuilders)	1.6	17
Tarnopolsky et al., 1988[65]	N = 6 males (bodybuilders)	2.7	17
Faber et al., 1986[157]	N = 76 males (bodybuilders)	2.4	22
Short and Short, 1983[154]	N = 30 males (footballers)	2.5	18
	N = 6 males (bodybuilders)	2.3	20
Burke et al., 1991[158]	N = 18 males (weight lifters)	1.9	18
Burke and Read, 1988[159]	N = 56 males (footballers)	1.5	15
Kleiner et al., 1990[160]	N = 8 females (bodybuilders)	2.8	37
	Overall mean	2.0 (0.5)	19 (6)

Note: Values are mean (SD). Trained = weight trained four times per week for more than 2 years; % EIN = % energy intake.

TABLE 7.3
Habitual Protein Intakes of Male and Female Endurance Athletes

Reference	Subjects	Protein (g/kg/day)	(% EIN)
Carter et al., 2001[155]	N = 8 males	1.7	16
	N = 8 females	1.3	17
Tarnopolsky et al., 1997[75]	N = 8 males	1.9	17
	N = 8 females	1.2	14
Tarnopolsky et al., 1995[74]	N = 7 males	1.8	15
	N = 8 females	1.0	12
Tarnopolsky et al., 1988[65]	N = 6 males	1.5	11
Phillips et al., 1993[41]	N = 6 males	1.9	15
	N = 6 females	1.0	13
Tarnopolsky et al., 1990[64]	N = 6 males	1.2	12
	N = 6 females	1.7	13
Saris et al., 1989[83]	N = 5 males	2.2	15
Deuster et al., 1986[87]	N = 51 females	1.6	13
Ellsworth et al., 1985[156]	N = 13 males	2.1	14
Nelson et al., 1986[84]	N = 17 EUM	1.0	15
	N = 11 AMEN	0.7	15
Marcus et al., 1985[85]	N = 6 EUM	1.3	17
	N = 11 AMEN	1.0	15
Drinkwater et al., 1984[88]	N = 13 EUM	1.1	13
	N = 14 AMEN	1.2	16
Approximate mean	Males	1.8 (0.4)	14 (2)
	Females	1.2 (0.3)	14 (2)

Note: Values are mean (SD). EUM = eumenorrheic; AMEN = amenorrheic females; EIN = energy intake.

Partially adapted from Tarnopolsky, M., *Nutrition*, 20, 662, 2004.

In summary, the majority of strength and endurance athletes consume adequate protein and energy to meet their needs. Even when one takes into account the modest increases required by certain athletes (see below), most athletes are still above these levels. It appears that the human body homeostatically adapts to exercise by matching protein and energy intakes to cover any increase in demand from the activity in question. In some groups, there are extrinsic pressures to restrict intake for weight class or aesthetic reasons. In fact, certain groups may not even be attaining the recommended intake levels for sedentary individuals. Each athlete must be considered as an individual when determining the adequacy of dietary protein and energy intakes. The identification of the at risk groups above may help the nutritionist or coach to be aware of those who may need special nutritional counseling.

7.7 DIETARY PROTEIN REQUIREMENTS FOR ATHLETES

In most countries there are no specific allowances for an effect of physical exercise on protein requirements. It is sometimes stated that these are not required because all athletes consume more energy and subsequently achieve adequate protein intakes. Others have argued that moderate exercise does not increase the requirement for dietary protein,[66,80,145] and therefore there is no need to provide specific protein requirements for athletes. However, these studies were undertaken using exercise intensities that would be considered recreational by most standards. Clearly, an elite athlete is performing daily exercise at a much higher intensity and for a longer duration than the novice. Therefore, it is critical to quantify the state of training and the daily volume for any study looking at protein requirements in athletes. Although most athletes consume enough protein to cover any potential increase in dietary need, there are individuals who may not even meet minimal requirements, and it is this group for whom an awareness of protein requirements is useful. For example, a person who is performing regular strenuous activity while on an energy-restrictive diet may wish to know the minimal protein intake for optimal functional status.

7.7.1 PROTEIN REQUIREMENTS FOR ENDURANCE ATHLETES

Given that amino acids can be oxidized as energy during exercise, it is theoretically possible that this may impact on the need for extra dietary protein. The determination of dietary protein requirements for endurance athletes is a function of the duration and intensity of exercise, gender, age, training status, and habitual energy and CHO intake. In a simplistic approach to determining protein requirements, it is possible to calculate the estimated need for dietary protein by an athlete from first principles. For example, if a 70-kg male was running for 1.5 h at 70% VO_{2peak} and protein accounted for 5% of the total energy expenditure, he would oxidize about 15 g of protein. If his basal protein requirement was 0.86 g/kg/day (60 g), this would represent an additional 25% increase in his daily protein requirement (1.07 g/kg/day). Most male and female endurance athletes habitually consume more protein than this (Table 7.3). These calculations are only rough estimates and most studies have used NBAL to try to quantify dietary protein requirements for endurance athletes.

Two often-quoted studies from the mid-1970s determined NBAL following the initiation of an endurance exercise program on a constant protein intake,[73] and while consuming two different protein intakes.[161] In a group of males starting an endurance exercise program they found that a protein intake of 1.5 g/kg/day was adequate to maintain a positive NBAL, whereas 1.0 g/kg/day was inadequate.[161] In addition, they also found that the subjects on a constant protein intake showed progressive adaptation to the moderate exercise program by improving NBAL over the course of about 1 week.[73] These latter findings suggested that there were adaptive changes to the stress of exercise (e.g., an increase in amino acid reutilization efficiency), and therefore, an increased protein intake was needed only at the initiation of an endurance exercise program. This is similar to our findings in men and women following a modest training program.[40] An improvement in NBAL with moderate-intensity endurance exercise training is due to a lower resting,[144] and exercise-induced,[40] amino acid oxidation.

With moderate-intensity endurance exercise ($\leq 50\%$ VO_{2peak}), there does not appear to be an increase in protein requirements.[80,162] At these modest exercise intensities, protein utilization is enhanced[80] and energy deficits are better tolerated.[162] In another study of endurance exercise at moderate intensity (46% VO_{2peak}), El-Khoury and colleagues[66] used a combined isotopic tracer and nitrogen excretion method and found that a protein intake of 1 g/kg/day was adequate for young males. The improvement in NBAL observed by Gaine and colleagues[144] occurred in men and women with modest aerobic capacity (39 ml/kg/min) after 4 weeks of modest exercise training (4 to 5 times/week at 65 to 85% max HR). Likely the most comprehensive study of endurance exercise training and protein metabolism was completed by Forslund and colleagues.[96] They studied leucine oxidation, protein, carbohydrate, fat, and energy balance over a 24-h period in men performing low- to moderate-intensity exercise (90 min at 45 to 50% VO_{2peak}) while consuming a higher (2.5 g/kg/day) and lower (1.0 g/kg/day) protein intake.[96] Whole-body protein balance was slightly negative on the 1.0 g/kg/day diet and positive on the 2.5 g/kg/day diet.[96] These results suggest that people performing moderate-intensity exercise do not require an increase in dietary protein intake or, at most, it is only marginally above 1.0 g/kg/day.[96] However, most athletes exercise at intensities of 65 to 85% of VO_{2peak}, where there may be a negative impact on protein homeostasis and NBAL.

For well-trained and elite endurance athletes, there does appear to be an increase in protein requirements.[6,41,65,163-165] One study used NBAL to determine the protein requirements in a group of endurance-trained males who were young (27 years; VO_{2peak} = 65 ml/kg/min) or middle-aged (52 years; VO_{2peak} = 55 ml/kg/min).[159] They found that a protein intake of 0.94 g/kg/day was required for NBAL, and whole-body protein synthesis (glycine tracer) increased with increasing protein intakes (0.61 > 0.92 > 1.21 g/kg/day). When accounting for interindividual variability by adding two standard deviations to the zero NBAL intercept, the estimated protein requirement for these males was about 1.28 g/kg/day.[165] We performed an NBAL experiment in six elite male endurance athletes (VO_{2peak} = 76.2 ml/kg/min; training >12 h/week) to determine what we considered to be close to the upper limit of protein requirements for endurance athletes.[65] We determined the safe protein intake for the elite athletes to be 1.6 g/kg/day, whereas the estimate for a sedentary control group (N = 6) was 0.86 g/kg/day, which was very close to Canadian and U.S. recommendations.[65] In a simulated Tour de France cycling study, Brouns and colleagues[163] found that well-trained cyclists (VO_{2peak} = 65.1 ml/kg/min) required protein intakes of 1.5 to 1.8 g/kg/min to maintain NBAL. In a final study, Friedman and Lemon[164] calculated that the protein requirement for five well-trained runners was about 1.49 g/kg/day, using NBAL. Another study performed in our laboratory found that both male (VO_{2peak} = 59 ml/kg/min) and female (VO_{2peak} = 55 ml/kg/min) endurance athletes had a negative NBAL while consuming a dietary protein intake that was close to the Canadian, U.S., and Australian recommended intake (males = 0.94 g/kg/day; females = 0.80 g/kg/day).[41] Finally, a recent study by Gaine and colleagues[97] found that the zero intercept for NBAL in well-trained athletes (VO_{2peak}

= 70.6 ml/kg/min) was 1.2 g/kg/day, which would equate to a +2 SD value of 1.5 to 1.7 g/kg/day.

To summarize the available data, it appears that low- and moderate-intensity endurance exercise does not result in an increase in dietary protein requirements. At the initiation of an endurance exercise program there may be a transient increase in dietary protein need, yet the body rapidly adapts to the increase in need. For the well-trained athlete (training 4 to 5 days per week for >45 min at >60% VO_{2max}), there appears to be an increase of about 20 to 25% in dietary protein requirements. In the elite athlete, the increase in dietary protein requirements may be as high as 1.6 g/kg/day (or nearly twice the recommended intake for sedentary persons). Given that the fitness of the Tour de France cyclists[163] and that of the athletes in our study[65] are respectively among the most demanding and highest reported, this protein intake is probably the top limit of requirement needed. Clearly, there may be some more demanding events; however, the day-to-day training is not likely to exceed that reported for the athletes in these studies.[65,163] In spite of these elevated requirements, there is no need for supplementation with a mixed diet of adequate energy intake, providing 15% of the energy from protein. For example, with an energy intake of about 3500 kcal/day (which is still modest), this would amount to about 125 g protein per day or ~1.6 to 1.9 g/kg/day.

One final point about protein requirements for endurance athletes is the possibility of a gender difference. We first found a gender difference in protein metabolism in 1990,[64] whereby males increased urinary urea excretion on an exercise compared to rest day, whereas females did not. We concluded that this was due to a glycogen-sparing effect seen in the women.[64] In the study where we found that the recommended intake for protein was inadequate for well-trained endurance athletes, we also found that the females had a less negative NBAL and their basal leucine oxidation was lower than that of the males.[41] In a subsequent study, we also found that females had a lower leucine oxidation than males both at rest and during exercise before and after a 38-day training program.[40] These findings may indicate that the dietary protein recommendations for endurance athletes (Table 7.4) may be 10 to 20% lower for females than for males.

7.7.2 PROTEIN REQUIREMENTS FOR RESISTANCE ATHLETES

In contrast to endurance exercise, resistance exercise results in muscle hypertrophy[98,166] rather than an increase in amino acid oxidation and mitochondrial biogenesis.[40,56] If, for example, there are no changes in efficiency of amino acid retention, there must, at some point, be a protein intake in excess of basal requirements to provide the amino acids required for anabolism. The extent of this increased need is again a function of the basal state of training, the duration, and the intensity of the training program.

An early study used NBAL and lean mass measurements to estimate the protein requirements during an isometric exercise training program.[167] They found that a daily protein intake of 1.0 g/kg (egg white and milk) was required to maintain positive NBAL and lean mass accretion in males performing isometric exercise for 75 min/day.[167] The equivalent protein intake from a mixed source would be about

TABLE 7.4
Estimated Protein Requirements for Athletes

Group	Protein Intake (g/kg/day)
Sedentary men and women	0.80–1.0
Elite male endurance athletes	1.6
Moderate-intensity endurance athletes[a]	1.2
Recreational endurance athletes[b]	0.80–1.0
Football, power sports	1.4–1.7
Resistance athletes (early training)	1.5–1.7
Resistance athletes (steady state)	1.0–1.2
Female athletes	~15% lower than male athletes

[a] Exercising approximately four to five times per week for 45 to 60 min.
[b] Exercising four to five times per week for 30 min at <55% VO_{2peak}.

Partially adapted from Tarnopolsky, M., *Nutrition*, 20, 662, 2004.

1.2 g/kg/day. Similar results were found in young males performing circuit training with both endurance and resistance exercise where even after a 40-day adaptation period protein requirements were ~1.4 g/kg/day.[168]

Modest-intensity resistance exercise programs can attenuate nitrogen loss at protein intakes close to the RDA for protein intake in older adults.[145] This phenomenon has also been observed in young men training with a protein intake of ~0.8 g/kg/day.[169] The ability to achieve NBAL (through increased nitrogen utilization efficiency) with modest resistance exercise may be indicative of accommodation and not adaptation because of the lower protein intake (~0.8 g/kg/day).[145] Campbell and colleagues[145] also found that whole-body protein synthesis in the group consuming protein at 0.8 g/kg/d was lower than for the group who consumed protein intakes of 1.6 g/kg/day. We performed an NBAL experiment in six well-trained bodybuilders (>2 years training experience) and six sedentary individuals and found that the protein requirement for the trained bodybuilders was only 12% greater than that for the sedentary controls.[65] We also found that the bodybuilders in this study were habitually consuming protein intakes of ~2.7 g/kg/day.[65] However, the error of the NBAL method was demonstrated in this study because if the positive NBAL on the high protein intake were extrapolated to net protein retention (assuming no change in breakdown), there would have been a 200 g/day increase in lean body mass each day. Some lay reports have used these data in support of the high protein intakes consumed by the bodybuilders. However, the magnitude of the positive NBAL cannot be directly extrapolated to an increase in lean mass for two reasons. First, there is an inherent error in the technique, which overestimates NBAL at high nitrogen intakes,[147] and second, protein synthesis and breakdown change in parallel.[13]

We followed up on our observations with two studies to more accurately characterize the impact of resistance training on dietary protein needs. In the first we reasoned that the protein requirements would be highest during the early adaptation period to unaccustomed training, since most of the myofibrillar protein accretion occurs within the first several months following the initiation of a resistance exercise program. Therefore, we exposed 12 young males to 2 months of a supervised resistance exercise program (6 days per week, 2 h/day, 70 to 85% 1RM) and measured NBAL, muscle mass, muscle protein, and strength before and after a 1-month period, where they were randomized to receive protein at 1.44 and 2.6 g/kg/day. We calculated the estimated protein requirement during this period to be ~1.65 g/kg/day.[98] Strength, muscle protein, and lean mass gains following training were not different between the two protein intakes.[98] We went on to use the conceptual framework put forth by Young et al.[147] and studied the protein kinetic response to graded protein intakes in young males who were performing weight training and high-intensity sprinting/power activities (e.g., football and rugby).[53] In this study we randomly allocated six sedentary males and seven athletes to receive a diet supplying protein at each of three levels (recommended intake, ~0.86 g/kg/day; moderate, ~1.4 g/kg/day; and high, ~2.4 g/kg/day). We measured NBAL, whole-body protein synthesis, leucine oxidation, and protein breakdown.[53] We calculated the estimated safe protein intake to be 0.89 g/kg/day for the sedentary group and 1.76 g/kg/day for the athletes.[53] The whole-body protein synthesis was greater for the athletes than for the sedentary controls at all protein intakes. Furthermore, whole-body protein synthesis was lower at 0.86 g/kg/day than at 1.4 and 2.8 g/kg/day, and appeared to plateau at around 1.4 g/kg/day for the athletes. At protein intakes of 2.8 g/kg/day, leucine oxidation increased nearly twofold, which provided evidence that protein intake above the requirement is merely oxidized for energy.[53]

7.8 POTENTIAL SIDE EFFECTS OF EXCESSIVE PROTEIN INTAKE

In general, there are probably few side effects arising from daily protein intakes under 2.0 g/kg/day in healthy people. Perhaps the most definite effect of a very high protein diet would be the cost of protein supplements or protein-rich foods. Even with dietary protein, the ultimate cost to produce a kilogram of beef is more than an isoenergetic amount of wheat. Furthermore, most meat products also contain significant amounts of fat, which, if taken at a high enough level, may render the diet atherogenic. Again, these are not likely to be a problem with protein intakes below 2.0 g/kg/day.

Although it is probable that most people can safely maintain very high protein intakes for long periods, there are several caveats that must be considered. First, a high-protein diet can increase urinary calcium excretion (from the sulfur-containing amino acids), which may be a concern for the female athlete with a low energy intake and amenorrhea. Second, high protein intakes in conjunction with preexisting renal disease may accelerate the progression of the disease.[149] Third, rodents fed very high protein intakes have been found to exhibit morphological changes in the liver mitochondria, which could be pathological.[170] Finally, some problems could theoretically occur if the protein is taken as an amino acid supplement. One possible problem relates to contamination of purified amino acids, as in the case of L-tryptophan supplements that were manufactured in Japan and caused a life-threatening disorder called eosinophilia-myalgia syndrome.[171,172] Some sources state that this occurred as a result of a high-performance liquid chromatography purified contaminant present from a bacterial processing method.[173] In addition to the expense involved, large doses of purified amino acids could potentially be carcinogenic and mutagenic. Such warnings are noted on the Materials Safety Data Sheet labels of purified chemical-grade laboratory amino acids, although these problems have not been substantiated in humans. Even if purified amino acids are safe, they are expensive and the efficacy is equivocal;[174,175] however, recent work does suggest that the addition of leucine to post-exercise supplements may confer metabolic advantages,[105] which could translate into enhanced performance. Although essential amino acids appear to be the most potent in stimulating post-exercise protein synthesis,[54] this response does not appear to be greater than the consumption of high biological value proteins.[108] Furthermore, the consumption of a drink containing exclusively essential amino acids may exclude amino acids that could enhance other aspects of the adaptation to exercise (such as proline for connective tissue adaptations) or arginine and glycine (for creatine synthesis).

7.9 SUMMARY

Protein is an important component of the diet and is involved in almost every structural and functional component of the human body. In general, endurance exercise may impact on the need for dietary protein by increasing the oxidation of amino acids. Resistance exercise may also have an impact through the need for amino acids to support muscle hypertrophy. At the onset of an endurance exercise program there is a negative effect on NBAL, yet with time the body adapts to the stress and NBAL and leucine oxidation are attenuated. After endurance exercise training, the amount of amino acid oxidized at the same absolute exercise intensity is reduced, yet the capacity of the body to oxidize amino acids is increased. However, only in the elite athlete (who is training very hard every day) is there a significant impact upon dietary protein requirements, with a maximal requirement of ~1.6 g/kg/day. For the resistance-trained athlete, there also appears to be a homeostatic adaptation to the stress of the exercise, where very well-trained athletes require only marginally more protein than sedentary persons, and those in the early stages of very intensive resistance exercise may require up to 1.7 g/kg/day. A dietary protein intake that represents 15% of the total energy intake with an energy-sufficient diet should cover the requirements for nearly all strength and endurance athletes. Given the increase in energy intake by most athletes, there is no need to use protein supplements to attain these levels. However, athletes on a low-energy diet or a low-CHO diet could have an inadequate protein intake to cover their needs. The timing of nutrient delivery appears to be important for resistance athletes, where an immediate post-exercise (or pre-/during exercise) intake of CHO and protein will lead to a more positive protein NBAL, probably by reducing protein breakdown (CHO) and stimulating synthesis (protein).

REFERENCES

1. Harris, H.A., Nutrition and physical performance: the diet of Greek athletes, *Proc Nutr Soc*, 25, 87, 1966.
2. von Liebig, J., *Animal Chemistry or Organic Chemistry in its Applications to Physiology*, London: Taylor & Watson, 1842.
3. Cathcart, E.P., Influence of muscle work on protein metabolism, *Physiol Rev*, 5, 225, 1925.
4. Lemon, P.W., Effects of exercise on dietary protein requirements, *Int J Sport Nutr*, 8, 426, 1998.
5. Rennie, M.J. and Tipton, K.D., Protein and amino acid metabolism during and after exercise and the effects of nutrition, *Annu Rev Nutr*, 20, 457, 2000.
6. Tarnopolsky, M., Protein requirements for endurance athletes, *Nutrition*, 20, 662, 2004.
7. Pellett, P.L., Protein requirements in humans, *Am J Clin Nutr*, 51, 723, 1990.
8. Fischer, C.P., Plomgaard, P., Hansen, A.K., Pilegaard, H., Saltin, B., and Pedersen, B.K., Endurance training reduces the contraction-induced interleukin-6 mRNA expression in human skeletal muscle, *Am J Physiol Endocrinol Metab*, 287, E1189, 2004.
9. Tipton, K.D., Ferrando, A.A., Williams, B.D., and Wolfe, R.R., Muscle protein metabolism in female swimmers after a combination of resistance and endurance exercise, *J Appl Physiol*, 81, 2034, 1996.
10. Bolster, D.R., Pikosky, M.A., Gaine, P.C. et al., Dietary protein intake impacts human skeletal muscle protein fractional synthetic rates after endurance exercise, *Am J Physiol Endocrinol Metab*, 289, E678, 2005.
11. Chesley, A., MacDougall, J.D., Tarnopolsky, M.A., Atkinson, S.A., and Smith, K., Changes in human muscle protein synthesis after resistance exercise, *J Appl Physiol*, 73, 1383, 1992.
12. Biolo, G., Maggi, S.P., Williams, B.D., Tipton, K.D., and Wolfe, R.R., Increased rates of muscle protein turnover and amino acid transport after resistance exercise in humans, *Am J Physiol*, 268, E514, 1995.
13. Phillips, S.M., Tipton, K.D., Aarsland, A., Wolf, S.E., and Wolfe, R.R., Mixed muscle protein synthesis and breakdown after resistance exercise in humans, *Am J Physiol*, 273, E99, 1997.
14. Miller, B.F., Olesen, J.L., Hansen, M. et al., Coordinated collagen and muscle protein synthesis in human patella tendon and quadriceps muscle after exercise, *J Physiol*, 567, 1021, 2005.
15. Hildebrandt, A.L., Pilegaard, H., and Neufer, P.D., Differential transcriptional activation of select metabolic genes in response to variations in exercise intensity and duration, *Am J Physiol Endocrinol Metab*, 285, E1021, 2003.
16. Mahoney, D.J., Parise, G., Melov, S., Safdar, A., and Tarnopolsky, M.A., Analysis of global mRNA expression in human skeletal muscle during recovery from endurance exercise, *FASEB J*, 19, 1498, 2005.
17. Mahoney, D.J. and Tarnopolsky, M.A., Understanding skeletal muscle adaptation to exercise training in humans: contributions from microarray studies, *Phys Med Rehabil Clin N Am*, 16, 859, 2005.
18. Frosig, C., Jorgensen, S.B., Hardie, D.G., Richter, E.A., and Wojtaszewski, J.F., 5'-AMP-activated protein kinase activity and protein expression are regulated by endurance training in human skeletal muscle, *Am J Physiol Endocrinol Metab*, 286, E411, 2004.

19. Atherton, P.J., Babraj, J., Smith, K., Singh, J., Rennie, M.J., and Wackerhage, H., Selective activation of AMPK-PGC-1alpha or PKB-TSC2-mTOR signaling can explain specific adaptive responses to endurance or resistance training-like electrical muscle stimulation, *FASEB J*, 19, 786, 2005.

20. Kim, P.L., Staron, R.S., and Phillips, S.M., Fasted-state skeletal muscle protein synthesis after resistance exercise is altered with training, *J Physiol*, 568, 283, 2005.

21. Timmons, J.A., Larsson, O., Jansson, E. et al., Human muscle gene expression responses to endurance training provide a novel perspective on Duchenne muscular dystrophy, *FASEB J*, 19, 750, 2005.

22. Coffey, V.G., Zhong, Z., Shield, A. et al., Early signaling responses to divergent exercise stimuli in skeletal muscle from well-trained humans, *FASEB J*, 20, 190, 2006.

23. Pilegaard, H., Osada, T., Andersen, L.T., Helge, J.W., Saltin, B., and Neufer, P.D., Substrate availability and transcriptional regulation of metabolic genes in human skeletal muscle during recovery from exercise, *Metabolism*, 54, 1048, 2005.

24. Keller, C., Steensberg, A., Pilegaard, H. et al., Transcriptional activation of the IL-6 gene in human contracting skeletal muscle: influence of muscle glycogen content, *FASEB J*, 15, 2748, 2001.

25. Bohe, J., Low, A., Wolfe, R.R., and Rennie, M.J., Human muscle protein synthesis is modulated by extracellular, not intramuscular amino acid availability: a dose-response study, *J Physiol*, 552, 315, 2003.

26. Pilegaard, H., Saltin, B., and Neufer, P.D., Effect of short-term fasting and refeeding on transcriptional regulation of metabolic genes in human skeletal muscle, *Diabetes*, 52, 657, 2003.

27. Febbraio, M.A., Hiscock, N., Sacchetti, M., Fischer, C.P., and Pedersen, B.K., Interleukin-6 is a novel factor mediating glucose homeostasis during skeletal muscle contraction, *Diabetes*, 53, 1643, 2004.

28. Cluberton, L.J., McGee, S.L., Murphy, R.M., and Hargreaves, M., Effect of carbohydrate ingestion on exercise-induced alterations in metabolic gene expression, *J Appl Physiol*, 99, 1359, 2005.

29. Balage, M., Sinaud, S., Prod'homme, M. et al., Amino acids and insulin are both required to regulate assembly of the eIF4E·eIF4G complex in rat skeletal muscle, *Am J Physiol Endocrinol Metab*, 281, E565, 2001.

30. Carroll, C.C., Fluckey, J.D., Williams, R.H., Sullivan, D.H., and Trappe, T.A., Human soleus and vastus lateralis muscle protein metabolism with an amino acid infusion, *Am J Physiol Endocrinol Metab*, 288, E479, 2005.

31. Mitch, W.E. and Goldberg, A.L., Mechanisms of muscle wasting. *N Engl J Med*, 335, 1897, 1996.

32. Lowell, B.B., Ruderman, N.B., and Goodman, M.N., Regulation of myofibrillar protein degradation in rat skeletal muscle during brief and prolonged starvation, *Metabolism*, 35, 1121, 1986.

33. Tidball, J.G., Inflammatory cell response to acute muscle injury, *Med Sci Sports Exerc*, 27, 1022, 1995.

34. Belcastro, A.N., Skeletal muscle calcium-activated neutral protease (calpain) with exercise, *J Appl Physiol*, 74, 1381, 1993.

35. Kameyama, T. and Etlinger, J.D., Calcium-dependent regulation of protein synthesis and degradation in muscle, *Nature*, 279, 344, 1979.

36. Zeman, R.J., Kameyama, T., Matsumoto, K., Bernstein, P., and Etlinger, J.D., Regulation of protein degradation in muscle by calcium. Evidence for enhanced nonlysosomal proteolysis associated with elevated cytosolic calcium, *J Biol Chem*, 260, 13619, 1985.

37. Medina, R., Wing, S.S., and Goldberg, A.L., Increase in levels of polyubiquitin and proteasome mRNA in skeletal muscle during starvation and denervation atrophy, *Biochem J*, 307 (Pt 3), 631, 1995.

38. Du, J., Wang, X., Miereles, C. et al., Activation of caspase-3 is an initial step triggering accelerated muscle proteolysis in catabolic conditions, *J Clin Invest*, 113, 115, 2004.

39. Smith, K. and Rennie, M.J., The measurement of tissue protein turnover, *Baillieres Clin Endocrinol Metab*, 10, 469, 1996.

40. McKenzie, S., Phillips, S.M., Carter, S.L., Lowther, S., Gibala, M.J., and Tarnopolsky, M.A., Endurance exercise training attenuates leucine oxidation and BCOAD activation during exercise in humans, *Am J Physiol Endocrinol Metab*, 278, E580, 2000.

41. Phillips, S.M., Atkinson, S.A., Tarnopolsky, M.A., and MacDougall, J.D., Gender differences in leucine kinetics and nitrogen balance in endurance athletes, *J Appl Physiol*, 75, 2134, 1993.

42. Lamont, L.S., McCullough, A.J., and Kalhan, S.C., Comparison of leucine kinetics in endurance-trained and sedentary humans, *J Appl Physiol*, 86, 320, 1999.

43. Boyer, B. and Odessey, R., Kinetic characterization of branched chain ketoacid dehydrogenase, *Arch Biochem Biophys*, 285, 1, 1991.

44. Boyer, B. and Odessey, R., Quantitative control analysis of branched-chain 2-oxo acid dehydrogenase complex activity by feedback inhibition, *Biochem J*, 271, 523, 1990.

45. Wolfe, R.R., Wolfe, M.H., Nadel, E.R., and Shaw, J.H., Isotopic determination of amino acid-urea interactions in exercise in humans, *J Appl Physiol*, 56, 221, 1984.

46. MacLean, D.A., Spriet, L.L., Hultman, E., and Graham, T.E., Plasma and muscle amino acid and ammonia responses during prolonged exercise in humans, *J Appl Physiol*, 70, 2095, 1991.

47. Tarnopolsky, M.A., Parise, G., Gibala, M.J., Graham, T.E., and Rush, J.W., Myoadenylate deaminase deficiency does not affect muscle anaplerosis during exhaustive exercise in humans, *J Physiol*, 533, 881, 2001.

48. Wagenmakers, A.J., Beckers, E.J., Brouns, F. et al., Carbohydrate supplementation, glycogen depletion, and amino acid metabolism during exercise, *Am J Physiol*, 260, E883, 1991.

49. Wagenmakers, A.J., Brookes, J.H., Coakley, J.H., Reilly, T., and Edwards, R.H., Exercise-induced activation of the branched-chain 2-oxo acid dehydrogenase in human muscle, *Eur J Appl Physiol Occup Physiol*, 59, 159, 1989.

50. Kasperek, G.J. and Snider, R.D., Effect of exercise intensity and starvation on activation of branched-chain keto acid dehydrogenase by exercise, *Am J Physiol*, 252, E33, 1987.

51. Kasperek, G.J., Dohm, G.L., and Snider, R.D., Activation of branched-chain keto acid dehydrogenase by exercise, *Am J Physiol*, 248, R166, 1985.

52. Bowtell, J.L., Leese, G.P., Smith, K. et al., Effect of oral glucose on leucine turnover in human subjects at rest and during exercise at two levels of dietary protein, *J Physiol*, 525 (Pt 1), 271, 2000.

53. Tarnopolsky, M.A., Atkinson, S.A., MacDougall, J.D., Chesley, A., Phillips, S., and Schwarcz, H.P., Evaluation of protein requirements for trained strength athletes, *J Appl Physiol*, 73, 1986, 1992.

54. Tipton, K.D., Ferrando, A.A., Phillips, S.M., Doyle, D., Jr., and Wolfe, R.R., Postexercise net protein synthesis in human muscle from orally administered amino acids, *Am J Physiol*, 276, E628, 1999.

55. Riddell, M.C., Partington, S.L., Stupka, N., Armstrong, D., Rennie, C., and Tarnopolsky, M.A., Substrate utilization during exercise performed with and without glucose ingestion in female and male endurance trained athletes, *Int J Sport Nutr Exerc Metab*, 13, 407, 2003.
56. Tarnopolsky, M.A., Atkinson, S.A., MacDougall, J.D., Senor, B.B., Lemon, P.W., and Schwarcz, H., Whole body leucine metabolism during and after resistance exercise in fed humans, *Med Sci Sports Exerc*, 23, 326, 1991.
57. Ferrando, A.A., Tipton, K.D., Doyle, D., Phillips, S.M., Cortiella, J., and Wolfe, R.R., Testosterone injection stimulates net protein synthesis but not tissue amino acid transport, *Am J Physiol*, 275, E864, 1998.
58. Balagopal, P., Ljungqvist, O., and Nair, K.S., Skeletal muscle myosin heavy-chain synthesis rate in healthy humans, *Am J Physiol*, 272, E45, 1997.
59. Moore, D.R., Phillips, S.M., Babraj, J.A., Smith, K., and Rennie, M.J., Myofibrillar and collagen protein synthesis in human skeletal muscle in young men after maximal shortening and lengthening contractions, *Am J Physiol Endocrinol Metab*, 288, E1153, 2005.
60. Young, V.R. and Munro, H.N., Ntau-methylhistidine (3-methylhistidine) and muscle protein turnover: an overview, *Fed Proc*, 37, 2291, 1978.
61. Rathmacher, J.A., Flakoll, P.J., and Nissen, S.L., A compartmental model of 3-methylhistidine metabolism in humans, *Am J Physiol*, 269, E193, 1995.
62. Phillips, S.M., Parise, G., Roy, B.D., Tipton, K.D., Wolfe, R.R., and Tamopolsky, M.A., Resistance-training-induced adaptations in skeletal muscle protein turnover in the fed state, *Can J Physiol Pharmacol*, 80, 1045, 2002.
63. Gibala, M.J., Tarnopolsky, M.A., and Graham, T.E., Tricarboxylic acid cycle intermediates in human muscle at rest and during prolonged cycling, *Am J Physiol*, 272, E239, 1997.
64. Tarnopolsky, L.J., MacDougall, J.D., Atkinson, S.A., Tarnopolsky, M.A., and Sutton, J.R., Gender differences in substrate for endurance exercise, *J Appl Physiol*, 68, 302, 1990.
65. Tarnopolsky, M.A., MacDougall, J.D., and Atkinson, S.A., Influence of protein intake and training status on nitrogen balance and lean body mass, *J Appl Physiol*, 64, 187, 1988.
66. El-Khoury, A.E., Forslund, A., Olsson, R. et al., Moderate exercise at energy balance does not affect 24-h leucine oxidation or nitrogen retention in healthy men, *Am J Physiol*, 273, E394, 1997.
67. Lamont, L.S., McCullough, A.J., and Kalhan, S.C., Gender differences in leucine, but not lysine, kinetics, *J Appl Physiol*, 91, 357, 2001.
68. Bowtell, J.L., Leese, G.P., Smith, K. et al., Modulation of whole body protein metabolism, during and after exercise, by variation of dietary protein, *J Appl Physiol*, 85, 1744, 1998.
69. Lamont, L.S., Patel, D.G., and Kalhan, S.C., Leucine kinetics in endurance-trained humans, *J Appl Physiol*, 69, 1, 1990.
70. Lemon, P.W., Nagle, F.J., Mullin, J.P., and Benevenga, N.J., *In vivo* leucine oxidation at rest and during two intensities of exercise, *J Appl Physiol*, 53, 947, 1982.
71. Haralambie, G. and Berg, A., Serum urea and amino nitrogen changes with exercise duration, *Eur J Appl Physiol Occup Physiol*, 36, 39, 1976.
72. Fielding, R.A., Meredith, C.N., O'Reilly, K.P., Frontera, W.R., Cannon, J.G., and Evans, W.J., Enhanced protein breakdown after eccentric exercise in young and older men, *J Appl Physiol*, 71, 674, 1991.

73. Gontzea, I., Sutzescu, P., and Dumitrache, S., The influence of adaptation to physical effort on nitrogen balance in man, *Nutr Reports Int*, 22, 231, 1975.
74. Tarnopolsky, M.A., Atkinson, S.A., Phillips, S.M., and MacDougall, J.D., Carbohydrate loading and metabolism during exercise in men and women, *J Appl Physiol*, 78, 1360, 1995.
75. Tarnopolsky, M.A., Bosman, M., MacDonald, J.R., Vandeputte, D., Martin, J., and Roy, B.D., Postexercise protein-carbohydrate and carbohydrate supplements increase muscle glycogen in men and women, *J Appl Physiol*, 83, 1877, 1997.
76. Nair, K.S., Halliday, D., and Griggs, R.C., Leucine incorporation into mixed skeletal muscle protein in humans, *Am J Physiol*, 254, E208, 1988.
77. MacDougall, J.D., Gibala, M.J., Tarnopolsky, M.A., MacDonald, J.R., Interisano, S.A., and Yarasheski, K.E., The time course for elevated muscle protein synthesis following heavy resistance exercise, *Can J Appl Physiol*, 20, 480, 1995.
78. Yarasheski, K.E., Zachwieja, J.J., and Bier, D.M., Acute effects of resistance exercise on muscle protein synthesis rate in young and elderly men and women, *Am J Physiol*, 265, E210, 1993.
79. Welle, S., Thornton, C., Jozefowicz, R., and Statt, M., Myofibrillar protein synthesis in young and old men, *Am J Physiol*, 264, E693, 1993.
80. Butterfield, G.E. and Calloway, D.H., Physical activity improves protein utilization in young men, *Br J Nutr*, 51, 171, 1984.
81. Chiang, A.N. and Huang, P.C., Excess energy and nitrogen balance at protein intakes above the requirement level in young men, *Am J Clin Nutr*, 48, 1015, 1988.
82. Roy, B.D., Luttmer, K., Bosman, M.J., and Tarnopolsky, M.A., The influence of postexercise macronutrient intake on energy balance and protein metabolism in active females participating in endurance training, *Int J Sport Nutr Exerc Metab*, 12, 172, 2002.
83. Saris, W.H., van Erp-Baart, M.A., Brouns, F., Westerterp, K.R., and Ten, H.F., Study on food intake and energy expenditure during extreme sustained exercise: the Tour de France, *Int J Sports Med*, 10 (Suppl 1), S26, 1989.
84. Nelson, M.E., Fisher, E.C., Catsos, P.D., Meredith, C.N., Turksoy, R.N., and Evans, W.J., Diet and bone status in amenorrheic runners, *Am J Clin Nutr*, 43, 910, 1986.
85. Marcus, R., Cann, C., Madvig, P. et al., Menstrual function and bone mass in elite women distance runners. Endocrine and metabolic features, *Ann Intern Med*, 102, 158, 1985.
86. Deuster, P.A., Kyle, S.B., Moser, P.B., Vigersky, R.A., Singh, A., and Schoomaker, E.B., Nutritional survey of highly trained women runners, *Am J Clin Nutr*, 44, 954, 1986.
87. Deuster, P.A., Kyle, S.B., Moser, P.B., Vigersky, R.A., Singh, A., and Schoomaker, E.B., Nutritional intakes and status of highly trained amenorrheic and eumenorrheic women runners, *Fertil Steril*, 46, 636, 1986.
88. Drinkwater, B.L., Nilson, K., Chestnut, C.H., Bremner, W.J., Shainholtz, S., and Southworth, M.B., Bone mineral content of amenorrhic and eumenorrheic athletes, *N Engl J Med*, 311, 277, 1984.
89. Nattiv, A., Agostini, R., Drinkwater, B., and Yeager, K.K., The female athlete triad. The inter-relatedness of disordered eating, amenorrhea, and osteoporosis, *Clin Sports Med*, 13, 405, 1994.
90. Elwyn, D.H., Gump, F.E., Munro, H.N., Iles, M., and Kinney, J.M., Changes in nitrogen balance of depleted patients with increasing infusions of glucose, *Am J Clin Nutr*, 32, 1597, 1979.

91. Lemon, P.W. and Mullin, J.P., Effect of initial muscle glycogen levels on protein catabolism during exercise, *J Appl Physiol*, 48, 624, 1980.
92. Welle, S., Matthews, D.E., Campbell, R.G., and Nair, K.S., Stimulation of protein turnover by carbohydrate overfeeding in men, *Am J Physiol*, 257, E413, 1989.
93. Krempf, M., Hoerr, R.A., Pelletier, V.A., Marks, L.M., Gleason, R., and Young, V.R., An isotopic study of the effect of dietary carbohydrate on the metabolic fate of dietary leucine and phenylalanine, *Am J Clin Nutr*, 57, 161, 1993.
94. van Hammont, D., Harvey, C.R., Massicotte, D., Frew, R., Peronnet, F., and Rehrer, N.J., Reduction in muscle glycogen and protein utilization with glucose feeding during exercise, *Int J Sport Nutr Exerc Metab*, 14, 350, 2005.
95. Roy, B.D., Tarnopolsky, M.A., MacDougall, J.D., Fowles, J., and Yarasheski, K.E., Effect of glucose supplement timing on protein metabolism after resistance training, *J Appl Physiol*, 82, 1882, 1997.
96. Forslund, A.H., Hambraeus, L., Olsson, R.M., El-Khoury, A.E., Yu, Y.M., and Young, V.R., The 24-h whole body leucine and urea kinetics at normal and high protein intakes with exercise in healthy adults, *Am J Physiol*, 275, E310, 1998.
97. Gaine, P.C., Pikosky, M.A., Martin, W.F., Bolster, D.R., Maresh, C.M., and Rodriguez, N.R., Level of dietary protein impacts whole body protein turnover in trained males at rest, *Metabolism*, 55, 501, 2006.
98. Lemon, P.W., Tarnopolsky, M.A., MacDougall, J.D., and Atkinson, S.A., Protein requirements and muscle mass/strength changes during intensive training in novice bodybuilders, *J Appl Physiol*, 73, 767, 1992.
99. Biolo, G., Tipton, K.D., Klein, S., and Wolfe, R.R., An abundant supply of amino acids enhances the metabolic effect of exercise on muscle protein, *Am J Physiol*, 273, E122, 1997.
100. Zorzano, A., Balon, T.W., Goodman, M.N., and Ruderman, N.B., Additive effects of prior exercise and insulin on glucose and AIB uptake by rat muscle, *Am J Physiol*, 251, E21, 1986.
101. Garlick, P.J. and Grant, I., Amino acid infusion increases the sensitivity of muscle protein synthesis *in vivo* to insulin. Effect of branched-chain amino acids, *Biochem J*, 254, 579, 1988.
102. Castellino, P., Luzi, L., Simonson, D.C., Haymond, M., and DeFronzo, R.A., Effect of insulin and plasma amino acid concentrations on leucine metabolism in man. Role of substrate availability on estimates of whole body protein synthesis, *J Clin Invest*, 80, 1784, 1987.
103. Tessari, P., Inchiostro, S., Biolo, G. et al., Differential effects of hyperinsulinemia and hyperaminoacidemia on leucine-carbon metabolism *in vivo*. Evidence for distinct mechanisms in regulation of net amino acid deposition, *J Clin Invest*, 79, 1062, 1987.
104. Svanberg, E., Zachrisson, H., Ohlsson, C., Iresjo, B.M., and Lundholm, K.G., Role of insulin and IGF-I in activation of muscle protein synthesis after oral feeding, *Am J Physiol*, 270, E614, 1996.
105. Koopman, R., Wagenmakers, A.J., Manders, R.J. et al., Combined ingestion of protein and free leucine with carbohydrate increases postexercise muscle protein synthesis *in vivo* in male subjects, *Am J Physiol Endocrinol Metab*, 288, E645, 2005.
106. Borsheim, E., Tipton, K.D., Wolf, S.E., and Wolfe, R.R., Essential amino acids and muscle protein recovery from resistance exercise, *Am J Physiol Endocrinol Metab*, 283, E648, 2002.
107. Borsheim, E., Cree, M.G., Tipton, K.D., Elliott, T.A., Aarsland, A., and Wolfe, R.R., Effect of carbohydrate intake on net muscle protein synthesis during recovery from resistance exercise, *J Appl Physiol*, 96, 674, 2004.

108. Tipton, K.D., Elliott, T.A., Cree, M.G., Wolf, S.E., Sanford, A.P., and Wolfe, R.R., Ingestion of casein and whey proteins result in muscle anabolism after resistance exercise, *Med Sci Sports Exerc*, 36, 2073, 2004.

109. Miller, S.L., Tipton, K.D., Chinkes, D.L., Wolf, S.E., and Wolfe, R.R., Independent and combined effects of amino acids and glucose after resistance exercise, *Med Sci Sports Exerc*, 35, 449, 2003.

110. Borsheim, E., Aarsland, A., and Wolfe, R.R., Effect of an amino acid, protein, and carbohydrate mixture on net muscle protein balance after resistance exercise, *Int J Sport Nutr Exerc Metab*, 14, 255, 2004.

111. Tipton, K.D., Rasmussen, B.B., Miller, S.L. et al., Timing of amino acid-carbohydrate ingestion alters anabolic response of muscle to resistance exercise, *Am J Physiol Endocrinol Metab*, 281, E197, 2001.

112. Elliot, T.A., Cree, M.G., Sanford, A.P., Wolfe, R.R., and Tipton, K.D., Milk ingestion stimulates net muscle protein synthesis following resistance exercise, *Med Sci Sports Exerc*, 38, 667, 2006.

113. Zawadzki, K.M., Yaspelkis, B.B., III, and Ivy, J.L., Carbohydrate-protein complex increases the rate of muscle glycogen storage after exercise, *J Appl Physiol*, 72, 1854, 1992.

114. Ivy, J.L., Katz, A.L., Cutler, C.L., Sherman, W.M., and Coyle, E.F., Muscle glycogen synthesis after exercise: effect of time of carbohydrate ingestion, *J Appl Physiol*, 64, 1480, 1988.

115. Berardi, J.M., Price, T.B., Noreen, E.E., and Lemon, P.W., Postexercise muscle glycogen recovery enhanced with a carbohydrate-protein supplement, *Med Sci Sports Exerc*, 38, 1106, 2006.

116. Jentjens, R.L., Van Loon, L.J., Mann, C.H., Wagenmakers, A.J., and Jeukendrup, A.E., Addition of protein and amino acids to carbohydrates does not enhance postexercise muscle glycogen synthesis, *J Appl Physiol*, 91, 839, 2001.

117. van, H.G., Shirreffs, S.M., and Calbet, J.A., Muscle glycogen resynthesis during recovery from cycle exercise: no effect of additional protein ingestion, *J Appl Physiol*, 88, 1631, 2000.

118. Roy, B.D. and Tarnopolsky, M.A., Influence of differing macronutrient intakes on muscle glycogen resynthesis after resistance exercise, *J Appl Physiol*, 84, 890, 1998.

119. Roy, B.D., Fowles, J.R., Hill, R., and Tarnopolsky, M.A., Macronutrient intake and whole body protein metabolism following resistance exercise, *Med Sci Sports Exerc*, 32, 1412, 2000.

120. Burke, L.M., Collier, G.R., Davis, P.G., Fricker, P.A., Sanigorski, A.J., and Hargreaves, M., Muscle glycogen storage after prolonged exercise: effect of the frequency of carbohydrate feedings, *Am J Clin Nutr*, 64, 115, 1996.

121. Burke, L.M., Collier, G.R., Beasley, S.K. et al., Effect of coingestion of fat and protein with carbohydrate feedings on muscle glycogen storage, *J Appl Physiol*, 78, 2187, 1995.

122. Haff, G.G., Stone, M.H., Warren, B.J. et al., The effect of carbohydrate supplementation on multiple sessions and bouts of resistance exercise, *J Strength Cond Res*, 13, 111, 1999.

123. Tipton, K.D., Borsheim, E., Wolf, S.E., Sanford, A.P., and Wolfe, R.R., Acute response of net muscle protein balance reflects 24-h balance after exercise and amino acid ingestion, *Am J Physiol Endocrinol Metab*, 284, E76, 2003.

124. Bhasin, S., Storer, T.W., Berman, N. et al., Testosterone replacement increases fat-free mass and muscle size in hypogonadal men, *J Clin Endocrinol Metab*, 82, 407, 1997.

125. Florini, J.R., Hormonal control of muscle growth, *Muscle Nerve*, 10, 577, 1987.
126. Griggs, R.C., Kingston, W., Jozefowicz, R.F., Herr, B.E., Forbes, G., and Halliday, D., Effect of testosterone on muscle mass and muscle protein synthesis, *J Appl Physiol*, 66, 498, 1989.
127. Bhasin, S., Storer, T.W., Berman, N. et al., The effects of supraphysiologic doses of testosterone on muscle size and strength in normal men, *N Engl J Med*, 335, 1, 1996.
128. Volek, J.S., Kraemer, W.J., Bush, J.A., Incledon, T., and Boetes, M., Testosterone and cortisol in relationship to dietary nutrients and resistance exercise, *J Appl Physiol*, 82, 49, 1997.
129. Kraemer, W.J., Marchitelli, L., Gordon, S.E. et al., Hormonal and growth factor responses to heavy resistance exercise protocols, *J Appl Physiol*, 69, 1442, 1990.
130. Biolo, G., Williams, B.D., Fleming, R.Y., and Wolfe, R.R., Insulin action on muscle protein kinetics and amino acid transport during recovery after resistance exercise, *Diabetes*, 48, 949, 1999.
131. Bennet, W.M., Connacher, A.A., Scrimgeour, C.M., Smith, K., and Rennie, M.J., Increase in anterior tibialis muscle protein synthesis in healthy man during mixed amino acid infusion: studies of incorporation of [1-13C]leucine, *Clin Sci* (Lond), 76, 447, 1989.
132. Moller-Loswick, A.C., Zachrisson, H., Hyltander, A., Korner, U., Matthews, D.E., and Lundholm, K., Insulin selectively attenuates breakdown of nonmyofibrillar proteins in peripheral tissues of normal men, *Am J Physiol*, 266, E645, 1994.
133. Newman, E., Heslin, M.J., Wolf, R.F., Pisters, P.W., and Brennan, M.F., The effect of systemic hyperinsulinemia with concomitant amino acid infusion on skeletal muscle protein turnover in the human forearm, *Metabolism*, 43, 70, 1994.
134. McNurlan, M.A., Essen, P., Thorell, A. et al., Response of protein synthesis in human skeletal muscle to insulin: an investigation with L-[2H5]phenylalanine, *Am J Physiol*, 267, E102, 1994.
135. Joint position statement: nutrition and athletic performance. American College of Sports Medicine, American Dietetic Association, and Dietitians of Canada, *Med Sci Sports Exerc*, 32, 2130, 2000.
136. Coyle, E.F., Physiological determinants of endurance exercise performance, *J Sci Med Sport*, 2, 181, 1999.
137. Berneis, K., Ninnis, R., Haussinger, D., and Keller, U., Effects of hyper- and hypoosmolality on whole body protein and glucose kinetics in humans, *Am J Physiol*, 276, E188, 1999.
138. Horton, T.J., Pagliassotti, M.J., Hobbs, K., and Hill, J.O., Fuel metabolism in men and women during and after long-duration exercise, *J Appl Physiol*, 85, 1823, 1998.
139. Friedlander, A.L., Casazza, G.A., Horning, M.A. et al., Training-induced alterations of carbohydrate metabolism in women: women respond differently from men, *J Appl Physiol*, 85, 1175, 1998.
140. Melanson, E.L., Sharp, T.A., Seagle, H.M. et al., Effect of exercise intensity on 24-h energy expenditure and nutrient oxidation, *J Appl Physiol*, 92, 1045, 2002.
141. Lamont, L.S., McCullough, A.J., and Kalhan, S.C., Gender differences in the regulation of amino acid metabolism, *J Appl Physiol*, 95, 1259, 2003.
142. Hamadeh, M.J., Devries, M.C., and Tarnopolsky, M.A., Estrogen supplementation reduces whole body leucine and carbohydrate oxidation and increases lipid oxidation in men during endurance exercise, *J Clin Endocrinol Metab*, 90, 3592, 2005.
143. Evans, W., Fisher, E.C., Hoerr, R.A., and Young, V.R., Protein metabolism and endurance exercise, *Phys Sports Med*, 11, 63, 1983.

144. Gaine, P.C., Viesselman, C.T., Pikosky, M.A. et al., Aerobic exercise training decreases leucine oxidation at rest in healthy adults, *J Nutr*, 135, 1088, 2005.

145. Campbell, W.W., Crim, M.C., Young, V.R., Joseph, L.J., and Evans, W.J., Effects of resistance training and dietary protein intake on protein metabolism in older adults, *Am J Physiol*, 268, E1143, 1995.

146. Elwyn, D.H., New concepts in nitrogen balance, *Can J Gastroenterol*, 4, 9A, 1990.

147. Young, V.R., Bier, D.M., and Pellett, P.L., A theoretical basis for increasing current estimates of the amino acid requirements in adult man, with experimental support, *Am J Clin Nutr*, 50, 80, 1989.

148. Young, V.R. and Bier, D.M., A kinetic approach to the determination of human amino acid requirements, *Nutr Rev*, 45, 289, 1987.

149. Brenner, B.M., Meyer, T.W., and Hostetter, T.H., Dietary protein intake and the progressive nature of kidney disease: the role of hemodynamically mediated glomerular injury in the pathogenesis of progressive glomerular sclerosis in aging, renal ablation, and intrinsic renal disease, *N Engl J Med*, 307, 652, 1982.

150. Itoh, R., Nishiyama, N., and Suyama, Y., Dietary protein intake and urinary excretion of calcium: a cross-sectional study in a healthy Japanese population, *Am J Clin Nutr*, 67, 438, 1998.

151. Drinkwater, B.L., Bruemner, B., and Chesnut, C.H., III, Menstrual history as a determinant of current bone density in young athletes, *JAMA*, 263, 545, 1990.

152. Brownell, K.D., Steen, S.N., and Wilmore, J.H., Weight regulation practices in athletes: analysis of metabolic and health effects, *Med Sci Sports Exerc*, 19, 546, 1987.

153. Tarnopolsky, M.A., Cipriano, N., Woodcroft, C. et al., Effects of rapid weight loss and wrestling on muscle glycogen concentration, *Clin J Sport Med*, 6, 78, 1996.

154. Short, S.H. and Short, W.R. Four-year study of university athletes' dietary intake, *J Am Diet Assoc*, 82, 632, 1983.

155. Carter, S.L., Rennie, C., and Tarnopolsky, M.A., Substrate utilization during endurance exercise in men and women after endurance training, *Am J Physiol Endocrinol Metab*, 280, E898, 2001.

156. Ellsworth, N.M., Hewitt, B.F., and Haskell, W.L., Nutrient intake of elite male and female Nordic skiers, *Phys Sports Med*, 13, 78, 1985.

157. Faber, M., Benade, A.J., and van, E.M., Dietary intake, anthropometric measurements, and blood lipid values in weight training athletes (body builders), *Int J Sports Med*, 7, 342, 1986.

158. Burke, L.M., Gollan, R.A., and Read, R.S., Dietary intakes and food use of groups of elite Australian male athletes, *Int J Sport Nutr*, 1, 378, 1991.

159. Burke, L.M. and Read, R.S., A study of dietary patterns of elite Australian football players, *Can J Sport Sci*, 13, 15, 1988.

160. Kleiner, S.M., Bazzarre, T.L., and Litchford, M.D., Metabolic profiles, diet, and health practices of championship male and female bodybuilders, *J Am Diet Assoc*, 90, 962, 1990.

161. Gontzea, I., Sutzescu, P., and Dumitrache, S. The influence of muscular activity on nitrogen balance and on the need of man for proteins, *Nutr Reports Int*, 10, 35, 1974.

162. Todd, K.S., Butterfield, G.E., and Calloway, D.H., Nitrogen balance in men with adequate and deficient energy intake at three levels of work, *J Nutr*, 114, 2107, 1984.

163. Brouns, F., Saris, W.H., Stroecken, J. et al., Eating, drinking, and cycling. A controlled Tour de France simulation study. Part II. Effect of diet manipulation, *Int J Sports Med*, 10 (Suppl 1), S41, 1989.

164. Friedman, J.E. and Lemon, P.W., Effect of chronic endurance exercise on retention of dietary protein, *Int J Sports Med*, 10, 118, 1989.

165. Meredith, C.N., Zackin, M.J., Frontera, W.R., and Evans, W.J., Dietary protein requirements and body protein metabolism in endurance-trained men, *J Appl Physiol*, 66, 2850, 1989.

166. Sale, D.G., MacDougall, J.D., Alway, S.E., and Sutton, J.R., Voluntary strength and muscle characteristics in untrained men and women and male bodybuilders, *J Appl Physiol*, 62, 1786, 1987.

167. Torun, B., Scrimshaw, N.S., and Young, V.R., Effect of isometric exercises on body potassium and dietary protein requirements of young men, *Am J Clin Nutr*, 30, 1983, 1977.

168. Consolazio, C.F., Johnson, H.L., Nelson, R.A., Dramise, J.G., and Skala, J.H., Protein metabolism during intensive physical training in the young adult, *Am J Clin Nutr*, 28, 29, 1975.

169. Hickson, J.F., Hinkelmann, K., and Bredle, D.L., Protein intake level and introductory weight training exercise on urinary total nitrogen excretions from untrained men, *Nutr Res*, 8, 725, 1988.

170. Zaragosa, R., Renau-Piqueras, J., Portoles, M., Hernandez-Yago, J., Jorda, A., and Grisolia, S., Rats fed prolonged high protein diets show an increase in nitrogen metabolism and liver megamitochondria, *Arch Biochem Biophys*, 258, 426, 1987.

171. Hertzman, P.A., Blevins, W.L., Mayer, J., Greenfield, B., Ting, M., and Gleich, G.J., Association of the eosinophilia-myalgia syndrome with the ingestion of tryptophan, *N Engl J Med*, 322, 869, 1990.

172. Teman, A.J. and Hainline, B., Eosinophilia-myalgia syndrome, *Phys Sports Med*, 19, 81, 1991.

173. Yamaoka, K.A., Miyasaka, N., Inuo, G. et al., 1,1'-Ethylidenebis(tryptophan) (peak E) induces functional activation of human eosinophils and interleukin 5 production from T lymphocytes: association of eosinophilia-myalgia syndrome with a L-tryptophan contaminant, *J Clin Immunol*, 14, 50, 1994.

174. Slavin, J.L., Lanners, G., and Engstrom, M.A., Amino acid supplements: beneficial or risky? *Phys Sports Med*, 16, 221, 1988.

175. Bucci, L.R., Hickson, J.F., Jr., Wolinsky, I., and Pivarnik, J.M., Ornithine supplementation and insulin release in bodybuilders, *Int J Sport Nutr*, 2, 287, 1992.

8 Whey, Casein, and Soy Proteins

Brian S. Snyder and Mark D. Haub

CONTENTS

8.1 INTRODUCTION

Athletes and weight trainers often use protein supplements in an attempt to maximize their gains and performance. There are a large variety of protein supplements available on the market today, with the main sources coming from milk or soy processing. These supplements may contain a mixture of whey, casein, or soy protein, or may contain a relatively pure protein from one source. Many protein supplements include other types of supplements, such as glutamine or maltodextrose; thus, it is best to read the label and fully understand the full composition of the protein supplement.

While there is not a consensus regarding the best supplements to ingest to maximize the goals of athletes, current research is attempting to address this issue. This chapter will explain the current processes used to make these protein supplements and their physiological effects. It has been shown that the digestion and absorption of protein sources may be one of the most important factors in determining how protein is assimilated. There have been a limited number of studies directly comparing whey, casein, and soy proteins regarding their effects on both acute and chronic protein synthesis and lean body mass. Aside from body composition changes, protein source plays a role in general health outcomes. This chapter will present a summary of these data and attempt to elucidate the protein source that may be best for athletes.

8.2 FOOD SOURCES AND SUPPLEMENTS

Whey, casein, and soy proteins are all naturally occurring proteins found in foods that are consumed every day. The primary whole food source of whey and casein intake is dairy milk. Whey and casein can also be separated from whole milk, concentrated, and made into a variety of supplements. Soy protein is derived from soybeans and used in a variety of products. There are also a variety of soy supplements and foods commercially available.

8.2.1 WHEY PROTEIN

Whole milk is approximately 87% water, with the remaining 13% as solids. The 13% solids are composed of 30% fat, 37% lactose, 27% protein, and 6% minerals. Of the 27% of milk that is protein, 20% is whey protein and 80% is casein protein. Thus, by consuming whole milk, an individual will ingest a larger portion of protein in the form of casein than whey. During the process of making cheese, whey protein is separated out into a liquid fraction and was originally thought to be a waste product.[1] However, whey is now considered to be a good source of protein and is commonly processed into protein powders and many other products.

Whey protein contains all 20 amino acids and contains the highest naturally occurring portion of the branched-chain amino acids (BCAAs) leucine, valine, and isoleucine.[2] Branched-chain amino acids are important for athletes and active individuals, as they are metabolized for energy in working muscle. Additionally, leucine has been found to play a crucial role in the regulation of protein synthesis.[3–5]

TABLE 8.1
Percentage w/w Amino Acid Values for Specific Subfractions of Whey Protein

Amino Acid	β-Lactoglobulin	α-Lactalbumin	Glycomacropeptide	Ion-Exchange Whey
Essential	48.1	47.2	47.0	42.1
BCAA	25.1	21.0	22.5	21.2
Isoleucine	6.2	6.4	11.9	4.7
Leucine	13.6	10.4	1.7	11.8
Valine	5.4	4.2	8.9	4.7
Lysine	10.5	10.9	5.8	9.5
Methionine	2.9	0.9	2.0	3.1
Phenylalanine	3.2	4.2	0.0	3.0
Threonine	4.4	5.0	16.7	4.6
Tryptophan	2.0	5.3	0.0	1.3
Histidine	1.5	2.9	0.0	1.7
Arginine	2.6	1.1	0.0	2.4
Alanine	5.4	1.5	6.4	4.9
Asparagine	3.1	9.7	5.1	3.8
Aspartic Acid	6.9	7.3	1.7	10.7
Cystine	2.8	5.8	0.0	1.7
Glutamine	6.3	4.5	3.8	3.4
Glutamic Acid	11.3	7.3	15.5	15.4
Glycine	0.9	2.4	0.0	1.7
Proline	4.2	1.4	11.7	4.2
Serine	3.3	4.3	7.8	3.9
Tyrosine	3.6	4.6	0.0	3.4

The whey protein fraction is composed of numerous individual proteins, including β-lactoglobulin, α-lactalbumin, bovine serum albumin, lactoferrin, immunoglobulins, lactoperoxidase enzymes, and glycomacropeptides[6,7] (see Table 8.1). β-Lactoglobulin is the most abundant protein in whey, accounting for 50 to 55%, and is very high in the BCAAs. The biological function of β-lactoglobulin is not fully understood, but it has been recognized for its ability to bind hydrophobic molecules. α-Lactalbumin is the second most abundant protein found in whey and accounts for 20 to 25%. It is also the primary protein found in breast milk and is high in tryptophan and BCAAs. It has been shown to bind calcium and potentially can increase calcium absorption. Immunoglobulins make up about 10 to 15% of the protein in whey. They may provide immunity-enhancing benefits and are the predominant protein found in colostrum. Lactoferrin makes up approximately 1 to 2% of whey protein and may help to reduce inflammation. The amount of these native proteins remaining intact in the final whey product depends on the processes used to separate out the fat and lactose and purify the proteins. Additionally, the health benefits of these protein fractions are derived mainly from the bioactive peptides that enter the blood.[1]

Treatment with strong acids and high heat tends to indiscriminately denature all of the protein fractions and essentially hydrolyze the proteins into smaller peptides and free amino acids. This procedure also has a tendency to oxidize cystine and methionine, destroy serine and threonine, and convert glutamine and asparagine to glutamate and aspartate, respectively.[8] A better method to hydrolyze proteins is by adding specific proteolytic enzymes to break down the proteins into small peptides. However, it has been shown[1] that many of the health benefits associated with whey protein intake are associated with their individual proteins and not necessarily the amino acid content. These health benefits will be discussed later in this chapter. On the other hand, individuals with milk allergies may be able to safely digest highly hydrolyzed whey protein as a protein source without adverse effects because the allergenic native proteins are no longer present.

There are a few main types of whey protein supplements available for use. The first is undenatured whey, which is basically purified whey protein with most of its individual proteins in their native or undenatured form. Originally, undenatured whey concentrates ranged from 25 to 40% protein, with the remaining percentage coming from fat, lactose, mineral, and ash. This type of whey is still used in some baking and other food product applications. Newer techniques such as ultrafiltration have been developed to make the current whey concentrates, which range from 50 to 89% protein. The other main type of whey protein is whey protein isolate, which is approximately 90 to 95% whey protein. It contains minimal fat, lactose, or minerals and may be the best choice for lactose-intolerant individuals. However, some companies are now adding lactase to their whey protein powders to help with lactose digestion.

As stated previously, the native protein fractions of whey protein are implicated as offering the most health benefits associated with whey protein intake. Separating the fat, lactose, and minerals from these protein fractions without denaturing them was rather difficult and expensive until recently. One of the easiest ways to purify whey protein is to treat it with high heat and acid conditions to precipitate the proteins in a denatured form. Whey protein processed in this manner is typically referred to as hydrolyzed whey. The resulting small peptides are absorbed even faster than the larger native proteins present in the whey fraction.[8]

Researchers have recently developed four main types of processes to separate and purify whey proteins in an attempt to leave them in their more biologically active native forms. The types are selective precipitation, membrane filtration (ultra-filtration), selective adsorption, and selective elution (ion exchange).[7]

Selective precipitation is a more advanced method of precipitating proteins out of solution than simply adding acid and heat or proteolytic enzymes. There are numerous fraction-specific methods currently in use to precipitate and purify the proteins without applying as much heat or acid, thus limiting the denaturing of the protein fractions.

Membrane filtration procedures are separated into two subcategories, ultrafiltration and cross-flow filtration, as seen on some nutrition labels. These procedures separate the whey proteins by molecular mass (typically 5000 to 1000 g/mol) and are used to produce most whey concentrates.[7] However, this process does not fully separate out the lactose and fat; thus, whey concentrates derived from this method typically have higher levels of these two macronutrients. This method typically allows a majority of the proteins to remain in their native forms and in their original frequency of unprocessed whey.

Selective absorption is a process used to separate one type of protein out of the whey protein mixture while leaving the other proteins in solution, but it has not yet been widely applied to commercially available products. With the recent findings of health benefits associated with some of the subfractions of whey and the recently developed large throughput of manufacturing, some companies will soon start marketing whey protein subfractions.

Selective elution, also known as ion exchange chromatography, is the process most often used to make whey protein isolates. Using selective elution, whey protein solution is applied to an ion exchange column so that all of the proteins bind to the column. The column is then rinsed and the individual proteins are eluded one by one to produce highly purified whey proteins. This process can be used to both concentrate and fractionate the proteins. If done carefully, the native protein structures can be retained. However, some of the smaller peptides such as lactoferrin may have a decreased concentration, while the β-lactoglobulin protein fraction tends to increase in whey protein isolates.

8.2.2 Casein Proteins

Casein is the other, larger, protein fraction of milk, accounting for approximately 80% of the milk proteins. Casein is the protein source of cheese and forms curds during processing because it exists as a micelle in milk. The clotting properties of casein cause it to be digested and released into the intestine slowly.[9 11] This slow release into the intestine and ultimately circulation leads to a muted peak in plasma amino acid content compared to whey and soy proteins, which will be explained in Section 8.3. In supplemental form, casein is often made into caseinates because the native casein does not dissolve well in solution and forms clumps or curds. It is most often combined with calcium for dietary supplements, resulting in calcium caseinates. Casein is made up of three protein fractions: α-casein, β-casein, and κ-casein.

8.2.3 Soy Proteins

Soy protein is a product derived from soybeans. Whole soybeans are 40% protein, with the remaining percentage of macronutrients in the form of fat and carbohydrates. Soy protein is a complete protein with a relatively high amount of BCAAs, albeit lower than whey proteins' BCAA content.[12] Soy protein is also lower in methionine and lysine content. The carbohydrate content of soybeans is made up of several sugars that humans cannot digest. Raffinose and stachose are two such sugars, and if consumed in high amounts, pass into the large intestine where bacteria digest them, producing flatulence.

Whole soybeans also contain a number of chemicals and proteins that would be harmful to humans if they were not removed prior to ingestion. Raw soybeans contain trypsin inhibitors. Trypsin is a protease that breaks proteins down into smaller peptides by cutting the large proteins after lysine or arginine residues. Inhibiting trypsin may thereby result in protein malabsorption. Soybeans contain biologically active molecules know as isoflavones, which are similar in structure to estrogen in humans.

There are a variety of isoflavones present in raw soy, specifically known as genistein, daidzin, and glycitin.[13] These isoflavones can have numerous effects in the body, including mimicking estrogen, antiestrogen effects, as well as some effects unrelated to estrogen.[13] These chemicals remain in soy products that are not washed with alcohol to remove these isoflavones.

There are many different processes that raw soybeans must undergo before they are ready to be consumed by humans in whole food products or as protein supplements. The soybeans are first picked and cleaned. They are then conditioned, cracked, de-hulled, and rolled into flakes. The soybean oil is then removed from the flakes and used for other food applications. The remaining soy flakes are dried, resulting in defatted soybean flakes. These flakes can then be further processed into a variety of usable soy products. The flakes are essentially ready to be processed into soy protein concentrates by adding flavorings and other vitamins, and potentially concentrating them further. The soy flakes can also be ground into soy flour. Soy protein isolates are derived from the soy protein concentrate by removing most of the carbohydrates and any remaining fat. A soy protein isolate is almost 90% protein on a moisture-free basis. The removal of the carbohydrates tends to also remove most of the beany flavor that soy concentrates tend to retain. Soy protein isolates also typically have the lowest concentration of isoflavones. Another product made from soybeans is texturized soy protein. This product is the typical protein source in imitation chicken, pork, or other meat products. Texturized soy protein is also used in numerous other soy protein products; these products tend to retain the original isoflavone content.

8.3 POSTPRANDIAL KINETICS

8.3.1 DIGESTION AND ABSORPTION

Proteins are hydrolyzed in the stomach by pepsin with the aid of hydrochloric acid to cause unfolding and breaking of the proteins into smaller peptides. The amount of time that a protein spends in the stomach is dependent upon a number of variables, including the type and form of protein consumed, the fat content of the meal, the fiber content of the meal, the surface area, and the total weight of the meal consumed. Once proteins are passed into the small intestine, they are absorbed throughout the entire length of the small intestine. Pancreatic enzymes such as trypsin and chymotrypsin hydrolyze the proteins even further into oligopeptides. Protein is primarily absorbed into the blood as oligopeptides. Free amino acids are also present in the small intestine and are absorbed by specific transporters, with neutral amino acids absorbed fastest, followed by basic and acidic amino acids. Thus, the composition, quality, and source of the amino acid load influence the appearance of those amino acids in the plasma pool. Once amino acids are absorbed into the blood, they circulate via the portal vein to the liver and then to the rest of the body. These amino acids are metabolized for energy, made into proteins, or released back into circulation.

The splanchnic handling of amino acids is very important to their appearance in peripheral circulation, and thus availability for protein synthesis in other tissues such as muscle.[14] The intestinal and liver tissues have a high demand, and turnover, for protein and have first access to ingested amino acids. Splanchnic tissue takes up much of the dietary amino acids early in the postprandial state, which can directly affect their availability to peripheral tissues.[14,15] In fact, splanchnic protein metabolism accounts for the majority of whole-body protein metabolism at rest even though muscle has more mass.[16] The splanchnic zone acts as a buffer to amino acid ingestion to keep the level of circulating urea and free amino acids in check to prevent hyperaminoacidemia.[17]

8.3.2 ABSORPTION OF WHEY, CASEIN, MILK, AND SOY PROTEINS

The amount of time that a protein takes to enter circulation is partly dependent upon the form of the protein. Whole foods are absorbed slowly, and hydrolyzed proteins, in the form of small peptides, are absorbed the fastest. It is generally thought that whey protein is a quickly absorbed protein due in part to the fact that it remains soluble in solution.[9] Casein is absorbed very slowly, most likely due to the fact that it tends to clot in the stomach, delaying gastric emptying.[9,18] Most other protein sources fall somewhere between whey and casein in their rate of appearance in systemic circulation, with a tendency to be slightly slower than whey. Milk proteins consist of approximately 80% casein and 20% whey and appear in a pattern similar to that of casein alone. Soy protein is mostly soluble and appears in circulation more like whey proteins than milk or casein proteins.[19] The intestinal half transit time of soy proteins is shorter than that of milk proteins, potentially playing a role in the reduced bioavailability of soy proteins.[12] It has also been shown that soy proteins are less digestible on a nitrogen basis.[12] The pattern of amino acids reaching the liver is more unbalanced in soy proteins than milk proteins due to the lower digestibility of the soy proteins.[12,20] Also, soy proteins tend to produce more urea than casein intake, indicating an increased oxidation of soy proteins and reduced availability of their amino acids for protein synthesis.[21] Soy proteins arrive quickly and in large amounts in the splanchnic region, most likely contributing to the increased urea production as the splanchnic region uses these amino acids.[17,21] The appearance of amino acids in the peripheral circulation are, for the most part, dependent upon the amino acids that have been ingested. However, this is not the case for amino acids that are highly metabolized in the splanchnic regions. There is a paucity of data directly comparing whey vs. soy regarding these postprandial properties. To fully elucidate the differences, it is necessary to directly compare whey and soy proteins considering that both whey and soy proteins exit the stomach quickly. Whey appears to have a slow and efficient intestinal absorption.[22]

8.3.3 HABITUAL PROTEIN INTAKE

In general, increases in habitual protein intake lead to increases in amino acid catabolism and deamination as well as an increase in the cycling protein gains and losses.[17] Interestingly, the amount of nitrogen loss, as urea or lack of absorption, with higher protein intakes may also depend on the form of protein ingested. It has been shown that soy protein leads to a greater loss of nitrogen than milk proteins.[17] In a study conducted by Morens et al.,[17] the net postprandial protein utilization was higher in the milk group (74%) than in the soy group (71%) at habitually normal protein intakes (1 g/kg/day), and this difference became even greater (71% vs. 61%) with habitually high protein intakes (2 g/kg/day).[17] Ingestion of habitual high protein diets resulted in a trend toward decreased circulating amino acids when fed the high-protein soy test meal. In fact, soy protein deamination was increased 54% between the normal protein and high protein intake.[17] This is critical as the availability of circulating amino acids is, in part, responsible for the rate of muscle protein synthesis, and soy protein may lead to reduced levels of circulating amino acids.[17]

8.4 PROTEIN SYNTHESIS

Skeletal muscle mass is maintained by a balance between muscle protein synthesis (muscle PS) and muscle protein breakdown (muscle PB), yielding an overall net protein state (NPS). This balance can be written as an algebraic equation where muscle PS – muscle PB = NPS. If muscle PS is greater than muscle PB, then NPS will be positive. A chronic positive NPS over time yields protein accretion, and likely increased muscle mass. Conversely, NPS will be negative if muscle PB is greater than muscle PS. If an individual is experiencing chronic negative NPS, he or she is losing muscle mass, as in older individuals with sarcopenia as well as disease and disuse states. However, in nondisease or disuse states, the main determinants of NPS are changes in muscle PS.[23] These changes are due to a variety of stimuli, including feeding and exercise. Additionally, amino acid availability, insulin, and total energy load are all key factors that influence PS.

8.4.1 AMINO ACID INFUSION

Muscle PS is the main determinant of net protein balance in healthy adults.[19,23] Numerous studies have shown that total body PS[9,22] and muscle PS[24,25] are increased in response to amino acid provision at rest. However, this increase in muscle PS is transient, even if circulating amino acid levels remain elevated.[23,25] This is why an additional stimulus, i.e., resistance exercise,[26–28] is needed to achieve increased muscle mass over time.[29] Much of the original muscle PS work was done using free amino acid infusions as the nitrogen source.[30] This early research suggests that as much as 80% of the effect of feeding amino acids on muscle PS is attributed to the amino acid content of the meal.[31–34] This point was refined and expanded in numerous recent studies. It appears that as long as the amino acid source contains all the essential amino acids (EAAs), it will increase muscle PS above baseline.

Some recent studies have compared providing a mixture of all 20 amino acids with EAAs only. Tipton et al. found that 40 g of mixed amino acids did not differ from 40 g of EAA in their ability to promote muscle PS after exercise.[35] Unpublished data discussed by both Drs. Robert Wolfe and Michael Rennie examined whether nonessential amino acids (NEAAs) are needed to increase muscle PS at rest. Muscle PS was measured in subjects given 30 g of a balanced mixture of EAAs and NEAAs over a 3-h period. The protocol was repeated using 14 g of EAAs only. There was no difference in muscle PS or NBS between the two groups.[23] Additionally, it has been shown that NEAAs do not induce increases in muscle PS at rest.[23] In fact, large doses of NEAAs sufficient to flood the system had no effect on muscle PS.[36] If only a single stimulatory amino acid is provided, i.e., valiene, leucine, phenylalanine, or threonine, an initial anabolic response is noted. However, this response is transient, as all other amino acids in the intracellular pool fall and muscle PS decreases.[36–38]

There are data that suggest there is an upper concentration of circulating amino acids above which additional increases in amino acid concentration have no effect on PS at rest. Rennie's group found that the system is saturated when the plasma amino acid concentration reaches approximately 2.5-fold normal circulating levels by means of amino acid infusion.[34] To further this point, the best relationship between exogenous amino acid provision and the stimulation of muscle PS was the concentration of extracellular EAAs. Increasing the extracellular EAA content resulted in the disappearance of amino acids from the intracellular space (most likely being incorporated into muscle),[34,39] suggesting that extracellular amino acid concentration, and not intracellular amino acid concentration, is the stimulus for increased muscle PS.[24,40,41] Further, a study conducted by Bohe et al.[24] supports the hypothesis that there is a curvilinear positive relationship between extracellular EAA and increased muscle PS and no relationship between muscle PS and intracellular EAA concentration. The extracellular availability is thought to signal for increased muscle PS, leading to increased uptake of amino acids as the intracellular amino acids are incorporated into protein.[42] Artificially reducing the plasma amino acid level has been studied by Wolfe's group through use of hemodialysis to reduce blood amino acid concentration in pigs by 50%.[23] When the amino acid concentration was reduced, there was a corresponding reduction of muscle PS. The inward transport of circulating amino acids was decreased while the intracellular concentrations remained constant. This change in muscle PS persisted for the entire 4-h hemodialysis procedure. Muscle PS returned to basal values when blood amino acid levels returned to normal shortly after conclusion of the hemodialysis. While the previous examples support a ceiling effect in a rested state, research is needed to determine if this occurs after exercise.

Muscle protein breakdown is a more complex and less studied side of the equation. It has been shown that provision of amino acids inhibits muscle PB,[43–45] but not as robustly as they stimulate muscle PS. This would make sense in protein sparing because the increased extracellualar amino acids may act as a signal that amino acids are available; thus PB is not needed to provide additional amino acids. However, many of the experiments showing this effect were either *in vitro*, conducted in nonhuman models, or conducted in individuals in extreme catabolic states such as burn victims.[23] Data regarding the control of muscle PB are equivocal, with some suggesting that in nondiseased human subjects, infusion or ingestion of amino acids has no effect on breakdown,[23,46,47] while others state the contrary.[9,22,46]

Muscle PB is the result of proteolysis. There are two main processes through which proteins in general may be degraded: the autophagic-lysomal pathway and the ubiquitin-proteosome pathway.[48] Both of these systems are present in skeletal muscle, yet their contribution to total PB is not yet fully understood. However, the autophagic-lysomal system is physiologically controlled by plasma and exogenous amino acids, which suggests its potential role in muscle PB. The autophagy system is a nonselective system, which is not specific for proteins alone but does metabolize protein into individual amino acids.

It appears that at rest, there is an upper limit of circulating amino acids beyond which additional amino acid provision will have no further effect on muscle PS. Data are lacking regarding this dose–response in conjunction with exercise. It also would appear that provisions of EAAs are sufficient to support acute changes in muscle PS. Whether EAAs, as opposed to a protein source containing all 20 amino acids, are optimal over time for maximizing muscle PS at rest or during exercise needs to be investigated further.

8.4.2 Whey vs. Casein at Rest

As discussed previously, whey, casein, and soy all have differing amino acid compositions and, seemingly more important, differing postprandial kinetics. The speed of amino acid absorption has a major impact on postprandial PS and PB responses of a meal. Whey protein is a very fast absorbed protein and, after ingestion, the appearance of circulating amino acids is rapid, increased, and transient. Whey protein has been shown to quickly and transiently increase whole-body PS as well as amino acid oxidation. Boirie et al. found that the increase in protein synthesis was 68% above baseline during the period from approximately 40 min to just after 140 min after ingesting a whey drink.[9] Casein is a slowly absorbed protein, and the appearance of postprandial circulating amino acids is slow, low, and prolonged. Casein tends to inhibit PB when consumed at rest and has a slight, but relatively long, increase in PS. The pattern of amino acid delivery with casein appears to lead to better leucine balance (net protein state) than whey at rest. It is interesting to note that casein ingestion does not lead to large increases in circulating levels of amino acids as was observed in many early amino acid infusion studies or whey ingestion studies. To further support these points, a study conducted by Dangin et al.[22] compared casein to a supplement containing amino acids in the same amount as native casein, and compared whey protein to that same dose of whey spread out over 13 small feedings every 20 min. All the feedings were composed of 30 g of protein. The two meals (casein and whey feedings every 20 min), which were designed to mimic casein, showed results that were similar to the previously listed results. The single whey feeding and casein amino acids group mimicked the previous results of whey protein.[22] It is of interest to note that the frequent whey feeding increased net leucine balance to 87 μmol/kg^{-1} and the casein feeding increased leucine balance to 38 μmol/kg^{-1}.[22] These authors did not statistically compare these values. Overall, it would appear that casein protein, and its slow absorption rate, leads to a greater positive net whole-body protein state than single feedings of whey protein or amino acids at rest. Additionally, frequent small feedings of whey proteins may lead to the greatest net leucine balance, indicative of the greatest protein accretion.

8.4.3 WHEY VS. CASEIN WITH EXERCISE

Contrary to the resting data, there is a much smaller body of literature examining the effects of whole food ingestion on the rates of protein synthesis after a resistance training bout. A recent study by Tipton et al.[49] examined casein or whey proteins with regard to their effects on muscle PS after resistance exercise. The main result of this study was that both casein and whey protein ingestion 1 h after resistance training lead to a positive amino acid balance, which can be translated to an acute increase in muscle PS.[49] These results differ from those of Boirie, Dangin, and co-workers,[9,22] suggesting that resistance training influences the use of amino acids. Although not statistically significant, it is interesting to note that the casein group did exhibit a greater phenylalanine balance (~35%) than the whey group. Additionally, the phenylalanine concentration remained elevated for a longer period in the casein group.[49] Conversely, net leucine balance was higher in the whey group. However, this may be attributed to the leucine content of the meal, such that whey protein has a greater leucine content than casein. Leucine taken up across the leg can be oxidized or used for protein synthesis, while muscle does not oxidize phenylalanine. Thus, phenylalanine may be a better marker of muscle PS. The whey group exhibited a higher insulin response than the casein group, which is likely due to the increased arterial leucine concentration. Additionally, it has been shown that leucine alone can stimulate PS. These differing results between casein and whey leave many questions to be answered. Overall, both casein and whey protein ingestion after resistance training elicit increased muscle PS. However, if there is a difference between these two protein sources, it appears to be small.

Demling and DeSanti[50] examined the effects of casein or whey on body composition and strength measures during 12 weeks of hypocaloric, high-protein diets, with resistance training, in overweight police officers. The protein supplements were hydrolysates. While both the casein and whey groups lost weight and gained lean mass, the casein group gained more lean mass. Additionally, the casein group had a greater increase in strength for the chest, shoulder, and legs.[50] It would appear that use of a casein supplement during weight loss and lean body mass gain in concert with resistance training leads to more accretion of lean body mass.

8.4.4 MILK

Elliot et al.[51] examined the effects of different milk compositions on the response of net muscle protein balance after resistance training. There were three groups who consumed either 237 g of fat-free milk, 237 g of whole milk, or 393 g of fat-free milk, which was isocaloric to the whole milk. The milk was ingested 1 h after the resistance training bout. All three milk compositions resulted in increased phenylalanine and threonine uptake, which is acutely indicative of increased protein synthesis. The group consuming the whole milk had the greatest threonine uptake, indicating increased protein synthesis compared to the other milk groups. It is of interest to note that whole-body leucine balance has been shown to be greater with the addition of carbohydrates and fat to a protein meal than protein alone in resting subjects.[52] Furthermore, the addition of fat and sucrose to milk proteins results in more protein uptake by the peripheral (i.e., muscle) tissues.[22,51,52] Also, the addition of fat to a protein meal after resistance training appears to increase muscle PS independent of total energy. There was no difference in the insulin response between the milk groups of the Elliot et al. study.[51]

8.4.5 MILK VS. SOY DURING REST AND EXERCISE

When comparing milk vs. soy, it has been shown that milk proteins are better at supporting protein anabolism in peripherial (i.e., muscle) tissues.[12,14,17,19] Soy proteins have been shown to be digested more rapidly and directed toward deamination as well as liver protein synthesis. This may be due to differing amino acid compositions of soy protein as well as its rapid delivery into circulation. Recently, Phillips et al.[19] compared both the acute and chronic effects of milk vs. hydrolyzed soy protein ingestion on post-exercise PS. To test the acute effects of milk and hydrolyzed proteins on net protein state, subjects consumed 18.2 g of protein from low-fat milk or from isoenergetic and isonitrogenous hydrolyzed soy protein beverage immediately after resistance training. The soy protein group showed a more rapid and transient hyperaminoacidemia than the milk group. The milk protein group had greater amino acid uptake, indicating a greater NPS than the soy group. It is important to note that the amino acid makeup of the two protein sources administered was similar.

The next step was to test the chronic effects of milk vs. hydrolyzed soy protein. Subjects consumed either low-fat milk or isocaloric and isonitrogenous hydrolyzed soy proteins immediately and at 1 h after resistance exercise bouts. A control group consumed maltodextrin equivalent in calories to the other drinks. The milk group gained more whole-body lean mass than the energy control group, but not statistically more than the soy group ($p = 0.11$) (personal communication). The increase in cross-sectional area of the vastus lateralis (quadricep) was greater in the milk group, although not statistically significant ($p = 0.08$).[19] Overall, it would appear that any difference in muscle PS exhibited by different sources of protein is small, yet may become relevant if a diet is solely of soy protein or over more than 12 weeks.

A potential underlying mechanism may be related to the isoflavone content of soy proteins. It has been shown that soy may play an inhibitory role in protein synthesis *in vitro* and in animal models.[53,54] It has been shown that the isoflavones present in varying concentrations in soy products are cytotoxic *in vitro*, partially due to their inhibition of protein tyrosine kinase and DNA topoisomerase activities. However, these mechanisms have not been elucidated in humans. The amount of soy isoflavones in the soy proteins administered or present in the blood have not been widely presented in these studies assessing PS.

8.4.6 SOY VS. WHEY

Brown et al.[55] conducted a study examining the chronic effects of soy or whey protein bars on lean body mass and antioxidant status. Subjects consumed three bars per day over 9 weeks with each protein bar adding an additional 11 g of protein to the subjects' habitual diet. The control group did complete the exercise protocol but did not consume a protein supplement. Both the whey and soy groups exhibited increases in percent lean body mass, while the control group did not significantly increase in percent lean body mass. There was not a difference between the soy and whey groups' increase in lean body mass.[55]

8.5 HEALTH BENEFITS OF WHEY, CASEIN, OR SOY PROTEINS

Many foods and supplements are now being examined as functional foods. Many of these foods have been used for their perceived health benefits for hundreds of years, and science is now elucidating the mechanisms eliciting their health benefits.

8.5.1 WHEY

Whey has been used as a functional food for many years in some cultures. As already mentioned, whey contains all of the essential amino acids and is a good source of the BCAAs. It is a protein source that can be used to support anabolism. It also contains colostrums, β-lactoglobulin, α-lactalbumin, bovine serum albumin, lactoferrin, immunoglobulin, lactoperoxidase enzymes, and glycomacropeptides. It is thought to provide antimicrobial activity and additional immune functions, prevent osteoporosis, increase glutathione, and may lead to better nitrogen retention in elderly women.[56]

Lactoferrin and glycomacropeptides seem to have bactericidal activity. Lactoferrin may be converted to lactoferricin in the stomach after ingestion, which has been shown to inhibit microorganism growth *in vitro* with mixed results in humans.[57] Lactoferrin may also have some antifungal properties. α-Lactalbumin may have a function in immune response as well, and the mechanisms of action are currently being elucidated.[58]

Whey protein concentrate is a good source of cystine, which is used to make glutathione (GSH).[59] GSH is a potent antioxidant and is important in neutralizing reactive oxygen species. There are some case studies that suggest that increased whey protein intake is protective against some cancers.

Immunoglobulins are present in milk and may transfer passive immunity to people who ingest them. Colostrum has the highest component of immunoglobulins and is present in milk, but whey protein still has immunoglobulins.

8.5.2 CASEIN

Casein has been shown to be a good source of protein and essential amino acids as well. Additionally, the β- and κ-caseins seem to inhibit the angiotensin converting enzyme. Hence, casein may play a role in reducing blood pressure in hypertensive individuals.[57] During the breakdown of κ-caseins, a small peptide is formed that has been shown to exhibit antithrombotic activity by inhibiting fibrinogen binding,[57] thereby potentially delaying atherogenesis. Casein also aids calcium absorption.[57] Thus, many supplement companies incorporate calcium caseinates to assist in calcium delivery with the intent of preventing osteoporosis.

8.5.3 Milk

Whole milk is composed of both whey and casein proteins and has been shown to be better at supporting muscle PS acutely compared to hydrolyzed soy protein.[19] Milk ingestion has also been associated with lower blood pressure and a reduced risk of hypertension.[1] Recently, increased intake of dairy products such as milk and yogurt has been shown to enhance weight loss.[60–63] However, the proposed mechanism that was shown to exist in animal models does not seem to transfer to humans. Thus, the mechanism for the associated weight loss appears to be calcium independent,[64] at least when calcium intake is adequate. In a multicenter trial,[65] milk intake without weight loss did not elicit favorable changes in metabolic outcomes.

8.5.4 Soy

There are numerous health benefits that have been attributed to increased soy protein intake. Unfortunately, the results of many of the studies on the topic are mixed. Additionally, mechanisms that work well in an animal model may not always transfer to human applications.

8.5.4.1 Vegetarians

Vegetarian athletes have a limited choice of protein sources, especially if they are vegan. These athletes would almost require the inclusion of soy protein in their diet to be able to consume an adequate protein intake. While it appears that soy protein may not be the ideal choice for maximal muscle PS, it has been shown to be viable as a sole source of dietary protein. Studies have been conducted where soy protein was used to replace other protein sources without negative effects on the subjects.[66–73] However, these tests were conducted in nonexercising individuals. As shown by Phillips, soy protein may not be the optimal choice for athletes and those seeking increased muscle mass. Additionally, because both resistance and cardiovascular exercise alone can decrease cardiovascular risks,[74] the benefits of including soy in the diet of an athlete may not be worth the potential decrease in attained muscle mass. However, sedentary persons may notice less of the diminished effect of soy protein intake than highly trained and competitive athletes.

8.5.4.2 Cardiovascular Risks

Soy protein intake has been touted for its effects on reducing blood cholesterol and improving risk factors for cardiovascular disease. The recommended daily intake to reap the benefits of soy protein was set at 25 g/day by the FDA following its review of the literature. However, the average dose in numerous clinical trials to elicit an approximate 3% reduction of LDL cholesterol was 50 g/day.[13] This value is double the FDA recommendation and may account for a quarter to one half of a person's daily total protein intake. It also appears that soy may be more effective at lowering cholesterol in hypercholesterolemic individuals.[75] It is of interest to note that soy isoflavones alone do not appear to affect blood lipid concentrations.[76] Inclusion of soy proteins as a trade for other, higher-fat sources of protein may be protective via decreasing the total and saturated fat intake regardless of the protein source. As we observed in older men,[77] the nonprotein macronutrients (carbohydrates, fiber, and saturated fat) were better predictors of lipoprotein lipid values than protein source (beef or soy).

8.5.4.3 Hot Flashes

Soy isoflavones have been shown to have weak estrogenic activity and may be able to mimic estrogen by binding estrogen receptors. The results of the body of literature regarding the effectiveness of isoflavone treatment of hot flashes are mixed. It appears that *in vivo*, some women may be more susceptible to the estrogenic activity of isoflavones than others.[13]

8.5.4.4 Cancer

The idea that soy protein and isoflavone intake are associated with reduced risk of cancer stemmed from the high consumption of soy products in Asian countries and some animal models that exhibited this relationship. Unfortunately, some studies have shown that soy intake decreases cancer risk, while others have shown no effect.[13,78–80] Some studies have even shown increased risk.[13,81,82] A new hypothesis is being tested that isoflavone intake may only be protective in adult life when consumed in adolescence.[13]

8.6 RECOMMENDATIONS

For most athletes, achieving competitive advantages and optimizing recovery and gains are the most important variables. Considering the intake of only one type of protein source (whey, casein, or soy), it would appear that casein leads to the optimal total body protein state at rest. However, following resistance exercise, it would appear that ingestion of a combination of whey and casein, or milk proteins, offers the most benefit to athletes attempting to increase strength, power, and lean mass. The addition of carbohydrates to an amino acid source or consuming milk in its whole form (with fat and carbohydrates) ellicits a greater increase in muscle PS. The precise dose and source of amino acids, carbohydrates, and fat to be ingested both before and after a resistance training bout has not been fully elucidated.

Milk itself and the protein components of milk are not agreeable with some athletes. In this case, hydrolyzed whey protein or casein supplements may afford similar results. It has been shown that soy protein can also support anabolism, but to a lesser degree. Thus, vegans should include soy protein in their diet to ensure an adequate protein intake. To fully clarify these conditions, more closely controlled clinical trials are needed.

Independent of the source of protein, the most important variables to consider are total caloric and protein intake, which must be adequate to support gains and maintenance of lean body mass. Additionally, an amino acid source must be ingested either shortly before or after resistance or endurance activities to change NPS from a negative to a positive state. Even a small amount of protein with adequate carbohydrates has been shown to be able to switch NPS from negative to positive after endurance and resistance training.

8.7 SUMMARY

The use of protein supplements is prevalent among athletes. The protein supplement that an athlete chooses can affect his or her training and maintenance of lean body mass. There are three main sources of protein used in these supplements, and their processing plays a role in their functionality. While there is not a consensus regarding which protein is optimal, evidence seems to indicate whey and casein provide better acute gains in muscle protein accretion. Long-term studies are limited, but the data appear to indicate a long-term benefit of whey and casein use. While the difference in protein accretion between soy and milk proteins appears to be small, it may have physiological relevance, especially if consumed over extended periods.

Future research is needed to compare the use of all of these different protein sources in controlled clinical trials from acute and chronic perspectives. The dose and macronutrient profile as well as timing of ingestion should also be considered. Additionally, a diet based solely on each supplement as a protein source would be an interesting and needed comparison to elucidate the magnitude of the differences. However, a study with this design would have limited applicability.

REFERENCES

1. Marshall, K. (2004). Therapeutic applications of whey protein. *Altern Med Rev* 9: 136–156.
2. Bos, C., Gaudichon, C., and Tome, D. (2000). Nutritional and physiological criteria in the assessment of milk protein quality for humans. *J Am Coll Nutr* 19: 191S–205S.
3. Anthony, J.C., Anthony, T.G., and Layman, D.K. (1999). Leucine supplementation enhances skeletal muscle recovery in rats following exercise. *J Nutr* 129: 1102–1106.
4. Layman, D.K. (2002). Role of leucine in protein metabolism during exercise and recovery. *Can J Appl Physiol* 27: 646–663.
5. Norton, L.E. and Layman, D.K. (2006). Leucine regulates translation initiation of protein synthesis in skeletal muscle after exercise. *J Nutr* 136: 533S–537S.
6. Walzem, R.L., Dillard, C.J., and German, J.B. (2002). Whey components: millennia of evolution create functionalities for mammalian nutrition: what we know and what we may be overlooking. *Crit Rev Food Sci Nutr* 42: 353–375.
7. Etzel, M.R. (2004). Manufacture and use of dairy protein fractions. *J Nutr* 134: 996S–1002S.
8. Manninen, A.H. (2004). Protein hydrolysates in sports and exercise: a brief review. *J Sports Sci Med* 3: 60–63.
9. Boirie, Y., Dangin, M., Gachon, P., Vasson, M.P., Maubois, J.L., and Beaufrere, B. (1997). Slow and fast dietary proteins differently modulate postprandial protein accretion. *Proc Natl Acad Sci USA* 94: 14930–14935.
10. Mahe, S., Messing, B., Thuillier, F., and Tome, D. (1991). Digestion of bovine milk proteins in patients with a high jejunostomy. *Am J Clin Nutr* 54: 534–538.

11. Mahe, S., Roos, N., Benamouzig, R., Davin, L., Luengo, C., Gagnon, L., Gausserges, N., Rautureau, J., and Tome, D. (1996). Gastrojejunal kinetics and the digestion of [15N]beta-lactoglobulin and casein in humans: the influence of the nature and quantity of the protein. *Am J Clin Nutr* 63: 546–552.

12. Bos, C., Metges, C.C., Gaudichon, C., Petzke, K.J., Pueyo, M.E., Morens, C., Everwand, J., Benamouzig, R., and Tome, D. (2003). Postprandial kinetics of dietary amino acids are the main determinant of their metabolism after soy or milk protein ingestion in humans. *J Nutr* 133: 1308–1315.

13. Sacks, F.M., Lichtenstein, A., Van Horn, L., Harris, W., Kris-Etherton, P., and Winston, M. (2006). Soy protein, isoflavones, and cardiovascular health: an American Heart Association Science Advisory for professionals from the Nutrition Committee. *Circulation* 113: 1034–1044.

14. Fouillet, H., Gaudichon, C., Bos, C., Mariotti, F., and Tome, D. (2003). Contribution of plasma proteins to splanchnic and total anabolic utilization of dietary nitrogen in humans. *Am J Physiol Endocrinol Metab* 285: E88–E97.

15. Mariotti, F., Huneau, J.F., Mahe, S., and Tome, D. (2000). Protein metabolism and the gut. *Curr Opin Clin Nutr Metab Care* 3: 45–50.

16. Waterlow, J.C. (1995). Whole-body protein turnover in humans: past, present, and future. *Annu Rev Nutr* 15: 57–92.

17. Morens, C., Bos, C., Pueyo, M.E., Benamouzig, R., Gausseres, N., Luengo, C., Tome, D., and Gaudichon, C. (2003). Increasing habitual protein intake accentuates differences in postprandial dietary nitrogen utilization between protein sources in humans. *J Nutr* 133: 2733–2740.

18. Dangin, M., Boirie, Y., Guillet, C., and Beaufrere, B. (2002). Influence of the protein digestion rate on protein turnover in young and elderly subjects. *J Nutr* 132: 3228S–3233S.

19. Phillips, S.M., Hartman, J.W., and Wilkinson, S.B. (2005). Dietary protein to support anabolism with resistance exercise in young men. *J Am Coll Nutr* 24: 134S–139S.

20. Gaudichon, C., Bos, C., Morens, C., Petzke, K.J., Mariotti, F., Everwand, J., Benamouzig, R., Dare, S., Tome, D., and Metges, C.C. (2002). Ileal losses of nitrogen and amino acids in humans and their importance to the assessment of amino acid requirements. *Gastroenterology* 123: 50–59.

21. Luiking, Y.C., Deutz, N.E., Jakel, M., and Soeters, P.B. (2005). Casein and soy protein meals differentially affect whole-body and splanchnic protein metabolism in healthy humans. *J Nutr* 135: 1080–1087.

22. Dangin, M., Boirie, Y., Garcia-Rodenas, C., Gachon, P., Fauquant, J., Callier, P., Ballevre, O., and Beaufrere, B. (2001). The digestion rate of protein is an independent regulating factor of postprandial protein retention. *Am J Physiol Endocrinol Metab* 280: E340–E348.

23. Wolfe, R.R. (2002). Regulation of muscle protein by amino acids. *J Nutr* 132: 3219S–3224S.

24. Bohe, J., Low, A., Wolfe, R.R., and Rennie, M.J. (2003). Human muscle protein synthesis is modulated by extracellular, not intramuscular amino acid availability: a dose-response study. *J Physiol* 552: 315–324.

25. Bohe, J., Low, J.F., Wolfe, R.R., and Rennie, M.J. (2001). Latency and duration of stimulation of human muscle protein synthesis during continuous infusion of amino acids. *J Physiol* 532: 575–579.

26. Biolo, G., Maggi, S.P., Williams, B.D., Tipton, K.D., and Wolfe, R.R. (1995). Increased rates of muscle protein turnover and amino acid transport after resistance exercise in humans. *Am J Physiol* 268: E514–E520.

27. Phillips, S.M., Tipton, K.D., Aarsland, A., Wolf, S.E., and Wolfe, R.R. (1997). Mixed muscle protein synthesis and breakdown after resistance exercise in humans. *Am J Physiol* 273: E99–E107.

28. Phillips, S.M., Tipton, K.D., Ferrando, A.A., and Wolfe, R.R. (1999). Resistance training reduces the acute exercise-induced increase in muscle protein turnover. *Am J Physiol* 276: E118–E124.

29. Rennie, M.J., Wackerhage, H., Spangenburg, E.E., and Booth, F.W. (2004). Control of the size of the human muscle mass. *Annu Rev Physiol* 66: 799–828.

30. Bennet, W.M., Connacher, A.A., Scrimgeour, C.M., Smith, K., and Rennie, M.J. (1989). Increase in anterior tibialis muscle protein synthesis in healthy man during mixed amino acid infusion: studies of incorporation of [1-13C]leucine. *Clin Sci (Lond)* 76: 447–454.

31. Bennet, W.M., Connacher, A.A., Scrimgeour, C.M., Jung, R.T., and Rennie, M.J. (1990). Euglycemic hyperinsulinemia augments amino acid uptake by human leg tissues during hyperaminoacidemia. *Am J Physiol* 259: E185–E194.

32. Bennet, W.M., Connacher, A.A., Scrimgeour, C.M., and Rennie, M.J. (1990). The effect of amino acid infusion on leg protein turnover assessed by L-[15N]phenylalanine and L-[1-13C]leucine exchange. *Eur J Clin Invest* 20: 41–50.

33. Cheng, K.N., Dworzak, F., Ford, G.C., Rennie, M.J., and Halliday, D. (1985). Direct determination of leucine metabolism and protein breakdown in humans using L-[1-13C, 15N]-leucine and the forearm model. *Eur J Clin Invest* 15: 349–354.

34. Rennie, M.J., Bohe, J., and Wolfe, R.R. (2002). Latency, duration and dose response relationships of amino acid effects on human muscle protein synthesis. *J Nutr* 132: 3225S–3227S.

35. Tipton, K.D., Ferrando, A.A., Phillips, S.M., Doyle, D., Jr., and Wolfe, R.R. (1999). Postexercise net protein synthesis in human muscle from orally administered amino acids. *Am J Physiol* 276: E628–E634.

36. Smith, K., Reynolds, N., Downie, S., Patel, A., and Rennie, M.J. (1998). Effects of flooding amino acids on incorporation of labeled amino acids into human muscle protein. *Am J Physiol* 275: E73–E78.

37. Alvestrand, A., Hagenfeldt, L., Merli, M., Oureshi, A., and Eriksson, L.S. (1990). Influence of leucine infusion on intracellular amino acids in humans. *Eur J Clin Invest* 20: 293–298.

38. Smith, K., Barua, J.M., Watt, P.W., Scrimgeour, C.M., and Rennie, M.J. (1992). Flooding with L-[1-13C]leucine stimulates human muscle protein incorporation of continuously infused L-[1-13C]valine. *Am J Physiol* 262: E372–E376.

39. Bergstrom, J., Furst, P., and Vinnars, E. (1990). Effect of a test meal, without and with protein, on muscle and plasma free amino acids. *Clin Sci (Lond)* 79: 331–337.

40. Fox, H.L., Kimball, S.R., Jefferson, L.S., and Lynch, C.J. (1998). Amino acids stimulate phosphorylation of p70S6k and organization of rat adipocytes into multicellular clusters. *Am J Physiol* 274: C206–C213.

41. Kimball, S.R., Horetsky, R.L., and Jefferson, L.S. (1998). Signal transduction pathways involved in the regulation of protein synthesis by insulin in L6 myoblasts. *Am J Physiol* 274: C221–C228.

42. Wolfe, R.R. and Miller, S.L. (1999). Amino acid availability controls muscle protein metabolism. *Diabetes Nutr Metab* 12: 322–328.

43. Abumrad, N.N., Robinson, R.P., Gooch, B.R., and Lacy, W.W. (1982). The effect of leucine infusion on substrate flux across the human forearm. *J Surg Res* 32: 453–463.

44. Nagasawa, T., Kido, T., Yoshizawa, F., Ito, Y., and Nishizawa, N. (2002). Rapid suppression of protein degradation in skeletal muscle after oral feeding of leucine in rats. *J Nutr Biochem* 13: 121–127.

45. Nagasawa, T., Hirano, J., Yoshizawa, F., and Nishizawa, N. (1998). Myofibrillar protein catabolism is rapidly suppressed following protein feeding. *Biosci Biotechnol Biochem* 62: 1932–1937.

46. Biolo, G., Tipton, K.D., Klein, S., and Wolfe, R.R. (1997). An abundant supply of amino acids enhances the metabolic effect of exercise on muscle protein. *Am J Physiol* 273: E122–E129.

47. Biolo, G., Fleming, R.Y., Maggi, S.P., Nguyen, T.T., Herndon, D.N., and Wolfe, R.R. (2002). Inverse regulation of protein turnover and amino acid transport in skeletal muscle of hypercatabolic patients. *J Clin Endocrinol Metab* 87: 3378–3384.

48. Kadowaki, M. and Kanazawa, T. (2003). Amino acids as regulators of proteolysis. *J Nutr* 133: 2052S–2056S.

49. Tipton, K.D., Elliot, T.A., Cree, M.G., Wolf, S.E., Sanford, A.P., and Wolfe, R.R. (2004). Ingestion of casein and whey proteins results in muscle anabolism after resistance exercise. *Med Sci Sports Exerc* 36: 2073–2081.

50. Demling, R.H. and DeSanti, L. (2000). Effect of a hypocaloric diet, increased protein intake and resistance training on lean mass gains and fat mass loss in overweight police officers. *Ann Nutr Metab* 44: 21–29.

51. Elliot, T.A., Cree, M.G., Sanford, A.P., Wolfe, R.R., and Tipton, K.D. (2006). Milk ingestion stimulates net muscle protein synthesis following resistance exercise. *Med Sci Sports Exerc* 38: 667–674.

52. Fouillet, H., Gaudichon, C., Mariotti, F., Bos, C., Huneau, J.F., and Tome, D. (2001). Energy nutrients modulate the splanchnic sequestration of dietary nitrogen in humans: a compartmental analysis. *Am J Physiol Endocrinol Metab* 281: E248–E260.

53. Ji, S., Willis, G.M., Frank, G.R., Cornelius, S.G., and Spurlock, M.E. (1999). Soybean isoflavones, genistein and genistin, inhibit rat myoblast proliferation, fusion and myotube protein synthesis. *J Nutr* 129: 1291–1297.

54. Lohrke, B., Saggau, E., Schadereit, R., Beyer, M., Bellmann, O., Kuhla, S., and Hagemeister, H. (2001). Activation of skeletal muscle protein breakdown following consumption of soyabean protein in pigs. *Br J Nutr* 85: 447–457.

55. Brown, E.C., DiSilvestro, R.A., Babaknia, A., and Devor, S.T. (2004). Soy versus whey protein bars: effects on exercise training impact on lean body mass and anti-oxidant status. *Nutr J* 3: 22.

56. Arnal, M.A., Mosoni, L., Boirie, Y., Houlier, M.L., Morin, L., Verdier, E., Ritz, P., Antoine, J.M., Prugnaud, J. et al. (1999). Protein pulse feeding improves protein retention in elderly women. *Am J Clin Nutr* 69: 1202–1208.

57. Clare, D.A. and Swaisgood, H.E. (2000). Bioactive milk peptides: a prospectus. *J Dairy Sci* 83: 1187–1195.

58. Clare, D.A., Catignani, G.L., and Swaisgood, H.E. (2003). Biodefense properties of milk: the role of antimicrobial proteins and peptides. *Curr Pharm Des* 9: 1239–1255.

59. Bounous, G. (2000). Whey protein concentrate (WPC) and glutathione modulation in cancer treatment. *Anticancer Res* 20: 4785–4792.

60. Zemel, M. (2003). Calcium modulation of adiposity. *Obes Res* 11: 375–376.

61. Zemel, M.B. (2005). Calcium and dairy modulation of obesity risk. *Obes Res* 13: 192–193.

62. Zemel, M.B. (2005). The role of dairy foods in weight management. *J Am Coll Nutr* 24: 537S–546S.

63. Zemel, M.B., Richards, J., Milstead, A., and Campbell, P. (2005). Effects of calcium and dairy on body composition and weight loss in African-American adults. *Obes Res* 13: 1218–1225.

64. Haub, M.D., Simons, T.R., Cook, C.M., Remig, V.M., Al-Tamimi, E.K., and Holcomb, C.A. (2005). Calcium-fortified beverage supplementation on body composition in postmenopausal women. *Nutr J* 4: 21.

65. Barr, S.I., McCarron, D.A., Heaney, R.P., Dawson-Hughes, B., Berga, S.L., Stern, J.S., and Oparil, S. (2000). Effects of increased consumption of fluid milk on energy and nutrient intake, body weight, and cardiovascular risk factors in healthy older adults. *J Am Diet Assoc* 100: 810–817.

66. Beer, W.H., Murray, E., Oh, S.H., Pedersen, H.E., Wolfe, R.R., and Young, V.R. (1989). A long-term metabolic study to assess the nutritional value of and immunological tolerance to two soy-protein concentrates in adult humans. *Am J Clin Nutr* 50: 997–1007.

67. Istfan, N., Murray, E., Janghorbani, M., Evans, W.J. and Young, V.R. (1983). The nutritional value of a soy protein concentrate (STAPRO-3200) for long-term protein nutritional maintenance in young men. *J Nutr* 113: 2524–2534.

68. Istfan, N., Murray, E., Janghorbani, M., and Young, V.R. (1983). An evaluation of the nutritional value of a soy protein concentrate in young adult men using the short-term N-balance method. *J Nutr* 113: 2516–2523.

69. Scrimshaw, N.S., Wayler, A.H., Murray, E., Steinke, F.H., Rand, W.M., and Young, V.R. (1983). Nitrogen balance response in young men given one of two isolated soy proteins or milk proteins. *J Nutr* 113: 2492–2497.

70. Wayler, A., Queiroz, E., Scrimshaw, N.S., Steinke, F.H., Rand, W.M., and Young, V.R. (1983). Nitrogen balance studies in young men to assess the protein quality of an isolated soy protein in relation to meat proteins. *J Nutr* 113: 2485–2491.

71. Young, V.R., Puig, M., Queiroz, E., Scrimshaw, N.S., and Rand, W.M. (1984). Evaluation of the protein quality of an isolated soy protein in young men: relative nitrogen requirements and effect of methionine supplementation. *Am J Clin Nutr* 39: 16–24.

72. Young, V.R., Scrimshaw, N.S., Torun, B., and Viteri, F. (1979). Soybean protein in human nutrition: an overview. *J Am Oil Chem Soc* 56: 110–120.

73. Young, V.R., Wayler, A., Garza, C., Steinke, F.H., Murray, E., Rand, W.M., and Scrimshaw, N.S. (1984). A long-term metabolic balance study in young men to assess the nutritional quality of an isolated soy protein and beef proteins. *Am J Clin Nutr* 39: 8–15.

74. Banz, W.J., Maher, M.A., Thompson, W.G., Bassett, D.R., Moore, W., Ashraf, M., Keefer, D.J., and Zemel, M.B. (2003). Effects of resistance versus aerobic training on coronary artery disease risk factors. *Exp Biol Med* (Maywood) 228: 434–440.

75. Anderson, J.W., Johnstone, B.M., and Cook-Newell, M.E. (1995). Meta-analysis of the effects of soy protein intake on serum lipids. *N Engl J Med* 333: 276–282.

76. Weggemans, R.M. and Trautwein, E.A. (2003). Relation between soy-associated isoflavones and LDL and HDL cholesterol concentrations in humans: a meta-analysis. *Eur J Clin Nutr* 57: 940–946.

77. Haub, M.D., Wells, A.M., and Campbell, W.W. (2005). Beef and soy-based food supplements differentially affect serum lipoprotein-lipid profiles because of changes in carbohydrate intake and novel nutrient intake ratios in older men who resistive-train. *Metabolism* 54: 769–774.

78. Keinan-Boker, L., van Der Schouw, Y.T., Grobbee, D.E., and Peeters, P.H. (2004). Dietary phytoestrogens and breast cancer risk. *Am J Clin Nutr* 79: 282–288.

79. Linseisen, J., Piller, R., Hermann, S., and Chang-Claude, J. (2004). Dietary phy-toestrogen intake and premenopausal breast cancer risk in a German case-control study. *Int J Cancer* 110: 284–290.

80. Magee, P.J. and Rowland, I.R. (2004). Phyto-oestrogens, their mechanism of action: current evidence for a role in breast and prostate cancer. *Br J Nutr* 91: 513–531.

81. McMichael-Phillips, D.F., Harding, C., Morton, M., Roberts, S.A., Howell, A., Potten, C.S., and Bundred, N.J. (1998). Effects of soy-protein supplementation on epithelial proliferation in the histologically normal human breast. *Am J Clin Nutr* 68: 1431S–1435S.

82. Murata, M., Midorikawa, K., Koh, M., Umezawa, K., and Kawanishi, S. (2004). Genistein and daidzein induce cell proliferation and their metabolites cause oxidative DNA damage in relation to isoflavone-induced cancer of estrogen-sensitive organs. *Biochemistry* 43: 2569–2577.

9 Creatine

Richard B. Kreider

CONTENTS

9.1 INTRODUCTION

Creatine has become one of the most extensively studied and scientifically validated nutritional ergogenic aids for athletes. Additionally, creatine has been evaluated as a potential therapeutic agent in a variety of medical conditions. In terms of exercise, the energy supplied to rephosphorylate adenosine diphosphate (ADP) to adenosine triphosphate (ATP) during and following intense exercise is dependent to a large degree on the amount of phosphocreatine (PCr) stored in the muscle.[1,2] As PCr stores become depleted during intense exercise, energy availability deteriorates due to the inability to resynthesize ATP at the rate required.[1,2] Consequently, the ability to maintain maximal-effort exercise declines. Since the availability of PCr in the muscle may significantly influence the amount of energy generated during brief periods of high-intensity exercise, it has been hypothesized that increasing muscle creatine content via creatine supplementation may increase the availability of PCr and allow for an accelerated rate of resynthesis of ATP during and following high-intensity, short-duration exercises.[1–7] Theoretically, creatine supplementation during training may lead to greater training adaptations due to an enhanced quality and volume of work performed. In terms of potential medical applications, creatine is intimately involved in a number of metabolic pathways. Creatine deficiencies or lack of creatine availability has also been identified as a limiting factor in the pathology of a number of neurological and chronic diseases. For this reason, medical researchers have been investigating the potential therapeutic role of creatine supplementation in a variety of patient populations. The purpose of this chapter is to provide an overview of the available literature regarding the effects of creatine supplementation on muscle bioenergetics and training adaptations, potential medical uses of creatine, and medical safety of creatine.

9.2 REVIEW OF LITERATURE

9.2.1 CHEMICAL STRUCTURE AND SYNTHESIS

Creatine is an amino acid derivative synthesized from arginine, glycine, and methionine in the kidneys, liver, and pancreas (see Figure 9.1).[4,8] The metabolic fate of creatine is conversion to creatinine and excretion in the urine.[4]

9.2.2 BODY RESERVES

Approximately 95% of creatine is stored in the muscle. There is also a small amount of creatine (~5%) found in the brain and testes.[3,9] About two thirds of the creatine found in the muscle is stored as phosphocreatine (PCr), while the remaining amount

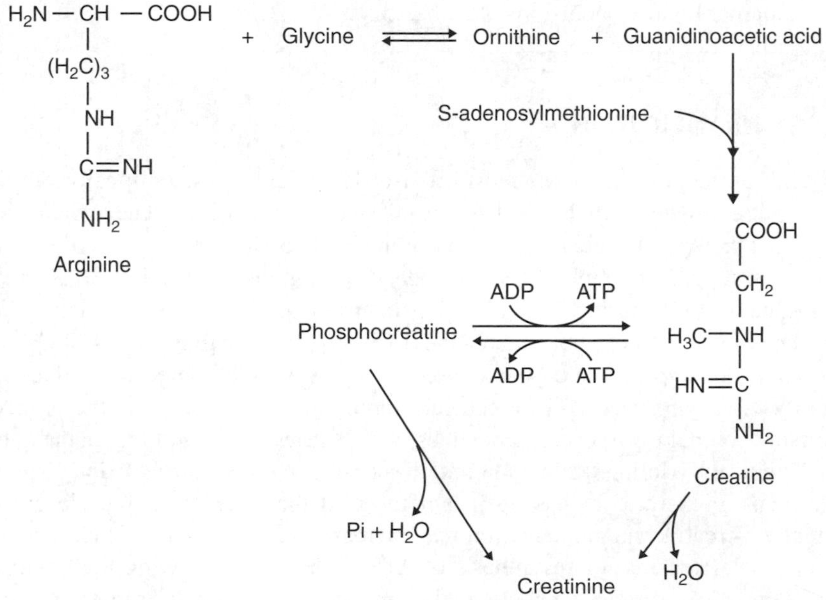

FIGURE 9.1 Chemical structure and biochemical pathway for creatine and creatinine synthesis. (From Paddon-Jones, D. et al., *J. Nutr.*, 134, 2888S–2894S, 2004.)

is stored as free creatine.[2] The total creatine pool (PCr + free creatine) in the muscle averages about 120 g for a 70-kg individual. However, the body has the capacity to store up to 160 g of creatine under certain conditions.[4,9] The body breaks down about 1 to 2% of the creatine pool per day (about 1 to 2 g/day) into creatinine in the muscle. The creatinine is then excreted in urine.[10] Creatine stores can be replenished by obtaining creatine in the diet or through endogenous synthesis of creatine from glycine, arginine, and methionine.[11,12] Normal dietary intake of creatine from food and creatine synthesis typically maintains creatine levels at about 120 g for a normal-size individual.[11,12] Vegetarians have been reported to have lower than normal muscle creatine stores.[13] Additionally, some people have been found to have creatine synthesis deficiencies, and therefore must depend on dietary or supplemental creatine intake to maintain normal muscle concentrations.[14,15]

9.2.3 DIETARY SOURCES

Table 9.1 presents a list of foods that contain relatively large amounts of creatine. Most dietary creatine is obtained from meat and fish. For example, there is about 1 to 2 g of creatine in a pound of uncooked beef and salmon.[3] Creatine can also be obtained in the diet from a number of dietary supplements. Since large amounts of fish and meat must be consumed in order to obtain gram quantities of creatine, dietary supplementation of creatine provides an inexpensive and efficient means of increasing dietary availability of creatine without excessive fat or protein intake.

TABLE 9.1
Creatine Content in
Selected Foods

Food	Creatine Content	
	g/lb	g/kg
Shrimp	Trace	Trace
Cod	1.4	3
Tuna	1.8	4
Salmon	2	4.5
Herring	3–4.5	6.5–10
Beef	2	4.5
Pork	2.3	5
Cranberries	0.01	0.02
Milk	0.05	0.1

Adapted from Balsom, P.D. et al., *Sports Med.*, 18, 268–280, 1994.

9.2.4 SUPPLEMENTATION PROTOCOLS

Sidebar 9.1 summarizes the various creatine supplementation protocols that have been studied over recent years. Most studies that have evaluated the effects of creatine monohydrate supplementation have utilized a creatine loading technique. This has typically involved ingesting 20 g/day of creatine (divided into four 5-g doses ingested throughout the day) for 5 to 7 days. More recently, researchers have suggested ingesting relative amounts of creatine (i.e., 0.3 g/kg/day), which would provide 15 to 30 g/day of creatine for 50- to 100-kg individuals.[5,12,16] Studies show that this protocol can increase muscle creatine and PCr by 10 to 40%.[5,16] Once muscle creatine stores are elevated, research indicates that you only need to ingest 3 to 5 g of creatine per day to maintain elevated creatine stores. Cessation of creatine maintenance doses after loading typically allows for creatine stores to return to normal within 4 to 6 weeks after loading. More recent studies indicate that it may only take 2 to 3 days to maximize creatine stores, particularly if creatine is ingested with carbohydrate or protein.[5,17,18] Additionally, a dose of 0.25 g/kg of fat-free mass (FFM) per day during the loading phase may be a sufficient method of increasing muscle creatine stores.[13] An alternative supplementation protocol is to ingest 3 g/day of creatine monohydrate for 28 days.[9] Studies show that this method can increase muscle concentrations of creatine as effectively as creatine loading techniques. However, this method would only result in a gradual increase in muscle creatine content compared to the more rapid loading method, and therefore may not promote as quick of an ergogenic benefit. Willoughby and Rosene[19,20] reported that 6 g/day of creatine during 12 weeks of resistance training was sufficient to promote positive changes in strength and muscle mass. Some athletes also cycle on and off creatine by taking loading doses of creatine monohydrate for 3 to 5 days every 3 to 4 weeks during training.[12,16] Theoretically, since it takes 4 to 6 weeks for elevated creatine stores to return to baseline, this protocol would be effective in increasing and maintaining elevated creatine stores over time.[12]

Sidebar 9.1: Creatine Supplementation Protocols

- Loading/Maintenance Protocol
  - Ingest 20 g/day divided into four equal doses for 5 to 7 days.
  - Ingest 0.3 g/kg/day (15 to 30 g/day for 50- to 100-kg individuals) for 5 to 7 days.
  - Ingest 0.25 g/kg of FFM per day for 5 to 7 days.
  - Ingest 3 to 5 g/day or 0.03 g/kg/day to maintain elevated stores.
- Low-Dose Protocol
  - Ingest 3 to 6 g/day during training.
- Cycling Protocol
  - Load/maintain during training and reduce/abstain between training periods.

9.2.5 Effects of Creatine Supplementation on Muscle Creatine Stores

Numerous studies indicate that dietary supplementation of creatine monohydrate increases muscle creatine and phosphocreatine content by 10 to 40%.[9,16] In simple terms, one can think of the normal creatine content of the muscle (about 120 g) as a gas tank that is normally about three fourths full. Creatine supplementation typically allows an individual to fill up his creatine storage tank up to 150 to 160 g (i.e., 20 to 30%). It should be noted that the amount of creatine retained in the muscle following creatine supplementation depends on the amount of creatine in the muscle before supplementation. Individuals with low creatine content in muscle prior to supplementation may increase creatine stores by 20 to 40%, while individuals with relatively high creatine levels before supplementation may experience only a 10 to 20% increase in muscle creatine content. Performance changes in response to creatine supplementation have been correlated with the magnitude of increase in muscle creatine levels.[21,22] Differences in intrasubject creatine retention have been described as creatine responders and non-responders. Subsequent research has shown that ingestion of creatine (5 g) with carbohydrate (20 to 95 g) or with 50 to 60 g carbohydrate and protein helps all subjects maximize creatine stores.[17,18,23,24] Once creatine levels are elevated and an individual stops taking creatine, studies indicate it may take 4 to 6 weeks before creatine levels return to baseline.[25,26] There is no evidence that muscle creatine levels fall below baseline after cessation of creatine supplementation, which might suggest a long-term suppression of endogenous creatine synthesis.[16,26,27]

9.2.6 Metabolic Role of Creatine

Most research on creatine has evaluated the effects of creatine supplementation on the content of high-energy phosphates within muscle and its role on exercise capacity and recovery following intense exercise that is dependent on the phosphagen energy system.[12,28] However, recent attention has also been paid to the role of creatine supplementation on creatine kinases (CKs) in muscle as well as the transfer of high-energy phosphates within the cell via what has been called the creatine phosphate shuttle[29–31] (Figure 9.2). CK is an important cellular enzyme that facilitates energy transduction in muscle cells by catalyzing the reversible transfer of a phosphate moiety between ATP and PCr.[32] There are several isoforms of CK which work simultaneously to form a rapid interconversion of PCr and ATP. In this regard, CK is composed of two subunit types, including M (muscle) and B (brain), with three isoenzymes, MM-CK, MB-CK, and BB-CK. In addition, a fourth CK isoenzyme (Mi-CK) is located on the outer side of the inner mitochondrial membrane.[32–34] CK activity is greatest in skeletal muscle and CK in the muscle exists almost exclusively in the MM form. MM-CK (also referred to as myofibrillar CK) is bound to the myofibrils and localized to the A-bands as well as distributed across the entire filament. MM-CK generates ATP from ADP. Mi-CK is found on the outer surface of the inner mitochondrial membrane and is functionally coupled to oxidative phosphorylation. Mi-CK, at the site of oxidative mitochondrial ATP generation, catalyzes the phosphorylation of creatine to PCr.[32–34] Fast-twitch fibers have greater

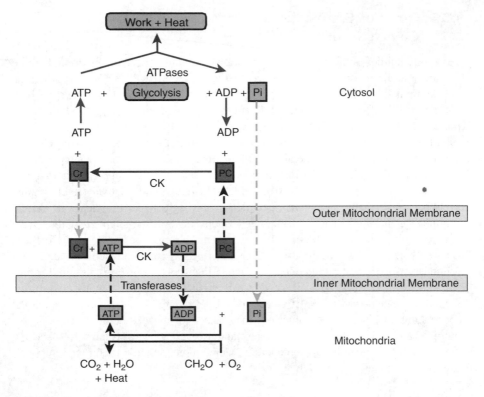

FIGURE 9.2 Basic diagram of the creatine phosphate shuttle.

CK activity, containing large amounts of MM-CK, than slow-twitch oxidative fibers, but the latter have a higher percentage of Mi-CK.[32–35] Recent studies suggest that dietary and muscle availability of creatine may influence CK activity in various healthy and diseased populations.[20,31,36–41]

From an ergogenic viewpoint, resynthesis of PCr could be the critical factor during sustained very high intensity exercise. Although the mechanisms are not clearly understood, a creatine phosphate shuttle may be the functional mechanism.[34,42] In addition to its role as an energy buffer, it has been proposed that the CK-PCr system functions in energy transport on the basis of the functional and physical association of CK isoenzymes with subcellular sites of ATP production and hydrolysis. In the creatine phosphate shuttle concept, PCr and Cr act as shuttle molecules between these sites.[35] One proposed shuttle is believed to be functionally coupled to glycolysis,[35] but others believe that the rapid resynthesis of PCr is likely to be oxidative in origin.[32,43,44] Mi-CK promotes the formation of PCr from creatine and from ATP formed via oxidative metabolism in the mitochondria.[34] van Deursen and others[35] note that PCr is presumed to diffuse from the mitochondria to the myofibrillar M-band, where it locally serves to replenish ATP with MM-CK as a catalyzing agent. Finally, Cr diffuses back to sites of ATP synthesis for rephosphorylation. The potential role of modulating CK activity and the shuttling of adenine nucleotides for synthesis and use have prompted a significant amount of research evaluating the potential clinical uses of creatine, as described in the following. Additionally, since creatine appears to play a role in shuttling of ATP from the mitochondria to the cytosol, it may also be involved in enhancing high-intensity aerobic exercise capacity.[31,34] Finally, creatine has been shown to have an important role in maintaining brain function and protecting neural activity in the brain following injury.[41,45–47]

9.2.7 THEORETICAL ERGOGENIC BENEFITS OF CREATINE SUPPLEMENTATION

Table 9.2 lists the types of exercise and sports that creatine supplementation has been suggested to influence, while Sidebar 9.2 lists the reported ergogenic benefits of creatine supplementation. Increasing muscle availability of creatine and PCr can affect exercise and training adaptations in several ways. First, increasing the availability of PCr in the muscle may help maintain availability of energy during high-intensity exercise like sprinting and intense weight lifting. Second, increasing the availability of PCr may help speed recovery between sprints or bouts of intense exercise. These adaptations would allow an athlete to do more work over a series of sprints or sets of exercise, theoretically leading to greater gains in strength, muscle mass, or performance over time. For this reason, creatine supplementation has primarily been recommended as an ergogenic aid for power/strength athletes or patients who need to increase strength, power, or maintain muscle mass. However, recent research indicates that endurance athletes may also benefit from creatine supplementation. In this regard, studies indicate creatine loading prior to carbohydrate loading promotes greater glycogen retention.[48] Additionally, studies indicate that ingesting creatine with carbohydrate during carbohydrate loading promotes greater creatine and glycogen retention.[18,49–51] Theoretically, this may improve glycogen availability for endurance athletes. Creatine has also been shown to improve repetitive sprint performance. Since endurance athletes employ interval training techniques in an attempt to improve speed and anaerobic threshold, creatine supplementation during training may improve interval training adaptations leading to improved performance. Finally, studies also indicate that creatine supplementation can help maintain body weight and muscle mass during training.[25,28,52–55] Since many endurance athletes have difficulty maintaining body mass during training, creatine supplementation may help maintain optimal body composition.

Sidebar 9.2: Potential Ergogenic Benefits of Creatine Supplementation

- Increased muscle mass and strength
- Increased single and repetitive sprint performance
- Enhanced glycogen synthesis
- Possible enhancement of aerobic capacity via greater shuttling of ATP from mitochondria and buffering of acidity
- Increased work capacity
- Enhanced recovery
- Greater training tolerance

TABLE 9.2
Examples of Sports Performance Theoretically Enhanced by Creatine Supplementation

Increased PCr
   Track sprints: 100, 200 m
   Swim sprints: 50 m
   Pursuit cycling
Increased PCr resynthesis
   Basketball
   Field hockey
   Football (American)
   Ice hockey
   Lacrosse
   Volleyball
Reduced muscle acidosis
   Downhill skiing
   Rowing
   Swim events: 100, 200 m
   Track events: 400, 800 m
Oxidative metabolism
   Basketball
   Soccer
   Team handball
   Tennis
   Volleyball
   Interval training in endurance athletes
Enhanced training
   Most sports
   Increased body mass/muscle mass
Bodybuilding
   Football (American, Australian)
   Heavyweight wrestling
   Power lifting
   Rugby
   Track/field events (shot put, javelin, discus)
   Weight lifting

Adapted from Williams, M.H. et al., *Creatine: The Power Supplement*, Human Kinetics Publishers, Champaign, IL, 1999.

9.2.8 EFFECTS OF CREATINE ON EXERCISE PERFORMANCE AND TRAINING ADAPTATIONS

As of this writing, there have been over 1000 articles published in the peer-reviewed scientific literature on creatine supplementation. Slightly over half of these studies have evaluated the effects of creatine supplementation on exercise performance. The majority of these studies (about 70%) indicate that creatine supplementation promotes a statistically significant improvement in exercise capacity.[28] This means that 95 times out of 100, if you take creatine as described in the study, you will experience a significant improvement in exercise performance. The average gain in performance from these studies typically ranges between 10 and 15%. For example, short-term creatine supplementation has been reported to improve maximal power/strength (5 to 15%), work performed during sets of maximal effort muscle contractions (5 to 15%), single-effort sprint performance (1 to 5%), and work performed during repetitive sprint performance (5 to 15%).[28] Long-term creatine supplementation appears to enhance the quality of training, generally leading to 5 to 15% greater gains in strength and performance.[28] Nearly all studies indicate that creatine supplementation increases body mass by about 1 to 2 kg in the first week of loading.[28] In training studies, subjects taking creatine typically gain about twice as much body mass or FFM (i.e., an extra 2 to 4 pounds of muscle mass during 4 to 12 weeks of training) than subjects taking a placebo. No study has reported that creatine supplementation significantly impairs exercise capacity, although some have suggested that weight gain may potentially impair performance in swimming or running. Although all studies do not report significant results, the preponderance of scientific evidence indicates that creatine supplementation appears to be an effective nutritional ergogenic aid for a variety of exercise tasks in a number of athletic and clinical populations.[12,28] The following highlights some of the recent research that has evaluated the effects of short- and long-term creatine supplementation on exercise performance and training adaptations.

9.2.8.1 Short-Term Supplementation

Numerous studies have been conducted to evaluate the effects of short-term creatine supplementation (3 to 7 days) on exercise performance. For example, Volek and colleagues[56] reported that creatine supplementation (25 g/day for 7 days) resulted in a significant increase in the amount of work performed during five sets of bench press and jump squats in comparison to a placebo group. Tarnopolsky and MacLennan[57] reported that creatine supplementation (20 g/day × 4 days) increased peak cycling power, dorsi-flexion maximal voluntary contraction (MVC) torque, and lactate in men and women with no apparent gender effects. Moreover, Wiroth and colleagues[58] reported that creatine supplementation (15 g/day × 5 days) significantly improved maximal power and work performed during 5 × 10 sec cycling sprints with 60-sec rest recovery in younger and older subjects.

Creatine supplementation has also been shown to improve exercise performance during various sport activities. For example, Skare and associates[59] reported that creatine supplementation (20 g/day) decreased 100-m sprint times and reduced the total time of 6 × 60 m sprints in a group of well-trained adolescent competitive runners. Mujika and colleagues[60] reported that creatine supplementation (20 g/day × 6 days) improved repeated sprint performance (6 × 15 m sprints with 30-sec recovery) and limited the decay in jumping ability in 17 highly trained soccer players. Similarly, Ostojic[61] reported that creatine supplementation (30 g/day for 7 days) improved soccer-specific skill performance in young soccer players. Theodorou et al.[62] reported that creatine supplementation (25 g/day × 4 days) significantly improved mean interval performance times in 22 elite swimmers. Mero and colleagues[63] reported that supplementation of creatine (20 g/day) for 6 days combined with sodium bicarbonate (0.3 g/kg) ingestion 2 h prior to exercise significantly improved 2 × 100 m swim performance. Finally, Preen and associates[64] evaluated the effects of ingesting creatine (20 g/day × 5 days) on resting and post-exercise creatine and PCr content as well as performance of an 80-min intermittent sprint test (10 sets of 5 or 6 × 6-sec sprints with varying recovery intervals). The authors reported that creatine increased resting and post-exercise creatine and PCr content, mean work performed, and total work performed during 6 × 6 sec sets with 54- and 84-sec recovery. In addition, work performed during 5 × 6 sec sprints with 24-sec recovery tended to be greater. While not all studies report significant effects from creatine supplementation, these findings and many others indicate that creatine supplementation can significantly improve performance of athletes in a variety of sport-related field activities.

9.2.8.2 Long-Term Supplementation

Theoretically, increasing the ability to perform high-intensity exercise may lead to greater training adaptations over time. Consequently, a number of studies have evaluated the effects of creatine supplementation on training adaptations. For example, Vandenberghe et al.[25] reported that in comparison to a placebo group, creatine supplementation (20 g/day × 4 days; 5 g/day × 65 days) during 10 weeks of training in women increased total creatine and PCr content, maximal strength (20 to 25%), maximal intermittent exercise capacity of the arm flexors (10 to 25%), and FFM by 60%. In addition, the researchers reported that creatine supplementation during 10 weeks of detraining helped maintain training adaptations to a greater degree. Noonan and collaborators[65] reported that creatine supplementation (20 g/day × 5 days; 0.1 or 0.3 g/kg/day of FFM × 51 days) in conjunction with resistance and speed/agility training significantly improved 40-yard dash time and bench press strength in 39 college athletes. Kreider and associates[54] reported that creatine supplementation (15.75 g/day × 28 days) during off-season college football training promoted greater gains in FFM and repetitive sprint performance in comparison to subjects ingesting a placebo. Likewise, Stone et al.[53] reported that 5 weeks of creatine ingestion (~10 or 20 g/day with and without pyruvate) promoted significantly greater increases in body mass, FFM, 1 RM bench press, combined 1 RM squat and bench press, vertical jump power output, and peak rate of force development during in-season training in 42 Division IAA college football players.

Volek and co-workers[52] reported that 12 weeks of creatine supplementation (25 g/day × 7 days; 5 g/day × 77 days) during periodized resistance training increased muscle total creatine and PC, FFM, types I, IIa, and IIb muscle fiber diameter, bench press and squat 1 RM, and lifting volume (weeks 5 to 8) in 19 resistance trained athletes. Kirksey and colleagues[66] found that creatine supplementation (0.3 g/kg/day × 42 days) during off-season training promoted greater gains in vertical jump height and power, sprint cycling performance, and FFM in 36 Division IAA male and female track and field athletes. Moreover, Jones and collaborators[67] reported that creatine (20 g/day × 5 days; 5 g/day × 10 weeks) promoted greater gains in sprint performance (5 × 15 sec with 15-sec recovery) and average on-ice sprint performance (6 × 80 m sprints) in 16 elite ice hockey players. Interestingly, Jowko et al.[68] reported that creatine supplementation (20 g/day × 7 days; 10 g/day × 14 days) significantly increased FFM and cumulative strength gains during training in 40 subjects initiating training. Additional gains were observed when 3 g/day of calcium beta-hydroxy-beta-methylbutyrate (HMB) was co-ingested with creatine. Finally, Willoughby and Rosene[19] reported that in comparison to controls, creatine supplementation (6 g/day × 12 weeks) during resistance training (6 to 8 repetitions at 85 to 90% × 3 weeks) significantly increased total body mass, FFM, and thigh volume, 1 RM strength, myofibrillar protein content, types I, IIa, and IIx myosin heavy-chain (MHC) mRNA expression, and MHC protein expression. In a subsequent paper, Willoughby and Rosene[20] reported that Cr supplementation (6 g/day × 12 weeks) increased M-CK mRNA expression apparently due to increases in the expression of myogenin and MRF-4. The researchers concluded that increases in myogenin and MRF-4 mRNA and protein may play a role in increasing myosin heavy-chain expression. These data indicate that creatine supplementation can directly influence muscle protein synthesis. Collectively, these studies and others provide strong evidence that creatine supplementation during intense resistance training leads to greater gains in strength and muscle mass.

9.2.9 POTENTIAL THERAPEUTIC USES OF CREATINE

Creatine and creatine phosphate are involved in numerous metabolic processes. Creatine synthesis deficiencies and abnormal availability of creatine and PCr have been reported to cause a number of medical problems. For this reason, the potential medical uses of creatine have been investigated since the mid-1970s. Initially, research focused on the role of creatine and creatine phosphate in reducing heart arrhythmias and improving heart function during ischemia events (i.e., lack of oxygen).[12] Initial studies also evaluated the effects of treating various medical populations who had creatine deficiencies (i.e., gyrate atrophy,[69–72] infants and children with low levels of PCr in the brain,[73–75] etc.). Interest in the potential medical uses of creatine has increased over the last 10 years. Researchers have been particularly interested in determining whether creatine supplementation may reduce rates of atrophy or muscle wasting, speed the rate of recovery from musculoskeletal and spinal cord injuries, and improve strength and muscle endurance in patients with various neuromuscular diseases.[12,16] For example, researchers have been evaluating whether creatine supplementation may improve clinical outcomes in patients with brain or spinal cord injuries,[47,76–79] muscular dystrophy,[40,80,81] myophathies,[38,82–85] Huntington's disease,[41,45,86,87] amyotrophic lateral sclerosis or Lou Gehrig's disease,[88–91] arthritis,[92] diabetes,[93] high cholesterol and triglyceride levels,[54,94] and elevated homocysteine levels.[95–98] Other studies have reported that creatine supplementation during training reduces injury rates in athletes[99–103] and allows athletes to tolerate intensified training to a greater degree.[104] Although more research is needed, some promising results have been reported in a number of clinically related studies, suggesting that creatine may have therapeutic benefits in certain patient populations.

9.2.10 MEDICAL SAFETY OF CREATINE

The only clinically significant side effect that has been consistently reported in the scientific and medical literature from creatine supplementation has been weight gain.[12,16,105] However, there have been a number of anecdotally reported side effects in the popular literature, such as gastrointestinal distress, muscle cramping, dehydration, and increased risk to musculoskeletal injury (i.e., muscle strains/pulls). Additionally, there has also been concern that short- or long-term creatine supplementation may increase renal stress or adversely affect the muscles, liver, or other organs of the body. One research group suggested that creatine supplementation may increase anterior compartment pressure in the leg, thereby increasing an individual's risk to developing anterior compartment syndrome (ACS).[106–109] Over the last few years, a number of studies have attempted to assess the medical safety of creatine. These studies indicate that creatine is not associated with any of these anecdotally reported problems, nor does it increase the likelihood of development of ACS.[100,110–118] In fact, there is recent evidence that creatine may lessen heat stress and reduce the susceptibility to musculoskeletal injuries among athletes engaged in training.[102,117,118] While people who take creatine may experience some of these problems, the incidence of occurrence in creatine users does not appear to be greater than subjects who take placebos, and in some cases has been reported to be less.[111]

Another concern that has been expressed is whether there are any long-term side effects of creatine supplementation. Athletes have been using creatine as a nutritional supplement since the mid-1960s. Widespread use as a dietary supplement began in the early 1990s. No clinically significant and reproducible side effects directly attributable to creatine supplementation have been reported in the scientific literature. Nevertheless, there are some concerns about the long-term side effects of creatine supplementation. Over the last few years, a number of researchers have begun to report long-term safety data on creatine supplementation. So far, no long-term side effects have been observed in athletes (up to 5 years), infants with creatine synthesis deficiency (up to 3 years), or in patient populations (up to 5 years).[12,111,112,115,116] One cohort of patients taking 1.5 to 3 g/day of creatine has been monitored since 1981 with no significant side effects.[69,70] Conversely, research has demonstrated a number of potentially helpful clinical uses of creatine in heart patients, infants and patients with creatine synthesis efficiency, patients suffering orthopedic injury, and patients with various neuromuscular diseases. Consequently, all available evidence suggests that creatine supplementation appears to be safe when taken within recommended guidelines.

9.2.11 ETHICAL CONSIDERATIONS

Several athletic governing bodies and special interest groups have questioned whether it is ethical for athletes to take creatine as a method of enhancing performance. Their rationale is that since studies indicate that creatine can improve performance and it would be difficult to ingest enough food in the diet alone to creatine load, that it is unethical to do so. Others argue that if you allow athletes to take creatine, they may be more predisposed to try other dangerous supplements or drugs. Still others have attempted to lump creatine in with anabolic steroids or banned stimulants and have called for a ban on the use of creatine and other supplements among athletes. Finally, fresh off of the ban of dietary supplements containing ephedra, some have called for a ban on the sale of creatine citing safety concerns. Creatine supplementation is not currently banned by any athletic organization, although the NCAA does not allow institutions to provide creatine or other muscle-building supplements to their athletes (e.g., protein, amino acids, HMB, etc). The International Olympic Committee considered these arguments and ruled that since creatine is readily found in meat and fish and there is no valid test to determine whether some athletes are taking creatine or not, there was no need to ban it. In my view, creatine loading is no different than carbohydrate loading. Many athletes ingest high-calorie concentrated-carbohydrate drinks in an effort to increase muscle glycogen stores or supplement their diet. If carbohydrate loading is not a banned practice, then creatine loading should not be banned. This is particularly true when one considers that creatine supplementation has been reported to decrease the incidence of musculoskeletal injuries,[99,100,112,119] heat stress,[99,117,118] provide neuroprotective effects,[37,45,47,76,78] and expedite rehabilitation from injury.[79,89,120] It could be argued that not allowing athletes to take creatine may actually increase the risk of athletic competition.

9.3 SUMMARY AND CONCLUSIONS

Creatine remains one of the most extensively studied nutritional ergogenic aids available for athletes. Hundreds of studies have reported that increasing muscle creatine stores through creatine supplementation can augment muscle creatine content, improve exercise and training adaptations, and provide some therapeutic benefit to some clinical populations. Consequently, creatine represents one of the most effective and popular nutritional ergogenic aids available for athletes. The future of creatine research is very promising. Researchers are attempting to determine ways to maximize creatine storage in the muscle, which types of exercise may obtain the greatest benefit from creatine supplementation, the potential medical uses of creatine, and the long-term safety and efficacy of creatine supplementation. Among these, the most promising area of research is determining the potential medical uses of creatine, particularly in patients with creatine synthesis deficiencies or neuromuscular diseases, or prevention of sarcopenia. Nevertheless, in regard to athletes, creatine has continually proved itself to be one of the most effective and safe nutritional supplements to increase strength, muscle mass, and performance. This is despite oftentime inaccurate and misleading information that has been written about creatine in the popular media over the last several years. Sidebar 9.3 describes some factors that Williams et al. suggested should be considered before taking creatine.[12] Research since this time has supported these conclusions and recommendations.

Sidebar 9.3: Should Athletes Take Creatine?

After extensively evaluating the literature, Williams et al.[12] concluded the following in their book, *Creatine: The Power Supplement* (available at http://www.humankinetics.com):

- Individuals contemplating creatine supplementation should do so after being informed of potential benefits and risks so that they may make an informed decision.
- Adolescent athletes involved in serious training should consider creatine supplementation only with approval/supervision of parents, trainers, coaches, and/or appropriate health professionals.
- If you plan to take creatine, purchase quality supplements from reputable vendors.
- Athletic administrators in organized sports who desire to establish policies on creatine supplementation for teams should base such policies on the scientific literature. Any formal administration policy should be supervised by a qualified health professional.
- Although more research is needed, available studies indicate that creatine supplementation appears to possess no health risk when taken at recommended doses and may provide therapeutic benefit for various medical populations.

REFERENCES

1. Chanutin, A., The fate of creatine when administered to man. *J Biol Chem*, 67: 29–34, 1926.
2. Hultman, E., J. Bergstrom, L. Spreit, and K. Soderlund, Energy metabolism and fatigue, in *Biochemistry of Exercise VII*, A. Taylor, P.D. Gollnick, and H. Green, Eds. Human Kinetics Publishers, Champaign, IL, 1990, pp. 73–92.
3. Balsom, P.D., K. Soderlund, and B. Ekblom, Creatine in humans with special reference to creatine supplementation. *Sports Med*, 18: 268–280, 1994.
4. Greenhaff, P., The nutritional biochemistry of creatine. *J Nutr Biochem*, 11: 610–618, 1997.
5. Greenhaff, P.L., Muscle creatine loading in humans: procedures and functional and metabolic effects, in *6th Internationl Conference on Guanidino Compounds in Biology and Medicine*. Cincinatti, OH, 2001.
6. Greenhaff, P., A. Casey, and A.L. Green, Creatine supplementation revisited: an update. *Insider*, 4: 1–2, 1996.
7. Harris, R.C., K. Soderlund, and E. Hultman, Elevation of creatine in resting and exercised muscle of normal subjects by creatine supplementation. *Clin Sci* (Colch), 83: 367–374, 1992.
8. Paddon-Jones, D., E. Borsheim, and R.R. Wolfe, Potential ergogenic effects of arginine and creatine supplementation. *J Nutr*, 134: 2888S–28894S, 2004.

9. Hultman, E., K. Soderlund, J.A. Timmons, G. Cederblad, and P.L. Greenhaff, Muscle creatine loading in men. *J Appl Physiol*, 81: 232–237, 1996.

10. Burke, D.G., T. Smith-Palmer, L.E. Holt, B. Head, and P.D. Chilibeck, The effect of 7 days of creatine supplementation on 24-hour urinary creatine excretion. *J Strength Cond Res*, 15: 59–62, 2001.

11. Williams, M.H. and J.D. Branch, Creatine supplementation and exercise performance: an update. *J Am Coll Nutr*, 17: 216–234, 1998.

12. Williams, M.H., R. Kreider, and J.D. Branch, *Creatine: The Power Supplement*. Human Kinetics Publishers, Champaign, IL, 1999, p. 252.

13. Burke, D.G., P.D. Chilibeck, G. Parise, D.G. Candow, D. Mahoney, and M. Tarnopolsky, Effect of creatine and weight training on muscle creatine and performance in vegetarians. *Med Sci Sports Exerc*, 35: 1946–1955, 2003.

14. DeGrauw, T.J., K.C. Cecil, G.S. Salomons, S.J.M. Van Dooren, N.M. Verhoeven, W.S. Ball, and C. Gadobs, The clinical syndrome of creatine transporter deficiency, in *6th Internationl Conference on Guanidino Compounds in Biology and Medicine*. Cincinatti, OH, 2001 (abstract).

15. Stockler, S. and F. Hanefeld, Guanidinoacetate methyltransferase deficiency: a newly recognized inborn error of creatine biosynthesis. *Wiener Klinische Wochenschrift*, 109: 86–88, 1997.

16. Kreider, R.B., B.C. Leutholtz, and M. Greenwood, Creatine, in *Nutritional Ergogenic Aids*, I. Wolinsky and J. Driskell, Eds. CRC Press, Boca Raton, FL, 2004, pp. 81–104.

17. Steenge, G.R., E.J. Simpson, and P.L. Greenhaff, Protein- and carbohydrate-induced augmentation of whole body creatine retention in humans. *J Appl Physiol*, 89: 1165–1171, 2000.

18. Green, A.L., E. Hultman, I.A. Macdonald, D.A. Sewell, and P.L. Greenhaff, Carbohydrate ingestion augments skeletal muscle creatine accumulation during creatine supplementation in humans. *Am J Physiol*, 271 (Pt 1): E821–E826, 1996.

19. Willoughby, D.S. and J. Rosene, Effects of oral creatine and resistance training on myosin heavy chain expression. *Med Sci Sports Exerc*, 33: 1674–1681, 2001.

20. Willoughby, D.S. and J.M. Rosene, Effects of oral creatine and resistance training on myogenic regulatory factor expression. *Med Sci Sports Exerc*, 35: 923–929, 2003.

21. Greenhaff, P.L., A. Casey, A.H. Short, R. Harris, K. Soderlund, and E. Hultman, Influence of oral creatine supplementation of muscle torque during repeated bouts of maximal voluntary exercise in man. *Clin Sci* (Colch), 84: 565–571, 1993.

22. Greenhaff, P.L., K. Bodin, K. Soderlund, and E. Hultman, Effect of oral creatine supplementation on skeletal muscle phosphocreatine resynthesis. *Am J Physiol*, 266 (Pt 1): E725–E730, 1994.

23. Greenwood, M., R.B. Kreider, C. Rasmussen, A.L. Almada, and C.P. Earnest, D-Pinitol augments whole body creatine retention in man. *J Exerc Physiol*, 4: 41–47, 2001 (online).

24. Kreider, R.B., D.S. Willoughby, M. Greenwood, G. Parise, E. Payne, and M.A. Tarnopolsky, Effects of serum creatine supplementation on muscle creatine content. *J Exerc Physiol*, 6: 24–33, 2003 (online).

25. Vandenberghe, K., M. Goris, P. Van Hecke, M. Van Leemputte, L. Vangerven, and P. Hespel, Long-term creatine intake is beneficial to muscle performance during resistance training. *J Appl Physiol*, 83: 2055–2063, 1997.

26. Candow, D.G., P.D. Chilibeck, K.E. Chad, M.J. Chrusch, K.S. Davison, and D.G. Burke, Effect of ceasing creatine supplementation while maintaining resistance training in older men. *J Aging Phys Act*, 12: 219–231, 2004.

27. Kreider, R., M. Greenwood, C. Melton, C. Rasmussen, E. Cantler, P. Milner, and A. Almada, Long-term creatine supplementation during training/competition does not increase perceptions of fatigue or adversely affect health status. *Med Sci Sport Exerc*, 34: S146, 2002.
28. Kreider, R.B., Effects of creatine supplementation on performance and training adaptations. *Mol Cell Biochem*, 244: 89–94, 2003.
29. Wallimann, T., M. Dolder, D. Neumann, and U. Schlattner, Compartmentation, structure, and function of creatine kinases: a rationale for creatine action, in *6th International Conference on Guanidino Compounds in Biology and Medicine*. Cincinatti, OH, 2001 (abstract).
30. Bessman, S. and F. Savabi, The role of phosphocreatine energy shuttle in exercise and muscle hypertrophy, in *Creatine and Creatine Phosphate: Scientific and Clinical Perspectives*, M.A. Conway and J.F. Clark, Eds. Academic Press, San Diego, CA, 1988, pp. 185–198.
31. Wallimann, T., M. Dolder, U. Schlattner, M. Eder, T. Hornemann, E. O'Gorman, A. Ruck, and D. Brdiczka, Some new aspects of creatine kinase (CK): compartmentation, structure, function and regulation for cellular and mitochondrial bioenergetics and physiology. *Biofactors*, 8: 229–234, 1998.
32. Clark, J.F., M.L. Field, and R. Ventura-Clapier, An introduction to the cellular creatine kinase system in contractile tissue, in *Creatine and Creatine Phosphate: Scientific and Clinical Perspectives*, M.A. Conway and J.F. Clark, Eds. Academic Press, San Diego, CA, 996, pp. 51–64.
33. Clark, J.F., Creatine and phosphocreatine: a review of their use in exercise and sport. *J Athl Train*, 32: 45–50, 1997.
34. Ma, T.M., D.L. Friedman, and R. Roberts, Creatine phosphate shuttle pathway in tissues with dynamic energy demand, in *Creatine and Creatine Phosphate: Scientific and Clinical Perspectives*, M.A. Conway and J.F. Clark, Eds. Academic Press, San Diego, CA, 1996, pp. 17–32.
35. van Deursen, J., A. Heerschap, F. Oerlemans, W. Ruitenbeek, P. Jap, H. ter Laak, and B. Weiringa, Skeletal muscles of mice deficient in muscle creatine kinase lack burst activity. *Cell*, 74: 621–631, 1993.
36. Askenasy, N. and A.P. Koretsky, Differential effects of creatine kinase isoenzymes and substrates on regeneration in livers of transgenic mice. *Am J Physiol*, 273 (Pt 1): C741–C746, 1997.
37. Wyss, M. and A. Schulze, Health implications of creatine: can oral creatine supplementation protect against neurological and atherosclerotic disease? *Neuroscience*, 112: 243–260, 2002.
38. Tarnopolsky, M.A., A. Parshad, B. Walzel, U. Schlattner, and T. Wallimann, Creatine transporter and mitochondrial creatine kinase protein content in myopathies. *Muscle Nerve*, 24: 682–688, 2001.
39. Hespel, P., B.O. Eijnde, W. Derave, and E.A. Richter, Creatine supplementation: exploring the role of the creatine kinase/phosphocreatine system in human muscle. *Can J Appl Physiol*, 26 (Suppl): S79–S102, 2001.
40. Felber, S., D. Skladal, M. Wyss, C. Kremser, A. Koller, and W. Sperl, Oral creatine supplementation in Duchenne muscular dystrophy: a clinical and 31P magnetic resonance spectroscopy study. *Neurol Res*, 22: 145–150, 2000.
41. Matthews, R.T., L. Yang, B.G. Jenkins, R.J. Ferrante, B.R. Rosen, R. Kaddurah-Daouk, and M.F. Beal, Neuroprotective effects of creatine and cyclocreatine in animal models of Huntington's disease. *J Neurosci*, 18: 156–163, 1998.

42. Newsholme, E. and I. Beis, Old and new ideas on the roles of phosphagens and the kinases, in *Creatine and Creatine Phosphate: Scientific and Clinical Perspectives*, M.A. Conway and J.F. Clark, Eds. Academic Press, San Diego, CA, 1996, pp. 3–15.

43. Blei, M.L., K.E. Conley, and M.J. Kushmerick, Separate measures of ATP utilization and recovery in human skeletal muscle. *J Physiol*, 465: 203–222, 1993.

44. Radda, G.K., Control of energy metabolism during energy metabolism. *Diabetes*, 45: S88–S92, 1996.

45. Ferrante, R.J., O.A. Andreassen, B.G. Jenkins, A. Dedeoglu, S. Kuemmerle, J.K. Kubilus, R. Kaddurah-Daouk, S.M. Hersch, and M.F. Beal, Neuroprotective effects of creatine in a transgenic mouse model of Huntington's disease. *J Neurosci*, 20: 4389–4397, 2000.

46. Dechent, P., P.J. Pouwels, B. Wilken, F. Hanefeld, and J. Frahm, Increase of total creatine in human brain after oral supplementation of creatine-monohydrate. *Am J Physiol*, 277 (Pt 2): R698–R704, 1999.

47. Hausmann, O.N., K. Fouad, T. Wallimann, and M.E. Schwab, Protective effects of oral creatine supplementation on spinal cord injury in rats. *Spinal Cord*, 40: 449–456, 2002.

48. Nelson, A.G., D.A. Arnall, J. Kokkonen, R. Day, and J. Evans, Muscle glycogen supercompensation is enhanced by prior creatine supplementation. *Med Sci Sports Exerc*, 33: 1096–1100, 2001.

49. van Loon, L.J., R. Murphy, A.M. Oosterlaar, D. Cameron-Smith, M. Hargreaves, A.J. Wagenmakers, and R. Snow, Creatine supplementation increases glycogen storage but not GLUT-4 expression in human skeletal muscle. *Clin Sci (Lond)*, 106: 99–106, 2004.

50. Op't Eijnde, B., E.A. Richter, J.C. Henquin, B. Kiens, and P. Hespel, Effect of creatine supplementation on creatine and glycogen content in rat skeletal muscle. *Acta Physiol Scand*, 171: 169–76, 2001.

51. Kehnder, M., J. Rico-Sanz, G. Kuhne, M. Dambach, R. Buchli, and U. Boutellier, Muscle phosphocreatine and glycogen concentrations in humans after creatine and glucose polymer supplementation measured noninvasively by 31P and 13C-MRS. *Med Sci Sports Exerc*, 30: S264, 1998.

52. Volek, J.S., N.D. Duncan, S.A. Mazzetti, R.S. Staron, M. Putukian, A.L. Gomez, D.R. Pearson, W.J. Fink, and W.J. Kraemer, Performance and muscle fiber adaptations to creatine supplementation and heavy resistance training. *Med Sci Sports Exerc*, 31: 1147–1156, 1999.

53. Stone, M.H., K. Sanborn, L.L. Smith, H.S. O'Bryant, T. Hoke, A.C. Utter, R.L. Johnson, R. Boros, J. Hruby, K.C. Pierce, M.E. Stone, and B. Garner, Effects of in-season (5 weeks) creatine and pyruvate supplementation on anaerobic performance and body composition in American football players. *Int J Sport Nutr*, 9: 146–165, 1999.

54. Kreider, R.B., M. Ferreira, M. Wilson, P. Grindstaff, S. Plisk, J. Reinardy, E. Cantler, and A.L. Almada, Effects of creatine supplementation on body composition, strength, and sprint performance. *Med Sci Sports Exerc*, 30: 73–82, 1998.

55. Earnest, C.P., P. Snell, R. Rodriguez, A. Almada, and T.L. Mitchell, The effect of creatine monohydrate ingestion on anaerobic power indices, muscular strength and body composition. *Acta Physiol Scand*, 153: 207–209, 1995.

56. Volek, J.S., W.J. Kraemer, J.A. Bush, M. Boetes, T. Incledon, K.L. Clark, and J.M. Lynch, Creatine supplementation enhances muscular performance during high-intensity resistance exercise. *J Am Diet Assoc*, 97: 765–770, 1997.

57. Tarnopolsky, M.A. and D.P. MacLennan, Creatine monohydrate supplementation enhances high-intensity exercise performance in males and females. *Int J Sport Nutr Exerc Metab*, 10: 452–463, 2000.

58. Wiroth, J.B., S. Bermon, S. Andrei, E. Dalloz, X. Hebuterne, and C. Dolisi, Effects of oral creatine supplementation on maximal pedalling performance in older adults. *Eur J Appl Physiol*, 84: 533–539, 2001.

59. Skare, O.C., Skadberg, and A.R. Wisnes, Creatine supplementation improves sprint performance in male sprinters. *Scand J Med Sci Sports*, 11: 96–102, 2001.

60. Mujika, I., S. Padilla, J. Ibanez, M. Izquierdo, and E. Gorostiaga, Creatine supplementation and sprint performance in soccer players. *Med Sci Sports Exerc*, 32: 518–525, 2000.

61. Ostojic, S.M., Creatine supplementation in young soccer players. *Int J Sport Nutr Exerc Metab*, 14: 95–103, 2004.

62. Theodorou, A.S., C.B. Cooke, R.F. King, C. Hood, T. Denison, B.G. Wainwright, and K. Havenetidis, The effect of longer-term creatine supplementation on elite swimming performance after an acute creatine loading. *J Sports Sci*, 17: 853–859, 1999.

63. Mero, A.A., K.L. Keskinen, M.T. Malvela, and J.M. Sallinen, Combined creatine and sodium bicarbonate supplementation enhances interval swimming. *J Strength Cond Res*, 18: 306–310, 2004.

64. Preen, D., B. Dawson, C. Goodman, S. Lawrence, J. Beilby, and S. Ching, Effect of creatine loading on long-term sprint exercise performance and metabolism. *Med Sci Sports Exerc*, 33: 814–821, 2001.

65. Noonan, D., K. Berg, R.W. Latin, J.C. Wagner, and K. Reimers, Effects of varying dosages of oral creatine relative to fat free body mass on strength and body composition. *J Strength Cond Res*, 12: 104–108, 1998.

66. Kirksey, K.B., M.H. Stone, B.J. Warren, R.L. Johnson, M. Stone, G. Haff, F.E. Williams, and C. Proulx, The effects of 6 weeks of creatine monohydrate supplementation on performance measures and body composition in collegiate track and field athletes. *J Strength Cond Res*, 13: 148–156, 1999.

67. Jones, A.M., T. Atter, and K.P. Georg, Oral creatine supplementation improves multiple sprint performance in elite ice-hockey players. *J Sports Med Phys Fitness*, 39: 189–196, 1999.

68. Jowko, E., P. Ostaszewski, M. Jank, J. Sacharuk, A. Zieniewicz, J. Wilczak, and S. Nissen, Creatine and beta-hydroxy-beta-methylbutyrate (HMB) additively increase lean body mass and muscle strength during a weight-training program. *Nutrition*, 17: 558–566, 2001.

69. Sipila, I., J. Rapola, O. Simell, and A. Vannas, Supplementary creatine as a treatment for gyrate atrophy of the choroid and retina. *N Engl J Med*, 304: 867–870, 1981.

70. Vannas-Sulonen, K., I. Sipila, A. Vannas, O. Simell, and J. Rapola, Gyrate atrophy of the choroid and retina. A five-year follow-up of creatine supplementation. *Ophthalmology*, 92: 1719–1727, 1985.

71. Heinanen, K., K. Nanto-Salonen, M. Komu, M. Erkintalo, A. Alanen, O.J. Heinonen, K. Pulkki, E. Nikoskelainen, I. Sipila, and O. Simell, Creatine corrects muscle 31P spectrum in gyrate atrophy with hyperornithinaemia. *Eur J Clin Invest*, 29: 1060–1065, 1999.

72. Nanto-Salonen, K., M. Komu, N. Lundbom, K. Heinanen, A. Alanen, I. Sipila, and O. Simell, Reduced brain creatine in gyrate atrophy of the choroid and retina with hyperornithinemia. *Neurology*, 53: 303–307, 1999.

73. Ensenauer, R., T. Thiel, K.O. Schwab, U. Tacke, S. Stockler-Ipsiroglu, A. Schulze, J. Hennig, and W. Lehnert, Guanidinoacetate methyltransferase deficiency: differences of creatine uptake in human brain and muscle. *Mol Genet Metab*, 82: 208–213. 2004.

74. Schulze, A., F. Ebinger, D. Rating, and E. Mayatepek, Improving treatment of guanidinoacetate methyltransferase deficiency: reduction of guanidinoacetic acid in body fluids by arginine restriction and ornithine supplementation. *Mol Genet Metab*, 74: 413–419, 2001.

75. Ganesan, V., A. Johnson, A. Connelly, S. Eckhardt, and R.A. Surtees, Guanidinoacetate methyltransferase deficiency: new clinical features. *Pediatr Neurol*, 17: 155–157, 1997.

76. Zhu, S., M. Li, B.E. Figueroa, A. Liu, I.G. Stavrovskaya, P. Pasinelli, M.F. Beal, R.H. Brown, Jr., B.S. Kristal, R.J. Ferrante, and R.M. Friedlander, Prophylactic creatine administration mediates neuroprotection in cerebral ischemia in mice. *J Neurosci*, 24: 5909–5912, 2004.

77. Brustovetsky, N., T. Brustovetsky, and J.M. Dubinsky, On the mechanisms of neuroprotection by creatine and phosphocreatine. *J Neurochem*, 76: 425–434, 2001.

78. Sullivan, P.G., J.D. Geiger, M.P. Mattson, and S.W. Scheff, Dietary supplement creatine protects against traumatic brain injury. *Ann Neurol*, 48: 723–729, 2000.

79. Jacobs, P.L., E.T. Mahoney, K.A. Cohn, L.F. Sheradsky, and B.A. Green, Oral creatine supplementation enhances upper extremity work capacity in persons with cervical-level spinal cord injury. *Arch Phys Med Rehabil*, 83: 19–23, 2002.

80. Tarnopolsky, M.A., Potential use of creatine monohydrate in muscular dystrophy and neurometabolic disorders, in *6th Internationl Conference on Guanidino Compounds in Biology and Medicine*. Cincinnati, OH, 2001 (abstract).

81. Tarnopolsky, M.A. and G. Parise, Direct measurement of high-energy phosphate compounds in patients with neuromuscular disease. *Muscle Nerve*, 22: 1228–1233, 1999.

82. Zange, J., C. Kornblum, K. Muller, S. Kurtscheid, H. Heck, R. Schroder, T. Grehl, and M. Vorgerd, Creatine supplementation results in elevated phosphocreatine/adenosine triphosphate (ATP) ratios in the calf muscle of athletes but not in patients with myopathies. *Ann Neurol*, 52: 126, 2002; discussion, 1206–1207.

83. Koumis, T., J.P. Nathan, J.M. Rosenberg, and L.A. Cicero, Strategies for the prevention and treatment of statin-induced myopathy: is there a role for ubiquinone supplementation? *Am J Health Syst Pharm*, 61: 515–519, 2004.

84. Borchert, A., E. Wilichowski, and F. Hanefeld, Supplementation with creatine monohydrate in children with mitochondrial encephalomyopathies. *Muscle Nerve*, 22: 1299–1300, 1999.

85. Tarnopolsky, M.A., B.D. Roy, and J.R. MacDonald, A randomized, controlled trial of creatine monohydrate in patients with mitochondrial cytopathies. *Muscle Nerve*, 20: 1502–1509, 1997.

86. Andreassen, O.A., A. Dedeoglu, R.J. Ferrante, B.G. Jenkins, K.L. Ferrante, M. Thomas, A. Friedlich, S.E. Browne, G. Schilling, D.R. Borchelt, S.M. Hersch, C.A. Ross, and M.F. Beal, Creatine increases survival and delays motor symptoms in a transgenic animal model of Huntington's disease. *Neurobiol Dis*, 83: 479–491, 2001.

87. Verbessem, P., J. Lemiere, B.O. Eijnde, S. Swinnen, L. Vanhees, M. Van Leemputte, P. Hespel, and R. Dom, Creatine supplementation in Huntington's disease: a placebo-controlled pilot trial. *Neurology*, 61: 925–930, 2003.

88. Andreassen, O.A., B.G. Jenkins, A. Dedeoglu, K.L. Ferrante, M.B. Bogdanov, R. Kaddurah-Daouk, and M.F. Beal, Increases in cortical glutamate concentrations in transgenic amyotrophic lateral sclerosis mice are attenuated by creatine supplementation. *J Neurochem*, 77: 383–390, 2001.

89. Tarnopolsky, M.A., Potential benefits of creatine monohydrate supplementation in the elderly. *Curr Opin Clin Nutr Metab Care*, 3: 497–502, 2000.

90. Drory, V.E. and D. Gross, No effect of creatine on respiratory distress in amyotrophic lateral sclerosis. *Amyotroph Lateral Scler Other Motor Neuron Disord*, 3: 43–46, 2002.

91. Mazzini, L., C. Balzarini, R. Colombo, G. Mora, I. Pastore, R. De Ambrogio, and M. Caligari, Effects of creatine supplementation on exercise performance and muscular strength in amyotrophic lateral sclerosis: preliminary results. *J Neurol Sci*, 191: 139–144, 2001.

92. Willer, B., G. Stucki, H. Hoppeler, P. Bruhlmann, and S. Krahenbuhl, Effects of creatine supplementation on muscle weakness in patients with rheumatoid arthritis. *Rheumatology* (Oxford), 39: 293–298, 2000.

93. Op't Eijnde, B., B. Urso, E.A. Richter, P.L. Greenhaff, and P. Hespel, Effect of oral creatine supplementation on human muscle GLUT4 protein content after immobilization. *Diabetes*, 50: 18–23, 2001.

94. Earnest, C.P., A. Almada, and T.L. Mitchell, High-performance capillary electrophoresis-pure creatine monohydrate reduced blood lipids in men and women. *Clin Sci*, 91: 113–118, 1996.

95. Brosnan, J.T., R.L. Jacobs, L.M. Stead, S. Ratnam, and M.E. Brosnan, Regulation of homocysteine metabolism: effects of insulin, glucagon and creatine. *FASEB J*, 15(4): A395, 2001.

96. Steenge, G.R., P. Verhoef, and P.L. Greenhaff, The effect of creatine and resistance training on plasma homocysteine concentration in healthy volunteers. *Arch Intern Med*, 161: 1455–1456, 2001.

97. McCarty, M.F., Supplemental creatine may decrease serum homocysteine and abolish the homocysteine 'gender gap' by suppressing endogenous creatine synthesis. *Med Hypotheses*, 56: 5–7, 2001.

98. Taes, Y.E., J.R. Delanghe, A.S. De Vriese, R. Rombaut, J. Van Camp, and N.H. Lameire, Creatine supplementation decreases homocysteine in an animal model of uremia. *Kidney Int*, 64: 1331–1337, 2003.

99. Greenwood, M., R.B. Kreider, C. Melton, C. Rasmussen, S. Lancaster, E. Cantler, P. Milnor, and A. Almada, Creatine supplementation during college football training does not increase the incidence of cramping or injury. *Mol Cell Biochem*, 244: 83–88, 2003.

100. Greenwood, M., R.B. Kreider, L. Greenwood, and A. Byars, Cramping and injury incidence in collegiate football players are reduced by creatine supplementation. *J Athl Train*, 38: 216–219, 2003.

101. Greenwood, M., J. Farris, R. Kreider, L. Greenwood, and A. Byars, Creatine supplementation patterns and perceived effects in select division I collegiate athletes. *Clin J Sport Med*, 10: 191–194, 2000.

102. Greenwood, M., R. Kreider, L. Greenwood, and A. Byars, Creatine supplementation does not increase the incidence of injury or cramping in college baseball players. *J Exerc Physiol*, 6: 16–22, 2003 (online).

103. Ortega Gallo, P.A., F. Dimeo, J. Batista, F. Bazan, L. Betchakian, C. Garcia Cambon, and J. Griffa, Creatine supplementation in soccer players, effects in body composition and incidence of sport-related injuries. *Med Sci Sports Exerc*, 32: S134, 2000.
104. Volek, J.S., N.A. Ratamess, M.R. Rubin, A.L. Gomez, D.N. French, M.M. McGuigan, T.P. Scheett, M.J. Sharman, K. Hakkinen, and W.J. Kraemer, The effects of creatine supplementation on muscular performance and body composition responses to short-term resistance training overreaching. *Eur J Appl Physiol*, 91: 628–637, 2004.
105. Kreider, R., C. Rasmussen, C. Melton, M. Greenwood, T. Stroud, J. Ransom, E. Cantler, P. Milnor, and A.L. Almada, Long-term creatine supplementation does not adversely affect clinical markers of health. *Med Sci Sports Exerc*, 32: S134, 2000.
106. Schroeder, C., J. Potteiger, J. Randall, D. Jacobsen, L. Magee, S. Benedict, and M. Hulver, The effects of creatine dietary supplementation on anterior compartment pressure in the lower leg during rest and following exercise. *Clin J Sport Med*, 11: 87–95, 2001.
107. Carper, M.J., J.A. Potteiger, J.C. Randall, D.J. Jacobsen, M.W. Hulver, and J.P. Thyfault, Lower leg anterior compartment pressure response prior to, during, and following chronic creatine supplementation. *Med Sci Sports Exerc*, 33: S207, 2001.
108. Hile, A.M., J.M. Anderson, K.A. Fiala, J.H. Stevenson, D.J. Casa, and C.M. Maresh, Creatine supplementation and anterior compartment pressure during exercise in the heat in dehydrated men. *J Athl Train*, 41: 30–35, 2006.
109. Watson, G., D.J. Casa, K.A. Fiala, A. Hile, M.W. Roti, J.C. Healey, L.E. Armstrong, and C.M. Maresh, Creatine use and exercise heat tolerance in dehydrated men. *J Athl Train*, 41: 18–29, 2006.
110. Yoshizumi, W.M. and C. Tsourounis, Effects of creatine supplementation on renal function. *J Herb Pharmcother*, 4: 1–7, 2004.
111. Kreider, R.B., C. Melton, C.J. Rasmussen, M. Greenwood, S. Lancaster, E.C. Cantler, P. Milnor, and A.L. Almada, Long-term creatine supplementation does not significantly affect clinical markers of health in athletes. *Mol Cell Biochem*, 244: 95–104, 2003.
112. Schilling, B.K., M.H. Stone, A. Utter, J.T. Kearney, M. Johnson, R. Coglianese, L. Smith, H.S. O'Bryant, A.C. Fry, R. Keith, and M.E. Stone, Creatine supplementation and health variables: a retrospective study. *Med Sci Sports Exerc*, 33: 183–188, 2001.
113. Earnest, C.P., A. Almada, and T.L. Mitchell, Influence of chronic creatine supplementation on hepatorenal function. *FASEB J*, 10: A790, 1996.
114. Poortmans, J.R., H. Auquier, V. Renaut, A. Durussel, M. Saugy, and G.R. Brisson, Effect of short-term creatine supplementation on renal responses in men. *Eur J Appl Physiol Occup Physiol*, 76: 566–567, 1997.
115. Poortmans, J.R. and M. Francaux, Long-term oral creatine supplementation does not impair renal function in healthy athletes. *Med Sci Sports Exerc*, 31: 1108–1110, 1999.
116. Robinson, T.M., D.A. Sewell, A. Casey, G. Steenge, and P.L. Greenhaff, Dietary creatine supplementation does not affect some haematological indices, or indices of muscle damage and hepatic and renal function. *Br J Sports Med*, 34: 284–288, 2000.
117. Kilduff, L.P., E. Georgiades, N. James, R.H. Minnion, M. Mitchell, D. Kingsmore, M. Hadjicharlambous, and Y.P. Pitsiladis, The effects of creatine supplementation on cardiovascular, metabolic, and thermoregulatory responses during exercise in the heat in endurance-trained humans. *Int J Sport Nutr Exerc Metab*, 14: 443–460, 2004.

118. Volek, J.S., S.A. Mazzetti, W.B. Farquhar, B.R. Barnes, A.L. Gomez, and W.J. Kraemer, Physiological responses to short-term exercise in the heat after creatine loading. *Med Sci Sports Exerc*, 33: 1101–1108, 2001.
119. Tyler, T.F., S.J. Nicholas, E.B. Hershman, B.W. Glace, M.J. Mullaney, and M.P. McHugh, The effect of creatine supplementation on strength recovery after anterior cruciate ligament (ACL) reconstruction: a randomized, placebo-controlled, double-blind trial. *Am J Sports Med*, 32: 383–388, 2004.
120. Hespel, P., B. Op't Eijnde, M. Van Leemputte, B. Urso, P.L. Greenhaff, V. Labarque, S. Dymarkowski, P. Van Hecke, and E.A. Richter, Oral creatine supplementation facilitates the rehabilitation of disuse atrophy and alters the expression of muscle myogenic factors in humans. *J Physiol*, 536 (Pt 2): 625–633, 2001.

10 Glucosamine and Chondroitin Sulfate

Catherine G.R. Jackson

CONTENTS

10.1 INTRODUCTION

Americans currently spend more money on natural remedies for osteoarthritis than for any other medical condition,[1] thus producing an extremely large and lucrative market for the multi-billion-dollar supplement industry. Osteoarthritis is destined to become one of the most prevalent and costly diseases in our society. It is estimated that currently over 21 million adults in the U.S. suffer from osteoarthritis; it is predicted that this number will double over the next 20 years. Increasing age, female gender, and obesity are risk factors. It is also known that athletes of all types frequently live with chronic joint pain often associated with overuse injuries; they present an additional multi-million-dollar market for the supplements. Glucosamine and chondroitin sulfate have been widely publicized in the popular media as being capable of decelerating the degenerative processes, decreasing pain, and maintaining and improving joint function in osteoarthritis and other conditions where joint pain is the result. However, studies have not been able to confirm these statements. There are numerous anecdotal reports to which supplement manufacturers refer. However, the majority of clinical trials have small sample sizes, little or no follow-up, and are sponsored by the supplement manufacturers.[2] Problems in evaluation of efficacy begin with classification of these agents, as they have been called drugs, nutriceuticals, food supplements, alternative therapy, homeopathic therapy, and complementary therapy. Individuals with joint pain now consume very large quantities of glucosamine and chondroitin primarily based on a great volume of media coverage as to their value. There is currently much controversy and confusion concerning the topic.

In osteoarthritis the chondrocytes and aqueous matrix decrease with age, which results in poor-quality cartilage. Bones may become exposed and rub together, which creates damage and pain. With time, bones chip and fracture, which can lead to bone growth, producing increased pain and lack of mobility. The individual finds that this disrupts daily life and activity makes symptoms worse. Patients feel unwell and depressed. Active individuals may terminate exercise completely, which increases the risks of inactivity-related chronic diseases.

Osteoarthritis affects approximately 12% of the U.S. population and is a common cause of age-related pain and physical disability. The condition itself, however, is poorly understood. The degenerative process is not slowed or reversed with current treatments, which include aspirin, acetaminophen, and nonsteroidal anti-inflammatory drugs (NSAIDs). Interestingly, the origin of pain caused by the condition is unclear and, upon investigation, is more often attributed to lesions or referred pain rather than articular problems, as there are no nerves in articular cartilage. The biochemistry of glucosamine has led to the suggestion that its use might stop and possibly reverse the degenerative process. However, evidence is questionable. Chard and Dieppe[3] showed great insight into the problem by commenting that glucosamine may become the first agent about which we have more published systematic reviews, editorials, meta-analyses, and comments than primary research papers. They identified only 24 primary research studies, but also found 9 reviews and numerous comments and editorials. Most primary research studies are poor, and positive results are invariably found in supplement manufacturer-sponsored research. Chard and Dieppe[3] also concluded that there is more hype than magic, rationales for use are unclear, best dose and route of administration are unknown, and published work does not allow conclusions about efficacy or effectiveness. However, since it is safe, toxicity concerns cannot be raised. There is a need for regulation, as there could be long-term side effects, while the length of treatment is not known. Other uses of the drugs are to treat migraines,[4] gastrointestinal disorders such as Crohn's disease, ulcerative colitis, atherosclerosis, and capsular contracture in breast implants.[5]

10.2 DESCRIPTION OF PRODUCTS

10.2.1 GLUCOSAMINE

Glucosamine is an amino monosaccharide (amine sugar) that can be found in chitin, glycoproteins, and the glycosaminoglycans (mucopolysaccharides), such as heparin sulfate and hyaluronic acid. Other chemical designations are 2-amino-2-deoxy-beta-D-glucopyranose, 2-amino-2-deoxyglucose, and chitosamine.[6] It is available over the counter as a nutritional supplement as glucosamine hydrochloride (glucosamine HCl), glucosamine sulfate, or N-acetyl-glucosamine. Research has used primarily the chloride and sulfate salts, which are those most commonly purchased.

The chemical structure of glucosamine is such that at physiologic and neutral pH the molecule has a positive charge. Negative anions are found in the salt forms, which neutralize the charge. In glucosamine sulfate the anion is sulfate, in glucosamine HCl the anion is chloride, and in N-acetylglucosamine the amino group is acetylated, which results in a neutral charge. All forms are water soluble. Nutritional supplements are usually derived from marine exoskeletons with the chitin extracted from seashells. There are also synthetic forms. Since glucosamine falls under the 1994 Dietary Supplement Health and Education Act (DSHEA) and is classified as a medicinal product, its manufacture is not regulated. As a result, there is no standardization of active ingredients, concentrations, or reporting requirements for labels. A consumer cannot know what is contained in the product as glucosamine is inherently unstable and must be combined with other ingredients for stability. Analysis of products consistently produces the result that many formulations do not contain ingredients listed on the label.[7]

10.2.2 CHONDROITIN SULFATE

Chondroitin sulfate is a heteropolysaccharide identified as a glycosaminoglycan (GAG). GAGs form the ground substance in connective tissue's extracellular matrix. The molecule itself is comprised of repeating linear units of D-galactosamine and D-glucuronic acid. It is found in human cartilage, cornea, bone arterial walls, and skin; this form is called chondroitin sulfate A (chondroitin 4-sulfate). Cartilage of humans, fish, and shark contains chondroitin sulfate C (chondroitin 6-sulfate). The two forms differ in the amino group of chondroitin sulfate A and in the sulfate group of chondroitin sulfate C. There is a B form called dermatan sulfate, which is found in heart valves, tendons, skin, and arterial walls. The molecular weights of all forms range from 5,000 to 50,000 daltons. It is available over the counter as a nutritional supplement, usually in an isomeric mixture of A and C forms. Nutritional supplements are derived from varied sources, such as pork by-products (ears, snout), bovine trachea cartilaginous rings, whale septum, and shark cartilage.[6]

10.3 MECHANISMS

10.3.1 GLUCOSAMINE

Glucosamine is produced within the body in small amounts in reactions involving glucose and glutamic acid. It is a small molecule (molecular weight = 179.17) that is easily absorbed *in vivo*. Humans may decrease production with aging. It is not found in any common foods and cannot be obtained externally. If the body is not synthesizing the substance, it needs to be taken as a supplement. It is found in abundance in cartilage, with small amounts measured in tendons and ligaments; it is an essential substrate matrix that is a component of cartilage.

It is still not clear what the actions are of glucosamine taken as a nutritional supplement. Purported effects are the promotion and maintenance of the structure and function of cartilage in the joints of the body. It has also been reported that glucosamine has anti-inflammatory effects. The biochemistry, however, has been known for quite some time. Glucosamine, a sugar and a sulfated amino monosaccharide, is involved in glycoprotein metabolism where it is found in proteoglycans as polysaccharide groups called GAGs. All GAGs contain derivatives of glucosamine or glactosamine. These polysaccharides comprise 95% of the ground substance in the intracellular matrix of connective tissue. One of the GAGs, hyaluronic acid, is essential for the function of articular cartilage and is responsible for shock absorbing and deformability functions.[6] *In vitro* studies show that it can alter chondrocyte metabolism; it is not clear whether oral glucosamine can reach chondrocytes *in vivo*.[8]

Over 90% of the studies in glucosamine pharmacokinetics have used animal models. It has been shown that about 90% of the salt is absorbed from the small intestine and transported to the liver. The majority is then catabolized in the first pass; seldom is it detected in serum after oral ingestion. Free glucosamine is not usually detected in plasma.[9,10] How much is taken into joints is not known for humans, while some uptake is seen in articular cartilage in animals.

10.3.2 CHONDROITIN SULFATE

It is still not clear what the actions are of chondroitin sulfate when taken as a nutritional supplement. Purported effects are the promotion and maintenance of the structure and function of cartilage in the joints of the body. It has also been reported that chondroitin sulfate has anti-inflammatory and pain relief effects. The biochemistry has been known for some time. Chondroitin sulfate is a GAG, previously described in the glucosamine mechanisms. It is essential for the structure and function of articular cartilage and provides the same properties as hyaluronic acid. While intra-articular injections of hyaluronic acid have been shown to relieve joint pain and improve mobility, the same has not yet been demonstrated for chondroitin sulfate. It is speculated that oral ingestion of chondroitin sulfate may lead to an increase in hyaluronic acid. Thus, cartilage breakdown would be inhibited.[6]

It has been shown that absorption is from the stomach and small intestine. High molecular weight forms are not significantly absorbed, while low molecular weight forms show significant absorption after oral ingestion. How much is taken into joints is not known for humans, while it is known that some does enter the joint space.

10.4   REVIEW OF RESEARCH STUDIES AND CLINICAL TRIALS

10.4.1   GLUCOSAMINE

Glucosamine was looked at for use in reducing the symptoms of osteoarthritis as early as 1969.[11] A number of years ago early studies showed, in 20 patients, that the use of glucosamine sulfate resulted in patients who experience lessening or disappearance of symptoms with use over 6 to 8 weeks[12] with no adverse reactions. Barclay and associates[13] reviewed the pharmacology and pharmacokinetics of glucosamine and evaluated the available literature regarding safety and efficacy. Of the literature published between 1965 and 1997, three critically evaluated studies were found that reported a decrease in the symptoms of osteoarthritis. However, flaws in the research designs precluded making positive recommendations for improvements in the symptoms of osteoarthritis with oral glucosamine use. Intramuscular glucosamine administration, however, is effective.[14] No statistically significant difference in glucosamine sulfate and placebo were found in managing pain, leading to the conclusion by one group that the supplement was no more effective than the placebo.[15]

A 12-week study of 2000 mg/day doses of glucosamine in subjects with articular cartilage damage and possible osteoarthritis showed self-reported improvement in symptoms. However, while clinical and functional test scores improved over the evaluation period in both the test and placebo groups, there were no significant differences between groups at the end of the study.[16] The trend reported was that improvement could be seen after 8 weeks. A 3-year prospective, placebo-controlled study evaluating the effect of glucosamine sulfate use on joint space narrowing in knee osteoarthritis did not find statistically significant results in the most severe cases. However, patients with less severe radiographic knee osteoarthritis showed a trend toward significant reduction in joint space narrowing.[17] It has been shown that a 3-year treatment of osteoarthritis with glucosamine sulfate use retarded the progression of knee osteoarthritis as determined by a lesser joint space narrowing than in the placebo group.[18] The authors suggested that this retardation of narrowing of joint space might modify and slow the disease process; however, joint space narrowing is not associated with pain.

Positive results are difficult to demonstrate (glucosamine hydrochloride). The objective measurement differences between groups are not usually statistically significant. Results are reported as positive trends[19] in objective measurements. More often than not, however, patients report that they feel better than at the start of the trial.[19] Glucosamine use was shown to preserve joint space in that significant narrowing did not occur. It was suggested that long-term use prevents joint structure changes and improves disease symptoms.[20] However, a change in joint space is not necessarily associated with a change in pain levels. Some have reported overall positive results.[21]

Literature reviews usually conclude that glucosamine may not only provide symptomatic pain relief, but also have a role in chondroprotection.[22] Even though no differences were found between the glucosamine and placebo groups, and positive results were modest, it was still concluded that glucosamine sulfate may be a safe and effective symptomatic slow-acting drug for osteoarthritis.[23] Glucosamine can be administered orally, intravenously, intramuscularly, and intra-articularly. Reviews of primarily European and Asian literature have suggested that glucosamine sulfate use may provide pain relief, reduce tenderness, and improve mobility in patients with osteoarthritis.[24] Studies in the U.S. do not support these conclusions.

10.4.2 CHONDROITIN SULFATE

A number of years ago, based on *in vitro* studies, chondroitin sulfate was identified as a supplement that may provide chondroprotection.[25] A multicenter randomized, double-blind, controlled study of 143 subjects with osteoarthritis that used three different formulations of chondroitin sufate showed that improvement of subjective symptoms was achieved after 3 months of treatment.[26] A single daily dose of 1200 mg was found to be just as effective as three 400-mg doses.

A meta-analysis of chondroitin sulfate supplementation found 16 publications that fit criteria for inclusion. Criteria included types of joint involvement studied, study designs, numbers of patients enrolled, and pain index variables analyzed.[27] It was concluded that chondroitin sulfate may be useful in osteoarthritis treatment; however, results of the published studies were clouded by concomitant use of analgesics or NSAIDs, thus making conclusions about benefits difficult.[27] Some have suggested that it can be used as an anti-inflammatory without dangerous effects on the stomach, platelets, and kidneys.[28]

Conte and co-workers[29] showed that single daily doses of 0.8 g and two daily doses of 0.4 g resulted in an increase of plasma concentration of chondroitin sulfate for a 24-h period, showing that there was bioavailability. In 20 male volunteers chondroitin sulfate plasma levels increased in all subjects and peaked after 2 h.[30] It is questionable, however, as to what level of chondroprotection can be achieved by orally administered chondroitin sulfate. Baici and co-workers[31] found no changes in serum concentrations of glycosaminoglycan concentraton before and after ingestion of chondroitin sulfate in six patients with rheumatoid arthritis and six patients with osteoarthritis. They suggested that claims for benefits were biologically and pharmacologically unfounded.

Uebelhart and co-workers[32] assessed the clinical, radiological, and biological efficacy and tolerance of chondroitin 4- and 6-sulfate with symptomatic knee osteoarthritis in 42 patients over the period of 1 year. They reported that the combined preparation was an effective and safe symptomatic slow-acting drug for the treatment of knee osteoarthritis in 42 patients. It was claimed that this was the first study to demonstrate that the natural course of the disease could be changed with symptomatic slow-acting drugs in osteoarthritis (SYSADOAs). Others have made the same suggestion.[32]

10.4.3 COMBINED GLUCOSAMINE AND CHONDROITIN SULFATE

There is some evidence that if positive results in mild to moderate symptoms of osteoarthritis are seen, combined preparations of low molecular weight chondroitin sulfate and glucosamine may be more effective with results reported as synergistic.[33] In 93 patients a combination preparation was found to be effective when a randomized, placebo-controlled study design was implemented.[33] Combination therapy relieved symptoms of knee osteoarthritis and was safe when tested in 34 young males with chronic pain and radiographic evidence of degenerative disease;[34] however, this group was not the older population usually seen with osteoarthritis.

Animal studies show that both chondroitin sulfate and glucosamine sulfate stimulate chondrocyte growth *in vitro* and in animal models.[35] However, no direct evidence that they cause regeneration of cartilage in osteoarthris has been produced. In knee osteoarthritis, glucosamine sulfate can be shown to prevent knee joint space narrowing, and chondroitin polysulfate has been shown to prevent the same in finger osteoarthritis, as seen on radiographs.[35] These effects are not evidence of regeneration of cartilage. Topical creams have been evaluated using glucosamine sulfate, chondroitin sulfate, and camphor, which show improvement in relieving pain after 4 weeks.[36]

Some literature reviews have shown that glucosamine and chondroitin sulfates offer safe and effective alternatives to NSAIDs, which may have serious and life-threatening adverse effects.[37] When glucosamine and chondroitin preparations were subjected to meta-analysis, 15 studies were found to fit rigorous criteria. These studies showed some degree of efficacy; trials reported moderate to large effects, but the authors reported that most studies had flawed designs.[38] Chondroitin sulfate is a much larger molecule than glucosamine and is poorly absorbed. Some claim that, in combination with glucosamine, there is no added benefit,[11] but admit to the lack of side effects with use. Manufacturers now use a low molecular weight chondroitin sulfate in the hopes of increasing absorbability.

Deal and Moskowitz[39] reviewed glucosamine, chondroitin sulfate, and collagen hydrolysate use in the symptomatic treatment of osteoarthritis. They came to conclusions similar to those of most researchers in that recommendations are difficult to make with the current status of non-FDA-evaluated supplements, particularly with long-term use. At a cost of $30 to $45 per month, older adults on limited incomes may have difficulty sustaining treatment. Some believe that current therapies have little benefit and great risk because of the lack of data in humans; chondroprotection is still questionable, but glucosamine and chondroitin sulfate show modest effectiveness when taken together.[40] Most conclude that there is a modest efficacy for glucosamine and chondroitin sulfate use; however, long-term safety is not yet proved.[41] Meta-analysis does, however, show some degree of positive results with both supplements,[42] claiming that they are effective and safe.[43]

The preliminary results of a multicenter, double-blind, placebo- and celecoxib-controlled Glucosamine/Chondroitin Arthritis Intervention Trial (GAIT) have been published.[44] Subjects included 1583 patients with osteoarthritis of the knee randomly assigned to one of five groups for 24 weeks. Orally administered treatments were (1) 500 mg of glucosamine hydrochloride three times daily, (2) 400 mg of sodium chondroitin sulfate three times daily, (3) 500 mg of glucosamine plus 400 mg of chondroitin sulfate three times daily, (4) 200 mg of celecoxib daily, or (5) placebo. Patients were further stratified based on WOMAC™ pain stratum as either mild or moderate to severe. The authors concluded that both glucosamine and chondroitin sulfate alone or in combination did not reduce pain effectively in the overall patient population. In the subgroup of individuals with moderate to severe knee pain, combined glucosamine and chondroitin sulfate were found to have some efficacy. Interestingly, there were positive effects noted in 60% of the patients in the placebo group. As would be expected, these results have led to further controversy and discussion of the methods used both in the design of the study and in the statistical analysis.[45,46]

10.5 SIDE EFFECTS

10.5.1 GLUCOSAMINE

There are no known or reported contraindications to glucosamine supplementation. Concerns have been expressed for the potential to increase insulin resistance if glucosamine is given intravenously, as it has been shown to do so in both normal and experimentally diabetic animals. However, this effect is not seen in oral preparations. Some researchers, however, do suggest that it is contraindicated in diabetes with concerns about its effect on insulin secretion.[43,47] Individuals who are diabetic or overweight should err on the side of caution and carefully monitor blood sugar levels if supplements are taken. Because there are no data, children and pregnant or nursing women should avoid consumption.[6]

Side effects are few and are usually mild digestive problems such as upset stomach, nausea, heartburn, and diarrhea. These suggest that glucosamine is better taken with food. Short-term adverse effects for glucosamine use also include headache, drowsiness, and skin reactions. No allergic reactions have been reported.[6] There are no known interactions with any other nutritional supplement, drug, herb, or food. There are no reports of overdosage. Biochemical, hemostatic, and hematological measurements indicate that it is safe.[48] The usual dose recommended for benefit is 1500 mg.

10.5.2 CHONDROITIN SULFATE

There are no known or reported contraindications to chondroitin sulfate supplementation. Concerns have been expressed for the theoretical possibility that chondroitin sulfate may have antithrombotic activity and should be avoided by those with hemophilia and those taking anticoagulants, such as warfarin. It may also be immunosuppressive.[49] Since the most common form sold is a salt, those on salt-restricted diets should use a salt-free supplement. Because there are no data, children and pregnant or nursing women should avoid consumption.[6]

Side effects are few and are usually mild digestive problems such as nausea, heartburn, and diarrhea. No allergic reactions have been reported.[6] There are no known interactions with any other nutritional supplement, drug, herb, or food. If chitosan is taken, it may decrease absorption. There are no reports of overdosage. Biochemical, hemostatic, and hematological measurements indicate that it is safe.[48] The usual dose recommended for benefit is 1200 mg.

10.6 USE IN SPORT AND EXERCISE

Much of the use in sport and exercise is based on the possibility that both glucosamine and chondroitin sulfate will be chondroprotective and will reduce inflammation and pain if injury occurs. People who exercise will use these supplements for varied reasons, and many use them more for prophylaxis than after an injury. There is a belief that these supplements will help avoid injury, will speed up healing if it occurs, and will be a useful adjunct if surgery has occurred.[50]

Exercisers by the nature of what they do put stress on chondral surfaces and wear and injury can occur. Those most interested in supplementation are runners and those involved in contact and cutting sports where ligaments can be injured.[50] Many athletes injure or tear menisci, and chondroprotection is desired. However, there are no data in athletes to support any claims of benefit. The research that has been done has used individuals with osteoarthritis, and the supplements have been an adjunct to other therapies used at the same time. Whether the effects will be the same in those without joint damage is not known.

It is known that there is widespread use of supplements among athletes even though there may be no evidence for efficacy.[51] When Olympic athletes were surveyed, it was found that supplement use is widespread. The most common drugs taken were NSAIDs, used by 100% of surveyed gymnasts. It has also been reported that glucosamine and chondroitin sulfate are frequently first taken by athletes to ameliorate the pain and swelling following injury.[52] After initial use, many athletes tend to become chronic users of these substances, and concerns have been expressed over increased risk of adverse effects on the gastrointestinal, hepatic, and renal systems. There is much anecdotal evidence to indicate that athletes take glucosamine and chondroitin sulfate even without injury.

The fact remains that consumption of these supplements appears to be safe, although long-term studies have yet to be performed. Athletes will have to judge for themselves, but there are no cautions for use. Knowing that the placebo effect is real, the mere consumption of a product purported to alleviate pain may have a positive effect.

10.7 SUMMARY AND RECOMMENDATIONS

Glucosamine and chondroitin sulfate have been used as nutriceuticals since 1969.[11] They are believed to ameliorate the symptoms of osteoarthritis by reducing inflammation and by aiding in the restoration of normal cartilage.[53,54] While animal studies have shown positive effects, research in humans is still equivocal. However, as yet, no firm conclusions can be made about these homeopathic remedies.[55] A recommendation for the use of a nonpharmacological treatment for symptomatic osteoarthritis of the hip and knee includes exercise, both aerobic and strength training, and diet. Exercise was found to be just as effective as NSAIDs for improvement in pain and function.[56] The results of this study suggest that, in particular groups of individuals, supplement and drug therapy could be reduced or eliminated.

There is no question that human research needs to be done, particularly in athletes who consume these supplements in large quantities with no knowledge of their effects in the long term. Although anecdotal evidence suggests that glucosamine sulfate and chondroitin sulfate are widely used to ameliorate the symptoms of osteoarthritis and may be effective in some cases, the American College of Rheumatology Subcommittee on Osteoarthritis continues to evaluate recommendations for use.[57] The National Institute of Arthritis and Musculoskeletal and Skin Diseases (NIAMS) in collaboration with the National Center for Complementary and Alternative Medicine (NCCAM) announced in 1999 a multicenter effort to study the effectiveness of glucosamine and chondroitin sulfate use in a large database of subjects.[57] Initial published results did not show efficacy in the overall population, but there is a suggestion that the supplements may be useful in moderate to severe evaluated pain.

Athletes consistently look for an advantage in their sport and for natural ways to enhance their performance. While glucosamine and chondroitin sulfate cannot be considered ergogenic aids with the current lack of human data on exercisers, their use cannot be precluded because of their safety. Since little harm can be done, athletes can safely consume these supplements if they believe there will be a benefit. They can be found in pills, powders, and beverages ("joint juice," "motion potion"). The greatest benefit, if it does indeed occur, seems to be found in preparations that contain both glucosamine and low molecular weight chondroitin sulfate. Athletes can safely consume these supplements and need to decide if the cost ($30 to $45 per month) is warranted in light of equivocal research and the fact that, if benefits are noted, it takes one to several months before they are observed.[11] The supplements need to be regulated as there could be long-term side effects and the length of treatment is not known.[4] Since athletes are healthy, effects may not be the same as in those with the diseased joints of osteoarthritis. An excellent book has been published that outlines regimens for reducing pain.[57] Anecdotally, the regimens recommended in this publication are reported to be successful. While athletes take supplements for osteoarthritis to aid their exercise, those with osteoarthritis may find that exercise itself is the "drug" that will benefit them the most.[56,58]

REFERENCES

1. Morelli, V., Naquin, C., and Weaver, V., Alternative therapies for traditional disease states: osteoarthritis. *Am. Fam. Physician*, 67, 339, 2003.
2. Brief, A.A., Maurer, S.G., and Di Cesare, P.E., Use of glucosamine and chondroitin sulfate in the management of osteoarthritis. *J. Am. Acad. Orthop. Surg.*, 9, 352, 2001.
3. Chard, J. and Dieppe, P., Glucosamine for osteoarthritis: magic, hype, or confusion? *Br. Med. J.*, 322, 1439, 2001.
4. Sutton, L., Rapport, L., and Lockwood, B., Gucosamine: con or cure? Part II. *Nutrition*, 18, 693, 2002.
5. Skillman, J.M., Ahmed, O.A., and Rowsell, A.R., Incidental improvement of breast capsular contracture following treatment of arthritis with glucosamine and chondroitin. *Br. J. Plast. Surg.*, 55, 454, 2002.
6. Hendler, S.S. and Rorvik, D., Eds., *PDR for Nutritional Supplements*, Thomson Healthcare, Montvale, NJ, 2001.
7. Abimbola, O., Cox, D.S., Liang, Z., and Eddington, N.D., Analysis of glucosamine and chondroitin sulfate content in marketed products and the Caco-2 permeability of chondroitin sulfate raw materials. *J. Am. Nutraceut. Assoc.*, 3, 37, 2000.
8. Towheed, T.E. and Anastassiades, T.P., Glucosamine and chondroitin for treating symptoms of osteoarthritis. Evidence is widely touted but incomplete. *JAMA*, 283, 1483, 2000.
9. Setnikar, I., Palumbo, R., Canali, S., and Zanolo, G., Pharmacokinetics of glucosamine in man. *Arzneimittelforschung*, 43, 1109, 1993.
10. Setnikar, I. and Rovati, L.C., Absorption, distribution, metabolism and excretion of glucosamine sulfate. A review. *Arzneimittelforschung*, 51, 699, 2001.

11. Sutton, L., Rapport, L., and Lockwood, B., Gucosamine: con or cure? *Nutrition*, 18, 534, 2002.
12. Pujalte, J.M., Llavore, E.P., and Ylescupidez, F.R., Double-blind evaluation of oral glucosamine sulfate in the basic treatment of osteoarthritis. *Curr. Med. Res. Opin.*, 7, 110, 1980.
13. Barclay, T.S., Tsourounis, C., and McCart, G.M., Glucosamine. *Ann. Pharmacother.*, 32, 574, 1998.
14. Reichelt, A., Forster, K.K., Fisher, M., Rovati, L.C., and Setnikar, I., Efficacy and safety of intramuscular glucosamine sulfate in osteoarthritis of the knee. A randomised, placebo-controlled, double-blind study. *Arzneimittelforschung*, 44(1), 75–80, 1994.
15. Hughes, R. and Carr, A., A randomized, double-blind, placebo-controlled trial of glucosamine sulphate as an analgesic in osteoarthritis of the knee. *Rheumatology*, 41, 279, 2002.
16. Braham, R., Dawson, B., and Goodman, C., The effect of glucosamine supplementation on people experiencing regular knee pain. *Br. J. Sports Med.* 37, 45, 2003.
17. Bruyere, O., Honore, A., Ethgen, O., Rovati, L.C., Giacovelli, G., Henrotin, Y.E., Seidel, L., and Reginster, J.Y., Correlation between radiographic severity of knee osteoarthritis and future disease progression. Results from a 3-year prospective, placebo-controlled study evaluating the effect of glucosamine sulfate. *Osteoarthritis Cartilage*, 11, 1, 2003.
18. Pavelka, K., Gatternova, J., Olejarova, M., Machacek, S., Giacovelli, G., and Rovati, L.C., Glucosamine sulfate use and delay of progression of knee osteoarthritis: a 3-year, randomized, placebo-controlled, double-blind study. *Arch. Intern. Med.*, 162, 2113, 2002.
19. Houpt, J.B., McMillan, R., Wein, C., and Paget-Dellio, S.D., Effect of glucosamine hydrochloride in the treatment of pain of osteoarthritis of the knee. *J. Rheumatol.*, 26, 2294, 1999.
20. Reginster, J.Y., Bruyere, O., Lecart, M.P., and Henrotin, Y., Naturocetic (glucosamine and chondroitin sulfate) compounds as structure-modifying drugs in the treatment of osteoarthritis. *Curr. Opin. Rheumatol.*, 15, 651, 2003.
21. Drovanti, A., Bignamini, A.A., and Rovati, A.L., Therapeutic activity of oral glucosamine sulfate in osteoarthritis: a placebo-controlled double-blind investigation. *Clin. Ther.*, 3, 260, 1980.
22. Phoon, S. and Manolios, N., Glucosamine. A neutraceutical in osteoarthritis. *Aust. Fam. Physician*, 31, 539, 2002.
23. Noack, W., Fischer, M., Forster, K.K., Rovati, L.C., and Setnikar, I., Glucosamine sulfate in osteoarthritis of the knee. *Osteoarthritis Cartilage*, 2, 51, 1994.
24. da Camara, C.C. and Dowless, G.V., Glucosamine sulfate for osteoarthritis. *Ann. Pharmacother.*, 32, 602, 1998.
25. Pipitone, V.R., Chondroprotection with chondroitin sulfate. *Drugs Exp. Clin. Res.*, 17, 3, 1991.
26. Bourgeois, P., Chales, G., Dehais, J., Delcambre, B., Kuntz, J.L., and Rozenberg, S., Efficacy and tolerability of chondroitin sulfate 1,200 mg/day vs. chondrotin sulfate 3 × 400 mg/day vs. placebo. *Osteoarthritis Cartilage*, 6 (Suppl. A), 25, 1998.
27. Leeb, B.F., Schweitzer, H., Montag, K., and Smolen, J.S., A meta-analysis of chondroitin sulfate in the treatment of osteoarthritis. *J. Rheumatol.*, 27, 205, 2000.
28. Ronca, F., Palmieri, L., Panicucci, P., and Ronca, G., Anti-inflammatory activity of chondroitin sulfate. *Osteoarthritis Cartilage*, 6 (Suppl. A), 14, 1998.

29. Conte, A., Volpi, N., Palmieri, L., Bahous, I., and Ronca, G., Biochemical and pharmacokinetic aspects of oral treatment with chondroitin sulfate. *Arzneimittelforschung*, 45, 918, 1995.

30. Volpi, N., Oral bioavailability of chondroitin sulfate (Chondrosulf) and its constituents in healthy male volunteers. *Osteoarthritis Cartilage*, 10, 768, 2000.

31. Baici, A., Horler, D., Moser, B., Hofer, H.O., Fehr, K., and Wagenhauser, F.J., Analysis of glycosaminoglycans in human serum after oral administration of chondroitin sulfate. *Rheumatol. Int.*, 12, 81, 1992.

32. Uebelhart, D., Thonar, E.J., Delmas, P.D., Chantraine, A., and Vignon, E., Effects of oral chondroitin sulfate on the progression of knee osteoarthritis: a pilot study. *Osteoarthritis Cartilage*, 6 (Suppl. A), 39, 1998.

33. Das, A. and Hammad, T.A., Efficacy of a combination of FCHG49 glucosamine hydrochloride, TRH122 low molecular weight sodium chondroitin sulfate and manganese ascorbate in the management of knee osteoarthritis. *Osteoarthritis Cartilage*, 8(5), 343, 2000.

34. Leffler, C.T., Philippi, A.F., Leffler, S.G., Mosure, J.C., and Kim, P.D., Glucosamine, chondroitin, and manganese ascorbate for degenerative joint disease of the knee or low back: a randomized double-blind, placebo-controlled pilot study. *Mil. Med.*, 164, 85, 1999.

35. Priebe, D., McDiarmid, T., Mackler, L., and Tudiver, F., Do glucosamine or chondroitin cause regeneration of cartilage in osteoarthritis? *J. Fam. Pract.*, 52, 237, 2003.

36. Cohen, M., Wolfe, R., Mai, T., and Lewis, D., A randomized, double blind, placebo controlled trial of a topical cream containing glucosamine sulfate, chondroitin sulfate, and camphor for osteoarthritis of the knee. *J. Rheumatol.*, 30, 523, 2003.

37. de los Reyes, G.C., Koda, R.T., and Lien, E.J., Glucosamine and chondroitin sulfates in the treatment of osteoarthritis: a survey. *Prog. Drug Res.*, 55, 81, 2000.

38. McAlindon, T.E., LaValley, M.P., Gulin, J.P., and Felson, D.T., Glucosamine and chondroitin for treatment of osteoarthritis: a systematic quality assessment and meta-analysis. *JAMA*, 283, 1469, 2000.

39. Deal, C.L. and Moskowitz, R.W., Nutraceuticals as therapeutic agents in osteoarthritis. The role of glucosamine, chondroitin sulfate and collagen hydrolysate. *Rheum. Dis. Clin. North Am.*, 25, 379, 1999.

40. Walker-Bone, K., 'Natural remedies' in the treatment of osteoarthritis. *Drugs Aging*, 20, 517, 2003.

41. McAlindon, T., Glucosamine and chondroitin for osteoarthritis? *Bull. Rheum. Dis.*, 50, 1, 2001.

42. Towheed, T.E., Published meta-analyses of pharmacological therapies for osteoarthritis. *Osteoarthritis Cartilage*, 10, 836, 2002.

43. McClain, D.A., Hexaosamines as mediators of nutrient sensing and regulation in diabetes. *J. Diabetes Complications*, 16, 72, 2002.

44. Clegg, D.O., Reda, D.J., Harris, C.L., Klein, M.A., O'Dell, J.R., Hooper, M.M., et. al., Glucosamine, chondroitin sulfate, and the two in combination for painful knee osteoarthritis. *N. Engl. J. Med.*, 354, 795, 2006.

45. Hochberg, M.C., Nutritional supplements for knee osteoarthritis: still no resolution. *N. Engl. J. Med.*, 354, 858, 2006.

46. Ernst, E., Vassiliou, V.S., and Pelletier, J.P., Glucosamine and chondroitin sulfate for knee osteoarthritis: correspondence. *N. Engl. J. Med.*, 354, 2184, 2006.

47. McClain, D.A. and Crook, E.D., Hexosamines and insulin resistance. *Diabetes*, 45, 1003, 1996.

48. Adebeowale, A., Cox, D.S., Liang, Z., and Eddington, N.D., Analysis of glucosamine and chondroitin sulfate content in marketed products and the Caco-2 permeability of chondroitin sulfate raw materials. *J. Am. Nutraceut. Assoc.*, 3, 37, 2000.
49. Volpi, N., Inhibition of human leukocyte elastase activity by chondroitin sulfates. *Chem. Biol. Interact.*, 105, 157, 1997.
50. Hungerford, D., Navarro, R., and Hammad, T., Use of nutraceuticals in the management of osteoarthritis. *J. Am. Nutraceut. Assoc.*, 3, 23, 2000.
51. Huang, S.H., Johnson, K., and Pipe, A.L. The use of dietary supplements and medications by Canadian athletes at the Atlanta and Sydney Olympic Games. *Clin. J. Sport Med.*, 16, 27, 2006.
52. Garsline, R.T. and Kaeding, C.C. The use of NSAIDs and nutritional supplements in athletes with osteoarthritis: prevalence, benefits and consequences. *Clin. Sports Med.*, 24, 71, 2005.
53. Morelli, V., Naquin, C., and Weaver, V., Alternative therapies for traditional disease states: osteoarthritis. *Am. Fam. Physician*, 67, 339, 2003.
54. Deal, C.L., Osteoporosis: prevention, diagnosis, and management. *Am. J. Med.*, 102, 35S, 1997.
55. Long, L. and Ernst, E., Homeopathic remedies for the treatment of osteoarthritis: a systematic review. *Br. Homeopath. J.*, 90, 37, 2001.
56. Bischoff, H.A. and Roos, E.M. Effectiveness and safety of strengthening, aerobic, and coordination exercises for patients with osteoarthritis. *Curr. Opin. Rheumatol.*, 15, 141, 2003.
57. Bucci, L., *Pain Free: The Definitive Guide to Healing Arthritis, Low-Back Pain and Sports Injuries through Nutrition and Supplements.* Summit Group, Fort Worth, TX, 1995.
58. O'Rourke, M., Determining the efficacy of glucosamine and chondroitin for osteoarthritis. *Nurse Pract.*, 26, 44, 2001.

11 Carnitine

Sara Chelland Campbell and Robert J. Moffatt

CONTENTS

11.1 INTRODUCTION

11.1.1 CARNITINE: A BRIEF HISTORY

The word carnitine is derived from the Latin word *carno* or *carnis*, which means flesh or meat. Carnitine was discovered in muscle extracts by Gulewitsch and Krimberg[1] as well as Kutscher[2] in 1905 and was first thought to be involved with muscle function. Gulewitsch and Krimberg[1] identified the structure of carnitine as 3-hydroxy-4-N-trimethyl-aminobutyric acid ($C_7H_{15}NO_3$), which was later confirmed in 1927 by Tomita and Sendju.[3] Following its discovery, its exact configuration was

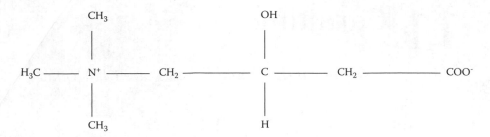

FIGURE 11.1 L-carnitine's chemical structure.

proposed in 1962[4] and became definite in 1997 as L- or R-3-hydroxy-4-N,N,N-trimethylaminobutyrate.[5] Initially carnitine was called vitamin B_T because of its necessity for growth in the yellow mealworm known as *Tenebrio molitor*. Subsequently, the distribution of carnitine in the organs of mammals, lower animals, plants, and microorganisms became well established[6] (Figure 11.1).

11.1.2 METABOLIC ACTIONS OF CARNITINE

The most widely investigated aspect of carnitine is the carnitine-dependent transport of fats to the intermitochondrial membrane; however, some other established roles include the preservation of membrane integrity, stabilization of a physiologic coenzyme A:acetyl-CoA ratio in the mitochondria, and the reduction of lactate production.[7,8]

Carnitine serves as a cofactor for several enzymes, including carnitine translocase and acylcarnitine transferases I and II, which are essential for the movement of activated long-chain fatty acids from the cytoplasm into the mitochondria (Figure 11.2). The translocation of fatty acids (FAs) is critical for the generation of adenosine triphosphate (ATP) within skeletal muscle, via β-oxidation. These activated FAs become esterified to acylcarnitines with carnitine via carnitine-acyl-transferase I (CAT I) in the outer mitochondrial membrane. Acylcarnitines can easily permeate the membrane of the mitochondria and are translocated across the membrane by carnitine translocase. Carnitine's actions are not yet complete because the mitochondrion has two membranes to cross; thus, through the action of CAT II, the acylcarnitines are converted back to acyl-CoA and carnitine. Acyl-CoA can be used to generate ATP via β-oxidation, Krebs cycle, and the electron transport chain. Carnitine is recycled to the cytoplasm for future use.

As previously mentioned, carnitine has a unique interaction with acyl-CoA in the mitochondria and is an important modulator of the acyl-CoA:free CoA ratio. This is demonstrated when acylcarnitines are formed. This relationship is defined by the rate of acyl-CoA production: if the acyl-CoAs are produced more rapidly than they are used, then the acyl-CoA within the intramitochondrial space is high compared to the free CoA concentration.[9,10] This imbalance can then be corrected because carnitine can bind the acyl-CoAs and the once elevated ratio can return to normal. The regulation of this ratio and the interaction of carnitine with acetyl-CoA may suppress the production of lactic acid during high-intensity exercise, primarily because it acts to inhibit the downregulation of the pyruvate dehydrogenase (PDH) caused by the increase in acetyl-CoA.[11]

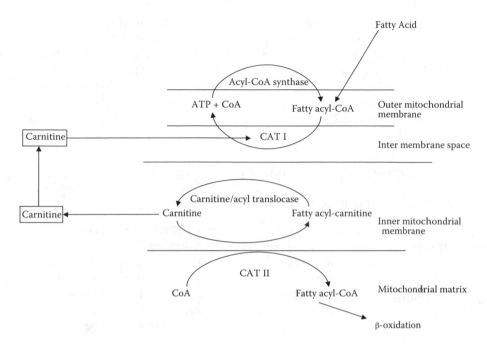

FIGURE 11.2 Roles of carnitine in the movement of long chain fatty acids into the mitochondrial matrix.

It is important to differentiate the two forms of carnitine, which are L-carnitine and D-carnitine (Dextro form). L-carnitine is the physiologically active form and is endogenously produced within the human, whereas D-carnitine is not physiologically active and is a synthetic.[12] Research has shown that subjects given D-carnitine saw a depletion of their endogenous stores of L-carnitine,[13,14] which may manifest itself as carnitine deficiency, especially during intense bouts of exercise.[15] Supplementation of D-carnitine is therefore not recommended because it may have a deleterious effect on the body as well as performance.

Carnitine plays a major role in substrate metabolism in healthy individuals, but there are individuals who have carnitine deficiencies, and in these individuals carnitine supplementation can be utilized as a therapeutic agent. Typically the daily average American diet has about 100 to 300 mg of carnitine.[16] The primary sources of carnitine are found in red meat and dairy products, whereas vegetables have very little L-carnitine; thus, vegetarian diets may contain miniscule amounts. Despite adequate intake of carnitine by the majority of the population, there is still a fraction of the population who have carnitine disturbances. This may be due to several metabolic abnormalities, which include defective carnitine synthesis, enhanced carnitine degradation, impaired transport of carnitine whether it is in or out of cells, and finally abnormal renal handling of carnitine.[17,18] These abnormalities manifest in a syndrome known as primary carnitine deficiency, the myopathic form having symptoms such as muscle fatigue, cramps, hypotona, and atrophy of the musculature, and the systemic form, the more severe form, having symptoms such as nausea, vomiting, and coma due to excessive fat storage because of reduced hepatic efficiency.[19–21]

Carnitine supplementation in these states has proven effective. For example, in cardiac diseases, the myocardium uses fatty acids as its primary source of fuel; therefore, a deficiency in carnitine may have a serious impact on heart rate and stroke volume and thus cardiac output. In fact, most research on these types of cardiac patients supports the use of carnitine as a supplement and furthermore has found that abnormal fatty acid metabolism is normalized.[22–25] The focus of this chapter, however, will be the effects and efficacy of carnitine supplementation in healthy populations, specifically as a potential ergogenic aid to athletic performance.

11.2 THE ROLE OF CARNITINE IN FAT METABOLISM

11.2.1 BIOSYNTHESIS OF CARNITINE

In humans carnitine is synthesized from the essential amino acids lysine and methionine.[12,26–28] Methionine contributes its methyl groups,[29–30] and the carbon and nitrogen moieties come from lysine.[31,32] In addition, ascorbic acid, iron, niacin, and vitamin B_6 are all requirements for the biosynthesis of carnitine[33] (Figure 11.3). The liver, kidney, heart, and skeletal muscle can convert the trimethyl lysine, which originates from digestion of proteins, to γ-butyrobetaine, but studies have shown that in humans only the liver and kidney can convert γ-butyrobetaine to carnitine.[10,12,34] This has several implications because the heart and skeletal muscles need carnitine but do not produce it; thus, carnitine's transport efficiency is critical, especially during activities such as exercise. Carnitine biosynthesis occurs at a rate of 2 μmol/kg of body weight/day, does not experience significant daily fluctuations, and seems to be related to the availability of N-trimethyllysine.[26]

As mentioned previously, the diet can provide a significant amount of carnitine, approximately 50% (100 to 300 mg/day) in the form of either free carnitine or short- and long-chain FAs.[35,36] This is true for individuals who consume large amounts of beef, pork, and lamb. In addition, this intake is sufficient to maintain normal carnitine homeostasis. Vegetarians who consume less than 0.5 μmol/kg of body weight/day must rely on endogenous production of carnitine to maintain homeostasis.[37]

Once carnitine is produced, the intracellular homeostasis is controlled by different membrane transporters called organic cation transporters (OCTNs), specifically OCTN2. OCTN2 acts to operate on both the intestinal and renal absorption of L-carnitine, in addition to playing a major role in tissue distribution and transport rates within circulation. This transporter has been implicated in the deficiencies mentioned earlier in this chapter, as research has shown that OCTN2 is directly inhibited by various agents and substances identified as causing systemic carnitine deficiencies.[38]

11.2.2 CARNITINE POOLS: DISTRIBUTION AND EXCRETION

In general, carnitine homeostasis is maintained several ways, including absorption from dietary sources, modest rates of biosynthesis, and reabsorption, which is very efficient.[26] Carnitine in its esterified forms as short- and long-chain acylcarnitines is found in several tissues and cellular fluid. In a healthy 70-kg adult the pool of

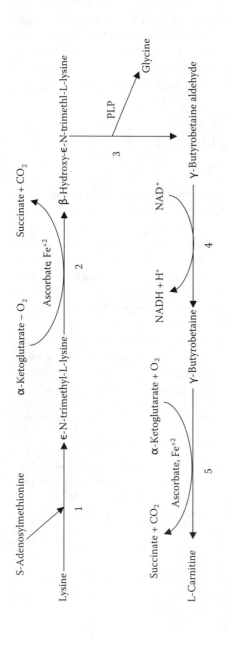

Enzymes utilized in carnitine's biosynthetic pathway

1 – Methylase

2 – Mitochondrial hydroxylase

3 – Aldolase

4 – Dehydrogenase

5 – Cytosolic hydroxylase

FIGURE 11.3 Carnitine biosynthesis.

carnitine is estimated to be about 100 mmol and is distributed between the skeletal and cardiac muscles (98%), liver and kidney (1.6%), and extracellular fluid (0.4%).[39]

Plasma carnitine concentrations in a normal U.S. population can range from 37 to 89 μM, with approximate concentrations for males ranging from 59.3 ± 11.9 μM and females 51.5 ± 11.6 μM. Studies have revealed that 54 to 87% of dietary carnitine is absorbed, which contributes to this plasma pool,[12,26] and furthermore during its metabolism and excretion it is highly conserved within the kidneys. Approximately 90 to 98% of ingested carnitine is reabsorbed in the renal tubules.[40] That which is not reabsorbed can be excreted via the feces (about 1 to 2%) or its typical elimination pathway through the urinary system (about 0.1 to 0.3%).[12]

11.3 CARNITINE UTILIZATION DURING EXERCISE

11.3.1 PYRUVATE DEHYDROGENASE COMPLEX

Research has postulated that there are a few interrelated pathways that can utilize carnitine to enhance the use of long-chain FAs while manipulating acetyl-CoA and pyruvate dehydrogenase (PDH). This would allow for the increased burning of fat as a fuel and the sparing of muscle glycogen during exercise. The rationale behind these assumptions is that *in vitro* experiments have shown that the activation of the pyruvate dehydrogenase complex (PDC) is inhibited by high ratios of acetyl-CoA:free CoA and NADH:NAD⁺.[41] Since carnitine is a known regulator of acetyl-CoA:free CoA via the formation of acylcarnitines, it is plausible to assume that carnitine may control the activity of the PDC.

This interaction can be illustrated during exercise when acetyl-CoA produced via the PDC and β-oxidation can be delivered to the Krebs cycle or accumulate in an acetyl-CoA and acylcarnitine pool. Carnitine can then accept the acetyl-CoA groups that continue to accumulate, directly affecting acetyl-CoA and carnitine status during exercise.

11.3.2 ACYLCARNITINES

It is important to exploit the role of the acylcarnitines because an increase in their formation is directly linked to an increase in acetyl-CoA while free carnitine levels decline in the muscle.[35] This yields no change in the overall carnitine level and maintenance of the acetyl-CoA:free CoA ratio. This will occur during all types and intensities of exercise. However, it is very important to also recognize follow-up *in vivo* studies examining muscle. They demonstrate that the full potential of PDC activity could be quickly reached and maintained.[42–44] Furthermore, PDC activity was still fully active with low lactate accumulation, which was to be expected. These results suggest that *in vivo* examinations give a more accurate portrayal of the intricate system and role of carnitine in metabolism and can give us hints into the effectiveness of carnitine as an ergogenic aid.

11.4 CARNITINE SUPPLEMENTATION

11.4.1 DOES CARNITINE SUPPLEMENTATION MAKE SENSE?

There are several rationales behind why carnitine might be a promising ergogenic aid. These reasons are related specifically to its proposed metabolic actions of being capable of transporting long-chain FAs into the mitochondria for utilization. The assumption is that more is better, and the more carnitine available for biological work, the more FAs that can be utilized for energy. To be more specific, this rationale is used to argue that there will be more FA oxidation since this oxidation is carnitine dependent, and that this will spare muscle glycogen. In addition, since carnitine promotes fat utilization, supplementation will then be successful in altering body composition to favor decreases in fat mass and aid in weight loss. Other rationales include increasing maximal oxygen consumption (VO$_2$ max), activating the PDC via the acetyl-CoA:free CoA ratio, replacing carnitine lost during exercise or redistributed to acylcarnitines, and, finally, allowing muscles to become more resistant to fatigue. All of these scenarios seem plausible and have been extensively researched as to their efficacy.

11.4.2 WHEN WOULD CARNITINE SUPPLEMENTATION BE EFFECTIVE?

When interpreting studies on carnitine, it is important to remember to focus on the changes that occur within the muscle because that is the major reservoir for carnitine. This will govern whether it is appropriate to supplement and how effective supplementation will be. The majority of research shows that carnitine is typically only effective during a primary or secondary carnitine deficiency when the body cannot maintain adequate levels of the metabolite,[16-24] although it is important to recognize that there are conflicting results regarding performance, specifically when examining the difference between exercise intensities.

The remainder of this chapter will focus on the exercise- and performance-related literature that has been completed. This body of literature will examine the possible role of carnitine as an ergogenic aid.

11.5 CARNITINE AND PERFORMANCE

11.5.1 DIETARY SUPPLEMENTATION AND BODY CARNITINE LEVELS

Research has provided many conflicting results when analyzing changes in body carnitine levels. This is primarily due to the fact that the methodology is inconsistent. Many of the studies have focused on blood or plasma levels of carnitine, but the primary action of carnitine occurs in the muscle. Therefore, those studies that reflect changes in muscle carnitine will most accurately reflect whether supplementation is necessary. Unfortunately, there are only a few studies that have reported muscle carnitine levels.[12,45-47] Those that have measured muscle levels find that supplementation with normal or low doses (approximately 1 to 6 g orally or intravenously) does not increase levels normally present in the muscle tissue. It seems as though there are only a couple of conditions where carnitine supplementation may actually act to increase concentrations within the muscle. These circumstances include a supraphysiological dose (100 mg/kg body weight). In addition, those individuals who are carnitine deficient will benefit from supplementation. Specifically, this is because those individuals already have low carnitine concentrations and supplementation will allow for the accumulation of the necessary carnitine content within the muscle to perform. These studies[12,45–47] emphasize that there is adequate carnitine within the muscle mitochondria to oxidize lipids, and furthermore that a carnitine deficiency will not occur as a result of aerobic exercise. In addition, when muscle carnitine levels were compared to plasma levels, it was found that the carnitine metabolic state, associated with exercise, was very poorly reflected by changes in both the plasma and urine.[46]

The general consensus is that individuals who abide by a standard diet will take in the necessary nutrients to maintain adequate levels of carnitine in the muscle. Furthermore, it is important to emphasize again that caution be exerted when analyzing the carnitine literature because individuals need to recognize the nature of the carnitine pools that were examined, whether in blood or muscle.

11.5.2 CARNITINE LEVELS AND ACUTE EXERCISE

Acute exercise is characterized by a single session that may be repeated for several days, not usually longer than a week. This type of exercise has been widely used in the scientific literature on carnitine to study the changes in carnitine concentrations that occur prior to and after a single exercise session. These types of studies are effective in quantifying carnitine concentrations within the body as well as providing an insight into its metabolism during exercise. Acute studies can set the framework for long-term research because the acute data are used to predict how carnitine will act with larger volumes of training.

Lennon et al.[48] examined subjects during submaximal cycle ergometry at 55% of VO_2 max and found that there was a significant decrease (about 20%) in muscle carnitine levels. They reported that as the muscle carnitine dropped there was a significant and concurrent increase in plasma carnitine from rest to the termination of 40 min of exercise. These results led the authors[48] to suggest that some acylcarnitines are lost to the plasma from the muscle during acute exercise bouts. They further suggested[48] that more intense exercise could severely deplete muscle carnitine levels.

Conflicting results were seen by Carlin et al.,[49] who found that with 90 min of cycling (50% VO_2 max) there were no decreases in total muscle carnitine levels, but increased levels of acylcarnitines and decreased free carnitine within the muscle were observed. Plasma levels of acylcarnitine were shown to increase progressively with exercise as a result of the decline in free carnitine, and not the transfer of carnitine from the muscle to the plasma.[49] Again, these studies help to illustrate the importance of measuring and analyzing carnitine pools separately. These results are supported by Harris et al.,[50] who found that both intermittent electrical stimulation and cycling resulted in no change in total muscle carnitine but a significant fall in free carnitine and a concurrent increase in acylcarnitine levels. In addition, Harris's group[50] was able to quantify that the resting mean carnitine concentration in muscle is approximately 20.0 mmol/kg dry muscle and that 77% of this was in the form of free carnitine and 19% was acylcarnitines. Their analysis helped make quantifying the concentrations more accurate as well as improved the validity of results.

To further examine the acute effects, Soop et al.[51] used femoral artery and vein catheters in seven healthy, moderately trained male cyclists who exercised for 2 h at 50% VO_2 max. The purpose was twofold: first, to examine fatty acid utilization during oral carnitine supplementation (5 g/day) during exercise and, second, to quantify and examine the changes that occur in plasma and muscle carnitine levels. Results from this study showed that despite a twofold increase in plasma carnitine levels with supplementation, there was no change in FA turnover, and thus no influence over substrate metabolism.[51] In addition, there were no differences between supplemented and nonsupplemented individuals with regard to plasma carnitine levels. In addition, free carnitine was observed to fall, but there was a release from the leg muscles during exercise. Furthermore, there was an increase in acylcarnitines in the plasma with no evidence of release from the leg muscles. Soop et al.[51] further conclude that there is an alternate site for acylation of carnitine, which they suggested is the liver. Keep in mind that these results do coincide with those of Lennon et al.[48] and Carlin et al.,[49] both of whom showed that there were increases in acylcarnitines and decreases in free carnitine. Soop et al.[51] have been able to shed more light on the intricate biochemical pathways that are involved in carnitine homeostasis during exercise. These results[48,49,51] support the notion that within the muscle adequate carnitine levels can be maintained during exercise and further deficiencies are not likely to occur in the muscle.

It seems evident from the numerous studies that there is no drastic effect on total muscle carnitine concentrations during acute exercise because of the redistribution that occurs; specifically, there is an increase in acylcarnitine and decrease in free carnitine concentrations. Thus, it seems likely that supplementation of carnitine for acute bouts of exercise will not be effective and is subsequently unnecessary.

11.5.3 CARNITINE AND HIGH-INTENSITY EXERCISE

It is evident that changes occur within the plasma and muscle with regard to free carnitine and acylcarnitine, but not necessarily total carnitine. The next logical step is to analyze the effect of intensity on carnitine concentrations. High-intensity exercise will decrease the free carnitine levels because of the reaction with acetyl-CoA. Furthermore, at very high intensities free carnitine will decrease to very low levels. Brass and Hiatt[52] have reported values as low as 0.5 to 1.0 mM/kg of wet muscle weight, which approach the concentration needed for half-maximal activity (0.25 to 0.45 mM/kg of wet muscle) of CAT. This decrease in free carnitine has been postulated to be the reason why exercise physiologists report a transition in substrate utilization between moderate- to high-intensity exercise.

Siliprandi et al.[53] supplemented with 2 g of carnitine before high-intensity exercise and found that PDH activity was stimulated and there was a reduction in both plasma lactate and pyruvate. In a similar study, Vecchiet et al.[54] administered L-carnitine or a placebo 1 h before cycle ergometer exercise. The exercise was a graded protocol designed to increase by 50 W every 3 min until exhaustion. Seventy-two hours later the subjects came in to repeat the trial; however, those who got carnitine first did their second trial with the placebo and vice versa. Results showed that VO_2 max increased while carbon dioxide production, pulmonary ventilation, and lactate production decreased.

Several authors have reported a decreased respiratory quotient (RQ) with car-nitine supplementation,[55–57] suggesting that carnitine influences substrate utilization. In support of this hypothesis, both Gorostiaga et al.[55] and Muller et al.[57] reported an increase in lipid utilization, therefore sparing carbohydrates and prolonging exercise time.

High-intensity exercise has been implicated in muscle soreness. Giamberardino et al.[58] examined the effects of carnitine on pain using the Visual Analog Scale, tenderness (pain thresholds), and creatine kinase (CK) release. Subjects were given 3 g/day of a placebo for 3 weeks, and then after a week, washout was given, 3 g/day of carnitine. Subjects performed a step test to stimulate eccentric muscular work during both supplementation periods. Results showed that carnitine supplementation reduced pain, tenderness, and CK release compared to placebo. These results are supported by Kraemer et al.,[59] who also found decreased muscle tissue damage as assessed by magnetic resonance imaging (MRI). Both authors suggest that carnitine supplementation is beneficial for hypoxic (high-intensity) exercise, perhaps due to its vasodilatory properties, and will reduce sarcolemma disruption and perceived muscle soreness.

Despite several studies showing the benefits of carnitine supplementation, there are several that do not show significant results. Hiatt et al.[46] set out to characterize carnitine at two different exercise intensities: 60 min at 50% lactate threshold (LT) and 30 min at a workload between LT and maximal work capacity for each individual. This was intended to reflect exercise intensities that primarily utilize FAs (50% LT) and carbohydrates (above LT to maximum) for energy production. Findings revealed that the lower-intensity exercise was not associated with changes in muscle carnitine metabolism as reflected by alterations in free carnitine and acylcarnitine.[46] In contrast, within 10 min of the high-intensity exercise, muscle acylcarnitine increased by 5.5-fold and free carnitine decreased by 66%. These changes remained over the duration of the high-intensity exercise and persisted for 60 min into recovery. The changes were seen in both long- and short-chain acylcarnitines. In addition, plasma acylcarnitine levels were also increased, suggesting that there is a redistri-bution of the carnitine pool that may persist even after recovery.[46] It is important to note that the authors did report that neither exercise bout was associated with changes in carnitine urinary excretion rates or plasma concentrations.

In support of this idea, Sahlin[60] examined carnitine concentrations during several exercise intensities (40, 75, and 100% VO_2 max). No changes were seen with cycling in total muscle carnitine concentration, acylcarnitine, or free carnitine during the low-intensity exercise (40% VO_2 max), but the high-intensity (75 and 100% VO_2 max) workout produced a significant increase in acylcarnitine from rest (6.9 ± 1.9 mmol/kg) to exercise (18.1 ± 1.0 mmol/kg). In addition, there was a concurrent decrease in free carnitine levels.[60] Decombaz et al.[47] took the next step and studied cross-country skiers who underwent prolonged strenuous exercise to determine if a carnitine deficiency developed. The exercise consisted of a ski race in the Swiss Alps with an average completion time of 13 hours 26 minutes. Carnitine intake was evaluated for 2 weeks prior to the race (average, 50 ± 4 mg/day) in these highly trained individuals. Again, there was no difference in total carnitine content from rest (17.9 ± 1.0 mmol/kg) to post-exercise (18.3 ± 0.8 mmol/kg). In addition, there was a 20% decline in free carnitine concentration that was offset by a 108% increase in acylcarnitine. The authors[47] concluded that carnitine deficiency would not develop in trained athletes with a moderate carnitine dietary intake.

There are varying results when analyzing the effects of carnitine on high-intensity exercise. Karlic and Lohninger[38] critically examined the effects of carnitine supplementation among athletes and reported that 305 subjects demonstrated improved exercise performance and maximum oxygen consumption while 70 did not. It is therefore important to evaluate the efficacy of supplementation on an individual basis, determining whether it will work for you.

11.5.4 INFLUENCE OF CHRONIC EXERCISE TRAINING ON CARNITINE STATUS

It is widely accepted that chronic-endurance aerobic training can induce changes within the skeletal muscle to enhance performance and increase endurance. Some of these changes include increased capillary density, increased enzymatic concentration, and an increase in the size and number of mitochondria. This is associated with an increased ability of the athlete to oxidize FAs, in the form of intramuscular triglycerides, for fuel. This phenomenon has led researchers to analyze the potential changes that might occur with carnitine concentrations in all pools, including urinary excretion, plasma, and muscle.

Several studies have documented that there are no differences in the resting plasma concentrations of carnitine between trained individuals and their sedentary counterparts.[28,61–63] This is practical because carnitine concentrations are governed by dietary intake, and as stated previously, the majority of the population has a diet containing sufficient precursors to promote adequate carnitine synthesis.[36] Similarly, it seems rather unlikely to lose carnitine in the urine, as it only contributes to approximately 1% of carnitine loss daily. The chance that a carnitine deficiency develops with training due to changes that occur within the plasma or urinary compartments is low because of the small fraction that they contribute to both exercise and daily excretion.

Since the muscle is the major pool for carnitine, it is important to pay particular attention to the results that have analyzed training and carnitine status. It is important to emphasize here that research findings regarding this topic are divergent in that there are researchers who support both sides of the question that asks whether training causes a change in carnitine concentration. There is literature to support that both changes occur as a result of training, as well as that which does not support changes. The discrepancy seems to be within the methodology of the studies, as there is little uniformity in measurements of carnitine with regard to what pool is studied or the techniques utilized to measure concentrations. In addition, there are differences in carnitine levels for each person within each muscle and levels vary between genders. Finally, the type of exercise does affect the extent of carnitine status, as presented in the previous section. All these possibilities present sources of error and must be thoroughly evaluated.

Lennon et al.[48] reported that males have significantly higher levels of muscle carnitine than females in both a high and moderate training group, and this is likely due to the increased muscle mass associated with the male. In addition, they report[48] that training status does not affect muscle carnitine concentrations in either the males or females.

Janssen et al.[64] further supported these findings with sedentary individuals who completed an 18- to 20-month marathon training program. Muscle carnitine was evaluated prior to, during, and after the completion of the marathon and was not affected during training, nor were sex-related differences observed.[65] In addition, running the marathon did not cause a significant decrease in muscle carnitine levels, suggesting that neither the training nor the strenuous exercise alters carnitine muscle levels. Finally, Decombaz et al.[47] measured the total muscle carnitine level of skiers for 2 years prior to an Alpine ski race and found that there were no significant changes over the course of their training regiment (mean, 17 vs. 16 μmol/g dry wt). It is important to point out that there were consistent individual variations (range, 12 to 22 μmol/g dry wt) that were stable for the course of the training. These results show that with training there is little variation in carnitine levels and that deficiencies will not occur as a result of this training, leading to the suggestion that the diet may provide a sufficient amount of precursors to synthesize adequate amounts of carnitine.

It is important to point out that there are studies that found differences in carnitine concentrations after training. One such study by Arenas et al.[66] found that endurance athletes showed a significant decrease in free and total muscle carnitine content after 4 months of training, and that these changes were not as severe as those seen in sprinters. The authors suggest[66] these differences were due to the endurance athletes having a higher concentration of type I muscle fibers, and thus a higher mitochondrial content than the type II fibers of the sprinters, leading to the conclusion that there was a wasting of the short-chain acylcarnitines, a result of chronic training, which would deplete the carnitine stores for subsequent training sessions. A limitation in this study was that the researchers did not separate the subjects by gender in their analysis and when reporting their findings. Furthermore, there was not an equal amount of males and females in both groups. The endurance group consisted of all males, whereas the sprint group had 5 females of 11 participants. It has been shown that there are significant differences between muscle carnitine levels in males and females.[48,67,68]

11.5.5 SUMMARY OF CARNITINE AND TRAINING EFFECTS

Exercise, whether it is acute or chronic, does not seem to influence the total muscle carnitine, but definite changes occur with regard to the accumulation of acylcarnitines and reduction in free carnitine. These changes are well documented[46,47,49–51,60,63,65] and provide a basis for the subsequent literature analyzing performance. The rationale is that despite the fact that exercise does not alter muscle carnitine concentration, supplementation may contribute to the already existing pool and furthermore influence performance. Carnitine supplementation has been postulated to influence performance by increasing the delivery of FAs into the mitochondria to prolong endurance exercise as well as delay fatigue by sparing muscle glycogen. Improving performance is a central theme in nutrition and sport and provides a basis for the implementation of a supplement to an individual's diet. It is therefore pertinent to examine the effects of supplementation on performance to validate the efficacy of an ergogenic aid.

11.5.6 CARNITINE SUPPLEMENTATION AND PERFORMANCE

Up to this point we have examined the influence of acute and chronic exercise on carnitine levels in the muscle, plasma, and urine. The literature is fairly consistent in that there does not seem to be a depletion of total muscle carnitine and that an acute bout or chronic training does not change these levels. It is important to now focus on the performance aspect of these and other studies. The intent is to ascertain whether carnitine supplementation enhances performance as measured by such variables as VO_2 max, RQ, exercise duration, blood lactate concentrations, substrate metabolism, and glycogen sparing. There have been several studies that measured all or some combination of these markers, and they will be presented in chronological order to help follow the progression of carnitine research.

An early study by Marconi et al.[62] used six competitive racewalkers and measured VO_2 max, blood lactate, and RQ. Subjects were supplemented with 4 g of oral carnitine for 2 weeks after which VO_2 max was found to be significantly increased from 54.5 ± 3.7 ml·kg·min^{-1} to 57.8 ± 4.7 ml·kg·min^{-1}. In addition, there were no significant changes in blood lactate accumulation or RQ at a fixed workload. The authors[62] speculated that this slight but significant increase in VO_2 max was due to the activation of substrate flow through the Krebs cycle. This simply means that with an increase in substrate flow through the Krebs cycle, there is a postulated increase in ATP production that allowed the subjects to increase VO_2 max. Subsequent studies[69] could not reproduce these results and found that 2 g of oral carnitine administered to separate groups for either 14 or 28 days produced no significant effects on either VO_2 max or lactate. It is important to note that the training statuses of the two groups were different, one being trained[62] and the other untrained.[69] However, neither study was able to alter blood lactate, RQ, heart rate (HR), or ventilation (V_E), suggesting that the increases in VO_2 max found in the Marconi study[62] may not be physiologically significant.

Angelini et al.[70] used a double-blind protocol to examine untrained subjects who were given either a placebo or carnitine supplementation (50 mg/kg/day) for 1 month during an exercise regiment. VO_2 max increased after the supplementation period, but it was not possible to determine whether the affect was due to the carnitine supplementation or the training regimen since untrained individuals can show significant improvements in VO_2 max within 30 days of aerobic training. Furthermore, Cooper et al.[65] showed that there was no significant improvement in marathon race time despite a daily supplementation of 4 g of oral carnitine for 10 days.

Oyono-Enguelle et al.[71] and Soop et al.[51] found no effect of carnitine supplementation for VO_2, volume of carbon dioxide (VCO_2), lactate, blood glucose at a fixed workload, or FA turnover. These studies used untrained[71] and moderately trained[51] individuals and supplemented 5 g orally for 10 days[71] and 2 g orally for 28 days,[51] respectively. Both studies concluded that in healthy subjects carnitine supplementation does not influence FA utilization, suggesting that the endogenous production of carnitine is sufficient to support exercise.

Gorostiaga et al.[55] utilized 10 endurance-trained subjects (8 marathoners, 1 cyclist, 1 jogger) and supplemented 2 g of oral carnitine for 28 days. Subjects exercised for 45 min at 66% of VO_2 max. Significant differences were observed between supplemented and nonsupplemented groups with respect to RQ during the 38- to 45-min interval (0.95 ± 0.01 vs. 0.98 ± 0.02, respectively), but not any of the earlier time intervals. There were no other changes reported in any of the other variables measured, which included VO_2 max, HR, blood glycerol, and resting blood FA concentrations. These results seem insignificant since other physiological parameters do not help to substantiate the reduction in RQ at one time interval.

In 1990, Siliprandi et al.[53] and Vecchiet et al.[54] examined the effects of 2 g of oral carnitine in a single dose approximately 1 h prior to cycle ergometer exercise. Carnitine supplementation was reported to reduce blood lactate and increase VO_2 max post-exercise. The authors claim that during this high-intensity exercise the PDC is stimulated, thereby reducing lactate production due to the alteration of the acetyl-CoA:free CoA ratio. These findings, however, were not supported, as Constantin-Teodosiu[42–44] showed that full activity of the PDC was reached within a minute of activation and is independent of carnitine supplementation.

Subsequent studies[45,72–77] have tried to extend carnitine research to cover varying lengths of time (7 to 14 days), utilize different exercise modalities, including swimming, and alter administration via either oral or intravenous doses. The variables measured included performance times, VO_2 max, VCO_2, substrate utilization, glycogen storage, blood lactate, and FA turnover. Findings from these experiments exhibit no support for the ergogenic benefits of carnitine on performance (Table 11.1). These physiological parameters are what govern our performance, and if a supplement is not successful in consistently altering these parameters, then the efficacy of carnitine as an ergogenic aid is diminished. It is important to note here that there have also been studies trying to elucidate carnitine as a weight-loss supplement due to its association with FA metabolism. The fact remains that these studies[78,79] show that carnitine is not a contributing factor to weight loss since many supplements are given with calorie-restricted diets and exercise programs that are in themselves effective tools in reducing weight and increasing muscle mass. Supplement companies then mask their results behind the truly effective tools in weight management.

11.6 RECOMMENDATIONS REGARDING CARNITINE SUPPLEMENTATION

Despite no nutritional deficiency of carnitine, several of the cofactors and precursors necessary for its production are essential. Thus, it should be emphasized that a well-balanced diet is vital for normal carnitine function. Carnitine supplementation,

TABLE 11.1
The Effects of Carnitine Supplementation on Performance

Reference	Subjects	Carnitine Dosage	Duration of Treatment	Dependent Variables	Effects of Carnitine
50	6 racewalkers	4 g, orally	14 days	VO_2 max, BLa–, RER	↑ VO_2 max, no change, BLa–, RER
57	3 M/6 F	2 g, orally	14 days	VO_2 max, BLa–	No change
60	10 M	2 g, orally	28 days	VO_2, VCO_2, RER, BLa–, plasma glucose	No effect of carnitine
47	7 M	5 g, orally	5 days	FFA, VO_2	No effect of carnitine
61	9 M/1 F	2 g, orally	28 days	RER, VO_2, HR, BLa–, plasma glucose	↓ RER, no other changes
62, 63	10 M	2 g, orally	1 h pre-exercise	VO_2 max, BLa–	↑ VO_2 max, ↓ BLa–
64	9 M	3 g, orally	7 days	RER, RPE, BLa–, HR, fat oxidation	No effect of carnitine
65	12 M	3 g, IV	40 min pre-exercise	VO_2, VCO_2, substrate oxidation	No change during exercise
66	20 M	2 g, 2 times/day, orally	7 days	Swim performance, BLa–	No effect of carnitine
41	8 M	6 g, orally	7–14 days	RER, FFA, VO_2	No effect of carnitine

however, is another issue. L-carnitine is very well tolerated, and there seems to be no toxicity and very few side effects even when taken in doses as large as 15 g/day.[28,80,81] The problem remains that even with supplementation there is not enough unequivocal evidence to support a necessity for supplementation. The vast majority of the research reveals no benefit to enhancing performance as a result of increased carnitine supplementation. In general, proper training and genetic endowment lead to athletic success, not supplementation, whether it be carnitine or any other supplement.[79] Despite the vast amount of literature on supplementation, it is still prominent to "prescribe" or recommend supplements as a way of enhancing performance.

In conclusion, the majority of studies reveal that carnitine supplementation does not seem to provide an ergogenic benefit to human performance. The body and diet are sufficient to provide enough carnitine to allow an individual to effectively regulate lipid metabolism both at rest and during various types of exercise.

11.7 SUMMARY

The role of carnitine in metabolism is very critical: it is a key component of the enzymes responsible for transporting long-chain FAs across the mitochondrial matrix where they can be used to produce energy. Carnitine is endogenously produced from the essential amino acids lysine and methionine in amounts that are sufficient to maintain homeostasis, when an individual's dietary intake includes a low to moderate amount of meat products. If there is a deficiency of carnitine, it is typically a result of impaired synthesis, increased degradation, inefficient transport, or abnormal renal handling. This can result in glucose dependency and perhaps even hypoglycemia. Skeletal musculature is weakened and may atrophy in addition to decreased myoglobin concentrations. Finally, cardiac muscle, which utilizes primarily FAs for fuel, may experience failure and frequent arrhythmias.

REFERENCES

1. Guleswitsch, W. and Krimberg, R., Zur Kenntnis der Extraktivstoffe der Muskeln. II. Mitteilung. Uber das Carnitin. *Hoppe Seylers Z. Physiol. Chem.*, 45, 326–330, 1905.
2. Kutscher, F., Uber Liebig's Fleischextrakt. Mitteilung I. *Z. Untersuch. Nahr. Genussem.*, 10, 528–537, 1905.
3. Tomita, M. and Sendju, Y., Uber die Oxyaminoverbindungen, welche die Biuretreaktion weigen. III. Spaltung der -Amino--oxybuttersaure in die opstich-aktiven Komponenten. *Hoppe Seylers Z. Physiol. Chem.*, 169, 263–277, 1927.
4. Kaneko, T. and Yoshida, R., On the absolute configuration of L-carnitine (vitamin B_T). *Bull. Chem. Soc. Jpn.*, 35, 1153–1155, 1962.
5. Bau, R., Schreiber, A., Metzenthin, T., Lu, R.S., Lutz, F., Klooster, W.T., Koetzle, T.F., Siem, H., Kleber, H.P., Brewer, F., and England, S., Neutron diffraction structure of (2R,3R)-L-(-)-[2-D] carnitine tetrachloroaurate, $[(CH_3)_3N\text{-}CH_2\text{-}CHOH\text{-}CHD\text{-}COOH]^+[AuCl_4]^-$: determination of the absolute stereochemistry of the crotonobetaine-to-carnitine transformation catalyzed by L-carnitine dehydratase from *Escherichia coli*. *J. Am. Chem. Soc.*, 119, 12055–12060, 1997.

6. Fraenkel, G., Blewett, M., and Coles, M., BT, a new vitamin of the B-group and its relation to the folic acid group, and other anti-anemia factors. *Nature*, 161, 981–983, 1948.
7. Siliprandi, N., Di Lisa, F., and Menabo, R., Clinical use of carnitine. Past, present and future. *Adv. Exp. Med. Biol.*, 273, 175, 1990.
8. Brevetti G., Chiariello, M., and Ferulano, G., Increases in walking distance in patients with peripheral vascular disease treated with L-carnitine: a double-blind, cross-over study. *Circulation*, 77, 767, 1988.
9. Siliprandi, N., Carnitine in physical exercise, in *Biochemical Aspects of Physical Exercise*, Benzi, G., Packer, L., and Siliprandi, N., Eds. Elsevier Science Publishers, Amsterdam, 1986, pp. 197–206.
10. Rebouche, C.J., Carnitine function and requirements during the life cycle. *FASEB J.*, 6, 3379–3386, 1992.
11. Jeukendrup, A.E., Regulation of fat metabolism in skeletal muscle. *Ann. N.Y. Acad. Sci.*, 967, 217, 2002.
12. Heinonen, O.J., Carnitine and physical exercise. *Sports Med.*, 22, 109–132, 1996.
13. Paulson, D.J. and Shug, A.L., Tissue specific depletion of L-carnitine in rat heart and skeletal muscle by D-carnitine. *Life Sci.*, 28, 2931–2938, 1981.
14. Negrao, C.E., Ji, L.L., Schauer, J.E., Nagel, F.J., and Lardy, H.A., Carnitine supplementation and depletion: tissue carnitines and enzymes in fatty acid oxidation. *J. Appl. Physiol.*, 63, 315–321, 1987.
15. Keith, R.E., Symptoms of carnitine-like deficiency in a trained runner taking DL-carnitine supplements. *JAMA*, 255, 1137, 1986.
16. DiPalma, J.R., L-carnitine: its therapeutic potential. *Am Fam. Physician*, 34, 127–130, 1986.
17. Engel, A.G., ReBouche, C.J., Wilson, D.M., Glasgow, A.M., Romshe, C.A., and Cruse, R.P., Primary systemic carnitine deficiency. II. Renal handling of carnitine. *Neurology*, 31, 819–825, 1981.
18. Borum, P.R., Carnitine function, in *Clinical Aspects of Human Carnitine Deficiency*, Borum, P.R., Ed. Pergamon, New York, 1986, pp. 16–27.
19. Engel, A.G. and Angelini, C., Carnitine deficiency of human skeletal muscle with associated lipid storage myopathy: a new syndrome. *Science*, 179, 899–902, 1973.
20. Pelligrini, G., Scarlato, G., and Moggio, M., A hereditary case in lipid storage myopathy with carnitine deficiency. *J. Neurol.*, 223, 73–84, 1980.
21. Ware, A.J., Burton, W.C., McGarry, J.D., Marks, J.F., and Weinburg, A.G., Systemic carnitine deficiency. Report of a fatal case with multisystemic manifestations. *J. Pediatr.*, 93, 959–962, 1978.
22. Bohles, H., The effects of preoperative L-C supplementation on myocardial metabolism during aorto-coronary bypass surgery. *Curr. Ther. Res.*, 39, 429–435, 1986.
23. Brooks, H., Goldberg, L., Holland, R., Klein, M., Sanzari, N., and DeFelice, S., Carnitine-induced effects on cardiac and peripheral hemodynamics. *J. Clin. Pharmacol.*, 17, 561–568, 1977.
24. DiPalma, J.R., Ritchie, D.M., and McMichael, R.F., Cardiovascular and antiarrhythmic effects of carnitine. *Arch. Int. Pharmacodyn. Ther.*, 217, 246–250, 1975.
25. Silverman, N.A., Schmitt, G., Vishwanath, M., Feinburg, H., and Levitsky, S., Effect of carnitine on myocardial function and metabolism following global ischemia. *Ann. Thorac. Surg.*, 40, 20–24, 1985.
26. Rebouche, C.J. and Seim, H., Carnitine metabolism and its regulation in microorganisms and mammals. *Ann. Rev. Nutr.*, 18, 39–61, 1998.
27. Beiber, L.L., Carnitine. *Ann. Rev. Biochem.*, 57, 261–283, 1988.

28. Ceretelli, P. and Marconi, C., L-carnitine supplementation in humans: the effects on physical performance. *Int. J. Sports Med.*, 11, 1–14, 1990.

29. Wolf, G. and Berger, C.R.A., Studies on the biosynthesis and turnover of carnitine. *Arch. Biochem. Biophys.*, 92, 360–365, 1961.

30. Bremer, J., Carnitine: metabolism and functions. *Physiol. Rev.*, 63, 1420–1480, 1983.

31. Tanphaichitr, V. and Broquist, H.P., Role of lysine and trimethyllysine in carnitine biosynthesis. II. Studies in rat. *J. Biol. Chem.*, 248, 2176–2181, 1973.

32. Cox, R.A. and Hoppel, C.L., Biosynthesis of carnitine and 4-N-trimethylaminobutyrate from lysine. *Biochem. J.*, 136, 1083–1090, 1973.

33. Broquist, H.P., Carnitine biosynthesis and function: introductory remarks. *Fed. Proc.*, 41, 2840–2842, 1982.

34. ReBouche, C.J. and Engel, A.G., Tissue distribution of carnitine biosynthetic enzymes in man. *Biochim. Biophys. Acta*, 630, 22–29, 1980.

35. Heinonen, O.J., Carnitine: Effect on Palmitate Oxidation, Exercise Capacity and Nitrogen Balance. An Experimental Study with Special Reference to Carnitine Depletion and Supplementation. Ph.D. dissertation, University of Turku, Finland, 1992.

36. Feller, A.G. and Rudman, D., Role of carnitine in human nutrition. *J. Nutr.*, 118, 541–547, 1988.

37. Lombard, K.A., Olson, A.L., Nelson, S.E., and ReBouche, C.J., Carnitine status of lactoovovegetarians and strict vegetarian adults and children. *Am. J. Clin. Nutr.*, 50, 301–306, 1989.

38. Karlic, H. and Lohninger, A., Supplementation of L-carnitine in athletes: does it make sense? *Nutrition*, 20, 709–715, 2004.

39. Engel, A.G. and ReBouche, C.J., Carnitine metabolism and inborn errors. *J. Inherit. Metab. Dis.*, 7, 38–43, 1984.

40. Frolich, J., Seccombe, D.W., and Hahn, P., Effect of fasting on free and esterified carnitine levels in human serum and urine: correlation with serum levels of free fatty acids and β-hydroxybutyrate. *Metabolism*, 27, 555–561, 1978.

41. Constantin-Teodosiu, D., Regulation of Pyruvate Dehydrogenase Complex Activity and Acetyl Group Formation in Skeletal Muscle during Exercise. Ph.D. dissertation, Huddinge University, Sweden, 1992.

42. Constantin-Teodosiu, D., Carlin, J.I., Cederblad, G., Hariss, R.C., and Hultman, E., Acetyl group accumulation and pyruvate dehydrogenase activity in human muscle during incremental exercise. *Acta Physiol. Scand.*, 143, 367–372, 1991.

43. Constantin-Teodosiu, D., Cederblad, G., and Hultman, E., PDC activity and acetyl group accumulation in skeletal muscle during prolonged exercise. *J. Appl. Physiol.*, 73, 2403–2407, 1992.

44. Constantin-Teodosiu, D., Cederblad, G., and Hultman, E., PDC activity and acetyl group accumulation in skeletal muscle during isometric contraction. *J. Appl. Physiol.*, 74, 1712–1718, 1993.

45. Vukovich, M.D., Costill, D.L., and Fink, W.J., Carnitine supplementation: effect on muscle carnitine and glycogen content during exercise. *Med. Sci. Sports Exerc.*, 26, 1122–1129, 1994.

46. Hiatt, W.R., Regensteiner, J.G., Wolfel, E.E., Ruff, L., and Brass, E.P., Carnitine and acylcarnitine metabolism during exercise in humans. *J. Clin. Invest.*, 84, 1167–1173, 1989.

47. Decombaz, J., Gmuender, B., Sierro, G., and Ceretelli, P., Muscle carnitine after strenuous endurance exercise. *J. Appl. Physiol.*, 72, 423–427, 1992.

48. Lennon, D.L., Stratman, F.W., Shrago, E., Nagle, F.J., Madden, M., Hanson, P., and Carter, A.L., Effects of acute moderate-intensity exercise on carnitine metabolism in men and women. *J. Appl. Physiol.*, 55, 489–495, 1983.

49. Carlin, J.I., Reddan, W.G., Sanjak, M., and Hodach R., Carnitine metabolism during prolonged exercise and recovery in humans. *J. Appl. Physiol.*, 61, 1275–1278, 1983.

50. Harris, R.C., Louise Foster, C.V., and Hultman, E., Acetylcarnitine formation during intense muscular contraction. *J. Appl. Physiol.*, 63, 440–442, 1987.

51. Soop, M., Bjorkman, O., Cederblad, G., Hagenfeldt, L., and Wahren, J., Influence of carnitine supplementation on muscle substrate and carnitine metabolism during exercise. *J. Appl. Physiol.*, 64, 2394–2399, 1988.

52. Brass, E.P. and Hiatt, W.R., The role of carnitine and carnitine supplementation during exercise in man and individuals with special needs. *J. Am. Coll. Nutr.*, 17, 207, 1998.

53. Siliprandi, N., DiLisa, F., Peiralisi, G., Ripari, P., Maccari, F., Menabo, R., Giamber-ardino, M.A., and Vecchiet, L., Metabolic changes induced by maximal exercise in humans following L-carnitine administration. *Biochem. Biophys. Acta*, 1034, 17–21, 1990.

54. Vecchiet, L., DiLisa, F., Peiralisi, G., Ripari, R., Menabo, R., Giamberardino, M.A., and Siliprandi, N., Influence of L-carnitine administration on maximal physical exercise. *Eur. J. Appl. Physiol.*, 61, 486–490, 1990.

55. Gorostiaga, E.M., Maurer, C.A., and Eclache, J.P., Decrease in RD during exercise following L-carnitine supplementation. *Int. J. Sports Med.*, 10, 71–80, 1989.

56. Wyss., V., Ganzit, G.P., and Rienzi, A., Effects of L-carnitine administration on VO_2 max and the aerobic-anaerobic threshold in normoxia and acute hypoxia. *Eur. J. Appl. Physiol. Occup. Physiol.*, 60, 1, 1990.

57. Muller, D.M., Seim, H., Kiess, W., Loster, II., and Richter T., Effects of oral L-carnitine supplementation on *in vivo* long-chain fatty acid oxidation in healthy adults. *Metabolism*, 51, 1389, 2002.

58. Giamberardino, M.A., Dragani, L., Valente, R., Di Lisa, F., Saggini, R., and Vecchiet, L., Effects of prolonged L-carnitine administration on delayed muscle pain and CK release after eccentric effort. *Int. J. Sports Med.*, 17, 203, 1996.

59. Kraemer, W.J., Volek, J.S., and French, D.N., The effects of L-carnitine L-tartarate supplementation on hormonal responses to resistance exercise and recovery. *J. Strength Cond. Res.*, 17, 455, 2003.

60. Sahlin, K., Muscle carnitine metabolism during incremental dynamic exercise in humans. *Acta Physiol. Scand.*, 138, 259–262, 1990.

61. Wagenmakers, A.J.M., L-carnitine supplementation and performance in man. *Med. Sci. Sports Exer.*, 32, 110–127, 1991.

62. Marconi C., Sassi, G., Carpenelli, A., and Ceretelli, P., Effects of L-carnitine loading on the aerobic and anaerobic performance of endurance athletes. *J. Sports Sci.*, 54, 131–135, 1985.

63. Borum, P.R., Plasma carnitine compartment and red blood cell carnitine compartment of healthy adults. *Am. J. Clin. Nutr.*, 46, 437–441, 1987.

64. Janssen, G.M.E., Scholte, H.R., Vaandrager, M.H.M., and Ross, J.D., Muscle carnitine level in endurance training and running a marathon. *Int. J. Sports Med.*, 10, S153–S155, 1989.

65. Cooper, M.B., Jones, D.A., Edwards, R.H.T., Corbucci, G.C., Montanari, G., and Trevisani, C., The effect of marathon running on carnitine metabolism and on some aspects of mitochondrial activities and antioxidant mechanisms. *J. Sport Sci.*, 4, 79–87, 1986.

66. Arenas, J., Ricoy, J.R., Encinas, A.R., Pola, P., D'Iddio, S., Zeviani, M., Didonato, S., and Corsi, M., Carnitine in muscle, serum and urine on non-professional athletes: effects of physical exercise, training and L-carnitine administration. *Muscle Nerve*, 14, 598–604, 1991.

67. Cederblad, G., Lindstedt, S., and Lundholm, K., Concentration of carnitine in human muscle tissue. *Clin. Chim. Acta*, 53, 311–321, 1974.

68. Harper, P., Wadstrom, C., and Cederblad, G., Carnitine measurements in liver, muscle tissue, and blood in normal subjects. *Clin. Chem.*, 39, 592–599, 1993.

69. Greig, C., Finch, K.M., Jones, D.A., Cooper, M., Sargeant, A.J., and Forte, C.A., The effect of oral supplementation with L-carnitine on maximum and submaximum exercise capacity. *Eur. J. Appl. Physiol.*, 56, 457–460, 1987.

70. Angelini, C., Vergani, L., and Costa, L., Use of carnitine in exercise physiology. *Adv. Clin. Enzymol.*, 4, 103–110, 1986.

71. Oyono-Enguelle, S., Freund, H., Ott, C., Gartner, M., Heitz, A., Marbach, J., Maccari, F., Frey, A., Bigot, H., and Bach, A.C., Prolonged submaximal exercise and L-carnitine in humans. *Eur. J. Appl. Physiol.*, 58, 53–61, 1988.

72. DeCombaz, J., Deriaz, O., Acheson, K., Gmuender, B., and Jequier, E., Effect of L-carnitine on submaximal exercise metabolism after glycogen depletion. *Med. Sci. Sports Exerc.*, 25, 733–740, 1993.

73. Natali, A., Santoro, D., Brandi, L.S., Faraggiana, D., Ciociaro, D., Pecori, N., Buzzigoil, G., and Ferrannini, E., Effects of hypercarnitinemia during increased fatty substrate oxidation in man. *Metabolism*, 42, 594–600, 1993.

74. Trappe, S.W., Costill, D.L., Goodpaster, B., Vukovich, M.D., and Fink, W.J., The effects of L-carnitine supplementation in performance during interval swimming. *Int. J. Sports Med.*, 15, 181–185, 1994.

75. Brass, E.P., Hoppel, C.L., and Hiatt, W.R., Effects of intravenous L-carnitine on carnitine homeostasis and fuel metabolism during exercise in humans. *Clin. Pharmacol. Ther.*, 55, 681–692, 1994.

76. Barnett, C., Costill, D.L., Vukovich, M.D., Cole, K.J., Goodpaster, B.H., Trappe, S.W., and Fink, W.J., Effect of L-carnitine supplementation on muscle and blood carnitine content and lactate accumulation during high-intensity spring cycling. *Int. J. Sports Nutr.*, 4, 280–288, 1994.

77. Colombani, P., Wenk, C., Kunz, I., Krahenbuhl, S., Kuhnt, M., Arnold, M., Frey-Rindova, P., Frey, W., and Langhans, W., Effects of L-carnitine supplementation on physical performance and energy metabolism of endurance trained athletes: a double-blind crossover study. *Eur. J. Appl. Physiol.*, 73, 434–439, 1996.

78. Gruneweld, K.K. and Bailey, R.S., Commercially marketed supplements for body-building athletes. *Sports Med.*, 15, 90–103, 1993.

79. Williams, M.H., Ergogenic and ergolytic substances. *Med. Sci. Sports Exerc.*, 24, S344–S348, 1992.

80. Snyder, T.M., Little, B.W., Roman-Campos, G., and McQuillen, J.B., Successful treatment of familial idiopathic lipid storage myopathy with L-carnitine and modified lipid diet. *Neurology*, 32, 1106–1115, 1982.

81. Waber, L.J., Valle, D., Neill, C., DiMauro, S., and Shug, A., Carnitine deficiency presenting as familial cardiomyopathy: a treatable defect in carnitine transport. *J. Pediatr.*, 101, 700–705, 1982.

12 β-Hydroxy-β-Methylbutyrate

Steven L. Nissen

CONTENTS

12.1 INTRODUCTION

Since the early 1960s, leucine and its keto acid, α-ketoisocaproate (KIC), have been the subject of research into the regulation of muscle protein synthesis and muscle protein breakdown.[1,2] However, in the early 1990s a downstream metabolite called β-hydroxy-β-methylbutyrate (HMB) was shown to have a positive effect on muscle protein[3] and was postulated to be responsible for the leucine effect on muscle protein metabolism.[4] Since the initial discovery, HMB has been studied extensively as an ergogenic aid in humans, especially related to exercise training.[3,5–12]

This chapter will focus on HMB and the benefits related to improving human performance and augmenting the effects of training. The areas that will be examined include magnification of the strength and fat-free mass gains associated with resistance training,[13] reduction of the muscle damage that occurs during intense exercise,[6,9] enhancement of indicators of endurance performance,[5] and how HMB combined with other nutrients can restore muscle mass lost from disease[14,15] and aging.[16] Lastly, the effects of HMB on cholesterol metabolism[4] and muscle proteolysis[3] will be addressed as a possible mechanism whereby HMB acts to increase lean tissue mass.

12.1.1 ENDOGENOUS PRODUCTION

Endogenous production of HMB occurs in muscle and liver[17,18] (Figure 12.1) and possibly other tissues. The first step in HMB formation is the transamination of leucine to KIC, which occurs in both the cytosol and mitochondria of muscle cells.[19] In the mitochondria, KIC is irreversibly oxidized to isovaleryl-CoA by the enzyme branched-chain α-keto acid dehydrogenase. Isovaleryl-CoA then undergoes further metabolic steps within the mitochondria (Figure 12.1), yielding β-hydroxy-β-methylglutaryl-CoA (HMG-CoA). Further metabolism by the enzyme HMG-CoA lyase results in the end products acetoacetate and acetyl-CoA. Approximately 90% of KIC is oxidized to isovaleryl CoA in liver mitochondria and ultimately to acetoacetate and acetyl-CoA.

In the cytosol of cells, the remaining ~10% of the KIC is oxidized to HMB[20–24] via the enzyme KIC dioxygenase. This enzyme requires molecular oxygen and iron,[24] and may be identical to p-phenylpyruvate dioxygenase, which is a key enzyme in the degradation of tyrosine converting 4-hydroxyphenylpyrvate to homogentisate.[25]

A second pathway in the production of HMB has also been postulated through the hydroxylation of methylcrotenoic acid (MCA), but only when biotin is deficient. It is proposed that MCA concentrations become elevated due to the low activity of the biotin-requiring enzyme MC-CoA carboxylase. HMB levels also increase,[26] suggesting that MCA may be hydrated to HMB by enol-CoA hydrase,[27] an enzyme of the isoleucine pathway. However, it is not clear whether MCA is directly converted to HMB during biotin deficiency, or if the rise in HMB is simply a result of feedback inhibition on the various enzymes along the pathway back to KIC.

Extrapolating from leucine turnover studies in pigs,[28] it is estimated that endogenous HMB production is equal to 0.2 to 0.4 g of HMB/day in a 70-kg man, depending on leucine intake. Furthermore, turnover of HMB is thought to be relatively rapid, as basal plasma concentrations in normal humans range from 1 to 4 nM.[29,30] Plasma levels of

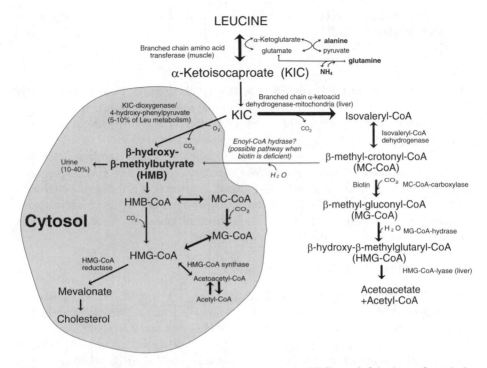

FIGURE 12.1 Overview of leucine, α-ketoisocaproate (KIC), and β-hydroxy-β-methyl-butyrate (HMB) metabolism.

HMB increase following ingestion of 1 g of HMB to approximately 115 nM, but are near basal levels 12 h later, again suggesting rapid metabolism.

12.1.2 FATE

HMB has two fates in the body: conversion to HMG-CoA[31–33] and excretion in the urine.[28–30] The metabolic pathway of HMB metabolism is conversion to HMG-CoA (Figure 12.1). In the cytosol, conversion of HMB to HMG-CoA occurs either through direct carboxylation or through dehydration of MCA-CoA (Figure 12.1). Subsequently, the cytosolic HMG-CoA produced can provide substrate for HMG-CoA reductase, which is the committed step in cellular cholesterol synthesis.[4] This fact has been hypothesized as a mechanism whereby HMB can affect cellular metabolism by providing a cholesterol precursor during times of elevated need.[4]

Urinary excretion of HMB in humans ranges from 10% to almost 50% of an exogenous HMB dosage.[4] Nissen et al.[3] reported that urine HMB excretion varied from 10 to 30 mg/day prior to supplementation, while supplementation of 1.5 and 3.0 g of HMB/day resulted in an increase in excretion to 450 to 500 mg/day and 950 to 1200 mg/day, respectively. Recent metabolic studies following ingestion of 1 g of HMB resulted in approximately 14% of the given dose being excreted in the urine. The percentage of the dosage excreted increased to 29% of the given dose after consumption of a single 3-g dose of HMB.[29] With both dosages of HMB given, most of the urinary excretion occurred within 6 h of the dosing, paralleling the increases in plasma HMB.[29]

12.1.3 ABSORPTION

Absorption of dietary HMB appears to be rapid and complete. Plasma HMB levels have been shown to be elevated as little as 30 min following consumption of 1 g of HMB.[29] Following a single 1-g oral dose of HMB, plasma HMB levels peaked at 115 nM at approximately 2 h postingestion, and after a single 3-g oral dose of HMB, plasma HMB levels peaked at 480 nM at approximately 1 h post ingestion.[29] Absorption is not increased by concurrent glucose ingestion (75 g); rather, HMB absorption is slightly slower when consumed with glucose, but overall it is the same either with or without concurrent glucose ingestion.[29] Data from our lab suggest the absorption of supplemental HMB is complete, as supplemental intake of 1.5 or 3 g of HMB did not appear to affect fecal HMB concentrations.

12.1.4 DIETARY AND SUPPLEMENTAL SOURCES

Most foods contain trace amounts of HMB. Fruits and vegetables have relatively low HMB concentrations ranging from 1 to 5 nmol/g, while most meats have higher concentrations ranging from 15 to 25 nmol/g.[34] However, some foods of plant origin have concentrations of HMB comparable to those seen in products of animal origin. For example, an herbal tea was found to contain 26 nmol HMB/g, while asparagus and squash have 22 nmol HMB/g.[35] Although diet is a source of HMB, endogenous production of HMB from leucine generally far exceeds dietary intake of HMB. Therefore, foods containing large concentrations of leucine would probably have a greater influence on the circulating concentrations of HMB in the body than the HMB found in most common foodstuffs. This was demonstrated in pigs when a meal supplemented with 50 g of leucine was consumed. Plasma HMB concentrations increased ten-fold over that of pigs fed a meal without supplemental leucine.[36] In humans given leucine intravenously, plasma HMB increased from 1.9 to 3.6 μM and plasma HMB rate of appearance increased from 0.19 to 0.27 μmol/kg/h.[37]

Supplemental HMB is commercially available as calcium β-hydroxy-β-methyl-butyrate-monohydrate, or $Ca(C_5H_9O_3)_2 \cdot H_2O$ (CaHMB; molecular weight = 292). Supplemental CaHMB is a white powder that is freely soluble in water and has a slightly bitter taste. HMB is chemically synthesized[38–42] and commercially sold under U.S. Patents 5,348,979, 5,360,613, and 6,103,764, which relate to nitrogen sparing, decreasing cholesterol, and increasing aerobic capacity, respectively. Based on previously reported data,[3] the recommended dosage is 3 g (as CaHMB) per day for a 70-kg man; therefore, HMB can easily be supplemented in the form of capsules or tablets, and thus individual dosage can be adjusted on a by-weight basis for significantly lighter or heavier individuals (38 mg of HMB/kg of body weight/day).

12.1.5 MECHANISM OF ACTION

Although the mechanism of action for HMB is not known, the primary working theory is that HMB acts by improving cell membrane integrity by supplying adequate substrate for cholesterol synthesis.[4] It is clear that HMB is converted to HMG-CoA in the cytosol, which can be used for cholesterol synthesis in cells.[4] In all cells, cholesterol is needed for the synthesis of new cell membranes as well as the repair of damaged membranes in maintaining proper cell function and growth.[43,44] Certain cells, such as muscle cells, require *de novo* synthesis of cholesterol for cell cholesterol functions. Therefore, during periods of increased stress on cells, such as occurs in muscle during intense exercise, the demand for cholesterol for growth or repair of cellular membranes may exceed that which can be made through normal endogenous production from available cellular HMG-CoA. Thus, supplemental HMB may help meet an increased demand for and maintain maximal cell function by supplying intracellular HMG-CoA for cholesterol synthesis. The cholesterol can then be used to build and stabilize muscle cell membranes. This theory is supported by observations on diverse cell functions such as immune function and milk fat synthesis, which also requires *de novo* synthesis of cholesterol in the cells.[4]

Another possible mechanism of action of supplemental HMB on muscle mass is that HMB somehow directly decreases muscle proteolysis or protein breakdown by having a direct effect on transcriptional or translational control of genes, enzyme activities, or other processes involved with proteolysis. When isolated chicken and rat muscles were studied *in vitro*, HMB addition to the muscle strip media decreased muscle proteolysis.[45] Further research *in vivo* has shown that HMB decreases muscle proteolysis through changes in the activity of the proteolytic enzymes such as thiol cathepsins and calpain II.[46] In humans undergoing an intense resistance exercise program, supplementing HMB resulted in a significant decrease in urinary 3-methylhistidine (3-MH), indicating decreased protein degradation during the first 2 weeks of the exercise program ($p < 0.04$ and $p < 0.001$ for weeks 1 and 2, respectively).[3] Therefore, increasing the circulating levels of HMB through supplementation may decrease the rate of muscle protein breakdown, which would be of benefit in unwanted catabolic conditions such as after heavy exercise or wasting conditions brought about by some diseases.

Both of the mechanisms proposed may contribute to the effects of HMB in helping maintain cellular function. The increase in cell function could be directly through an increase in cellular cholesterol, and thus stabilization of the cell membranes, or through a more positive protein balance by decreasing muscle protein breakdown. Whatever mechanisms are responsible for the effects of HMB, it appears HMB supplementation has a positive effect on minimizing cell damage and protein breakdown.[3,6,9,45]

12.2 APPLICATIONS

Supplemental HMB has been shown to augment the strength and fat-free mass gains associated with resistance training by approximately twofold.[13] Furthermore, HMB has been shown to have a positive effect not only in younger men and women resistance training,[8] but also in older adult men and women.[10] Other uses of HMB include improving indicators of endurance performance[5] and minimizing muscle damage that occurs during intense exercise.[6,9] HMB in combination with other nutrients has also been shown to have positive effects on muscle mass in nonexercising populations, such as those suffering from disease or age-related muscle loss.[14–16]

12.2.1 RESISTANCE TRAINING

There have been a total of nine peer-reviewed studies published so far with HMB in exercising humans. These are summarized in Table 12.1. From the original study investigating the effect of HMB on resistance training[3] to a meta-analysis on nutritional supplements,[13] HMB has been consistently shown to increase strength and fat-free mass gains in conjunction with a resistance training program.[8–11]

12.2.1.1 Increases Strength and Muscle Mass

In the first published study, Nissen et al.[3] reported a linear increase in lean body mass with HMB supplementation. Three weeks of HMB supplementation at 0, 1.5, or 3.0 g/day resulted in gains of 0.4, 0.8, and 1.2 kg of lean body mass, respectively. Furthermore, similar increases in total body strength were observed with the three levels of HMB supplementation. Total strength increased 338, 529, and 707 kg with 0, 1.5, and 3.0 g of HMB/day, respectively. Although positive changes were observed with the lower dose of 1.5 g of HMB/day, the dose of 3.0 g/day resulted in the greatest gains with resistance training. Later, in a study by Gallagher et al.,[9] it was concluded that a higher dose of HMB of up to 76 mg/kg of body weight/day (6 g/day) may result in some additional benefit, such as attenuating the creatine phosphokinase (CPK) levels during an intense training program. However, the higher dose did not appear to promote additional increases in one repetition maximum strength or fat-free mass.[7,9]

A meta-analysis by Nissen and Sharp[13] summarized the effects of HMB (and other nutritional supplements) on muscle mass and strength with resistance training. It was found that in conjunction with resistance training, supplementation of 3 g of HMB/day resulted in a net increase in lean mass of 0.28% per week and strength of 1.40% per week (Figure 12.2a and Figure 12.3a). When these results are expressed as an effect size, a method of data standardization, HMB resulted in a significant effect size of a net lean mass gain of 0.15 and strength gain of 0.19 (Figure 12.2b and Figure 12.3b). These effect size values indicate a highly positive effect of HMB supplementation on strength and muscle mass ($p < 0.01$). Table 12.1 summarizes the characteristics of all of the HMB studies included in the meta-analysis, including dosage used, age and gender of subjects, training status, training duration, and body composition method. The accumulative conclusion of the individual studies[3,8,9,11] along with the conclusion from the meta-analysis[13] clearly support the nutritional supplementation of HMB to augment strength and muscle mass gains from resistance training.

12.2.1.2 Effect of Gender and Training Status

Initially, most of the research performed on HMB supplementation with resistance training was conducted in college-aged men. However, Panton et al.[8] reported that men and women similarly respond to HMB supplementation. When corrected for the initial starting differences and expressed as a percent change, HMB supplementation resulted in similar improvements in strength, body composition, and degree of decrease in muscle damage with resistance training for both men and women.

TABLE 12.1
Summary of Characteristics of All Published Studies Using HMB with Resistance Training that Met the Specific Inclusion Criteria in a Meta-Analysis

Source HMB	Treatment (n)	Placebo (n)	Gender	Dosage/Day[a]	Age	Training Status[b]	Training (hours/week)	Duration (weeks)	Body Composition[c]
Gallagher et al.[9]	12	14	M	38 mg/kg	21.7	U	3	8	SF
Jowko et al.[11]	9	10	M	3 g	19–23	U	3	3	HW
Kreider et al.[7]	13	15	M	3 g	25.1	T	3	4	DEXA
Nissen et al. (short)[3]	15	6	M	3 g	19–22	U	3	3	TOBC
Nissen et al. (long)[3]	13	15	M	3 g	19–29	T	4	7	TOBC
Panton et al. (men)[8]	21	18	M	3 g	24.0	Both	3	4	HW
Panton et al. (women)[8]	18	18	F	3 g	27.0	Both	3	4	HW
Slater et al.[12]	9	9	M	3 g	–	T	3	6	DEXA
Vukovich et al.[10]	14	17	Both	3 g	70.1	U	2	8	DEXA
Average	13.8	13.6			29.2		3.0	5.2	

[a] Dosages are given in daily dosages.
[b] U = untrained (no previous resistance training in the last 3 months); T = trained (undergoing some form of resistance training prior to study).
[c] DEXA = dual-energy x-ray absorptiometry; HW = hydrostatic weighing; SF = skin-fold thickness; TOBC = total body electrical conductivity.

(a)

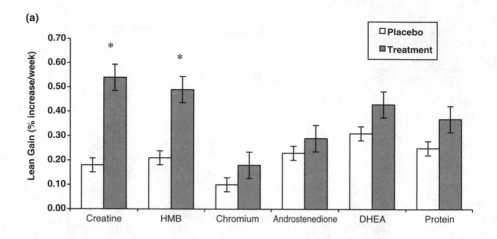

(b)

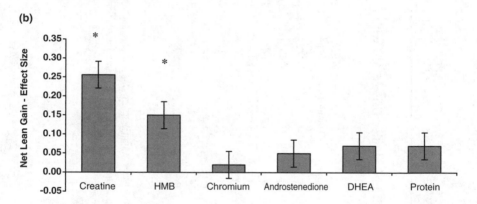

FIGURE 12.2 Comparison of the net lean mass gain of the placebo and treatment groups for each supplement. The upper panel (a) expresses lean gain as percent gained per week, while the lower panel (b) expresses the net effect size for each supplement. *, a significant effect of the treatment vs. the placebo ($p < 0.05$). (From Nissen, S.L. and Sharp, R.L., *J. Appl. Physiol.*, 94, 651–659, 2003.)

Furthermore, it was also reported that the response from HMB supplementation does not appear to be influenced by previous training status.[8] For example, HMB-supplemented trained men had about a 10-kg increase in chest press strength while HMB-supplemented untrained men had approximately a 9-kg increase. The study concluded that regardless of gender or training status, HMB supplementation increases strength gains from resistance training.

Vukovich et al.[10] also reported the effects of HMB in men and women. However, the study subjects were 70 years of age or older. Even older adult men and women were shown to respond equally to HMB supplementation (the study results are presented in the next section).

(a)

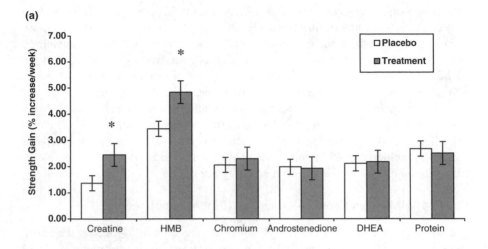

(b)

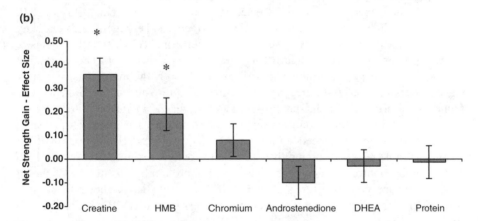

FIGURE 12.3 Comparison of the net strength gain of the placebo and treatment groups for each supplement. The upper panel (a) expresses strength gain as percent increased per week, while the lower panel (b) expresses the net effect size for each supplement. *, a significant effect of the treatment vs. the placebo ($p < 0.05$). (From Nissen, S.L. and Sharp, R.L., *J. Appl. Physiol.*, 94, 651–659, 2003.)

12.2.1.3 Benefit to Older Adults

Studies have also been conducted in elderly subjects participating in an exercise program, where it was shown that HMB supplementation improved body composition.[10] Seventy-year-old adult men and women were assigned to either 3 g of HMB or a placebo undergoing a 5 days/week exercise program for 8 weeks. The exercise program was a combination of both resistance training (2 days/week) and walking (3 days/week). After 8 weeks, HMB supplementation tended to increase fat-free mass gain ($p < 0.08$) and significantly decreased body fat ($p < 0.05$) compared to the placebo-supplemented subjects. In a second study in resistance training elderly subjects, strength gains during the study were similar between the HMB-supplemented group and the placebo-supplemented group.[47] However, HMB supplementation significantly improved functional ability as measured by a "get up and go" (GUG) test,[47] which measures the time to get up out of a chair, walk a set distance, turn around, and return to the chair and sit down again. Decreasing body fat and improving muscle function are both important findings in the elderly. Body fat, and in particular visceral fat storage, is linked to the development of insulin resistance (type II diabetes)[48] and cardiovascular disease.[49] Additionally, improving functional ability in the elderly should improve the quality of life and may result in decreasing falls, a common cause of injury in the elderly population.

12.2.1.4 HMB Compared to Other Nutritional Supplements

The previously mentioned meta-analysis by Nissen and Sharp[13] looked at the effects of common dietary supplements on lean mass and strength gains in conjunction with a resistance exercise program. A meta-analysis involves the scientific process of gathering and analyzing research results from all previous studies on a related topic to form a final conclusion. Peer-reviewed studies during the years 1967 to 2001 were included in the analysis of nutritional supplements and ergogenic aids marketed to improve the results from exercise or athletic performance. Criteria for inclusion in this meta-analysis were studies that were randomized and placebo controlled, were at least 3 weeks in duration, and performed full-body (all major muscle groups) resistance training at least twice per week. Over 250 researched supplements were found in the original search, and only 48 studies met the inclusion criteria for the meta-analysis. Interestingly, only six supplements had more than one published study (at least two studies were needed for inclusion). Creatine had 18 studies, HMB had 9 studies (Table 12.1), chromium had 12 studies, dehydroepiandrosterone (DHEA) had 2 studies, androstenedione had 3 studies, and protein had 4 studies. Of the six supplements analyzed, only creatine and HMB were statistically shown to augment strength and muscle mass gains. Furthermore, creatine and HMB gave statistically similar responses.

12.2.1.5 Combination of HMB and Creatine

Most commonly HMB is available singularly in capsule form. However, HMB is also found combined with other nutritional ingredients. The most popular of these products is a combination of HMB and creatine. As shown in a recent meta-analysis, creatine and HMB are the only two supplements that have been scientifically shown to individually increase strength and muscle mass.[13] One study measured the effect of a combination of creatine and HMB, and this combination was shown to work even better than each of the supplements alone.[11] This suggests creatine and HMB might work by different mechanisms. Lean mass and strength gains were significantly increased in the creatine, HMB, and combination of creatine and HMB groups, with the greatest increases reported in the subjects receiving the creatine and HMB combination. Therefore, the interaction between creatine and HMB results in an additive effect on lean body mass gain and strength with resistance training.

12.2.2 ENDURANCE

In addition to the studies supporting the use of HMB supplementation during resistance training, there is evidence to suggest that HMB can improve endurance as well. In a study by Vukovich and Dreifort,[5] competitive cyclists were randomly assigned in a double-blinded manner to one of three different supplementation periods (placebo, 3 g of HMB/day, or 3 g of leucine/day). Each cyclist completed each 2-week supplementation period with a 2-week washout period in-between periods. Maximal oxygen consumption and onset of blood lactate were measured prior to and after the 2 weeks of supplementation for each treatment. The cyclists maintained their current training volume throughout the study period. The results showed that HMB supplementation (3 g/day) resulted in a 3.6% increase in the time to reach VO_2 peak, while time to reach VO_2 peak decreased by -3.6% and -1.2% for the placebo and leucine treatments, respectively ($p < 0.05$). The onset of blood lactate accumulation was also delayed with HMB supplementation. At 2 mM blood lactate, VO_2 was significantly increased by 9.1% with HMB supplementation ($p < 0.05$), compared with 2.1% and 0.75% nonsignificant increases during the leucine and placebo supplementations, respectively. These findings suggest that HMB supplementation may improve the ability to exercise at a greater intensity for a longer duration. Similarly, O'Connor and Crowe[50] investigated the effects of HMB supplementation on the aerobic capacity of elite male rugby players. Although not significantly different, HMB supplementation resulted in a 2.3 ml/kg/min increase in aerobic power, while the control group experienced no change in aerobic power.[50] The results from this study need to be cautiously interpreted because the highly trained and motivated subjects were not blinded to the treatments.

Although not showing a significant effect on the indicators of endurance performance (VO_2 max/peak), studies by Knitter et al.[6] and Byrd et al.[51] reported that HMB supplementation can decrease the muscle damage and soreness associated with either prolonged or downhill running. In conclusion, HMB is one of the few, if not only, nutritional supplements shown to improve indicators of endurance performance.

12.2.3 MUSCLE DAMAGE

In studies investigating the effects of HMB on muscle damage either following a single bout of strenuous exercise[6,51] or during an intense resistance training program,[3,7–9,11] HMB supplementation has been shown to reduce the appearance of creatine phosphokinase (CPK) and lactate dehydrogenase (LDH), both indicators of muscle damage. Both CPK and LDH are muscle enzymes that appear in blood following muscle membrane damage or disruption, and the amount in blood is proportional to severity or magnitude of the muscle damage. Furthermore, supplementation of HMB also results in a significant decrease in plasma 3-MH, which is another marker used as an indicator of muscle breakdown or damage. While undergoing an intense resistance training program, subjects supplemented with HMB showed a decrease in 3-MH appearance in plasma during the first 2 weeks of the exercise program, which suggests a decrease in protein degradation.[3]

Knitter et al.[6] studied the effects of HMB on muscle damage following a single prolonged run. In this study, runners were recruited and assigned to either a placebo or 3 g of HMB/day. The subjects were asked to maintain their current running program during the supplementation period. After 6 weeks of supplementation and training, all subjects participated in a 20-km run. Blood was taken and analyzed for CPK and LDH before the run and at several time points after. Following the prolonged run, HMB supplementation resulted in a smaller increase in levels of CPK and LDH than the placebo-supplemented runners. In addition, Byrd et al.[51] examined the effect of HMB supplementation on muscle soreness and strength after downhill running. Following the downhill running protocol, HMB supplementation resulted in less perceived soreness and less strength loss, which may suggest a protective effect of HMB on muscle and less muscle damage occurring. Therefore, these results suggest that HMB appears to minimize the degree of muscle damage that occurs following intense, prolonged activity.

HMB supplementation has also been shown to minimize the muscle damage associated with an intense resistance training program. During the course of a 4-week weight training regimen in both men and women, HMB-supplemented subjects (n = 39) actually showed about a 2% decrease in CPK, while the placebo-supplemented subjects (n = 36) had a 26% increase in CPK levels due to the training intensity.[8] Similarly, Gallagher et al.[9] reported results from an 8-week resistance training program where subjects were assigned in a double-blind randomized fashion to receive either a placebo or HMB. This study also found significantly higher blood CPK levels in placebo-supplemented subjects during the start of the strenuous resistance training program than in those subjects taking HMB.[9] The findings from these studies in addition to several others[3,7,11] suggest HMB supplementation minimizes the muscle damage that occurs from repeated bouts of intense resistance exercise.

12.2.4 REVERSING UNWANTED MUSCLE LOSS (NONEXERCISE)

The *in vitro* data and clinical data in exercise suggest HMB could have a benefit in reducing muscle proteolysis, which should increase muscle mass in individuals suffering from unwanted muscle loss from disease or aging. Although not studied alone, a combination of HMB, arginine, and glutamine has been clinically examined in muscle-wasted AIDS[15] and cancer patients.[14] In each of the studies HMB was supplemented at 3 g/day, while arginine and glutamine were each supplemented at 14 g/day. The supplement was divided into two equal daily dosages. This combination of HMB and amino acids was shown to result in an increase in lean mass in wasting AIDS and cachexic cancer patients without the need for exercise. Both of the patient populations were in a highly catabolic state and were breaking down muscle tissue. Supplementing HMB to these patients is thought to minimize the protein breakdown they experience while the amino acids support immune, intestinal, and muscle protein synthesis. In the 8-week study in wasted

AIDS patients, the HMB-, arginine-, and glutamine-supplemented patients gained on average 2.5 kg of lean mass ($p < 0.01$), while the placebo-supplemented patients continued to lose lean mass and lost on average 0.7 kg during the study period. Similarly, cachexic cancer patients supplemented with the HMB, arginine, and glutamine mixture gained 1.4 kg of lean body mass in 8 weeks ($p < 0.05$), while the placebo-supplemented patients continued to lose an additional 1.1 kg of lean body mass. No exercise protocol was used in either of these studies with the nutritional mixture. Therefore, the nutritional mixture alone (HMB, arginine, and glutamine) resulted in increased cell function and restoration of muscle mass in catabolic patients losing muscle mass.

A combination of HMB, arginine, and lysine was shown to restore protein synthesis in older adult women (71.6 years of age), which resulted in significantly improved functionality, strength, and fat-free mass.[16] The HMB-, arginine-, and lysine-supplemented group significantly increased GUG performance time compared to the placebo-supplemented subjects. HMB, arginine, and lysine supplementation also resulted in increased leg and grip strength and tended to increase fat-free mass compared to the placebo-supplemented subjects. The resulting improvement in muscle mass, strength, and functionality has the potential to positively impact many aspects of daily activities of the ever-increasing elderly population.

12.2.5 WOUND HEALING

Similar to muscle-wasting conditions, HMB has been tested with two amino acids to determine if wound healing is improved.[52] Wound healing requires immune activation, cell proliferation, and protein synthesis,[53–55] and the combination of HMB with arginine and glutamine supports these cell functions. Williams et al.[52] studied the effects of HMB, arginine, and glutamine on wound healing, where a simulated model of wound healing was used. In this model, small subcutaneous catheters were inserted into the deltoid region of the subject's arm. After 2 weeks, the catheters were removed and analyzed for hydroxy-proline (OHP), an indicator of collagen synthesis. The researchers noted that the supplements were well tolerated and that no adverse events were reported during the supplementation period. The results showed that supplementation with HMB, arginine, and glutamine increased collagen synthesis by 67% over that of a placebo-supplemented group ($p < 0.03$). It was concluded from the study that the nutritional mixture of HMB, arginine, and glutamine would provide a safe nutritional means to increase wound healing in patients.

12.3 SAFETY

The safety of any supplement is a function of total dose, dosage schedule, and total time of consumption. Most supplements have not been systematically examined relative to safety and toxicity. In some regards, HMB is no different in that long-term, multiyear studies have not been completed. However, in each of the human efficacy studies, extensive safety data were collected.[56]

12.3.1 SAFETY AT RECOMMENDED DOSAGES

An analysis of the safety data available from nine published clinical studies on HMB was compiled and published by Nissen et al.[56] The nine studies included both young and elderly, males and females, ranging in age from 18 to 81 years, and the studies were from 3 to 8 weeks in length. Seven of the studies had a resistance exercise component, while one was in subjects who ran and another had no exercise component. In each of the studies, data were collected on emotional profile, adverse events, and blood chemistry and hematology. The following is a summary of the safety of consuming 3 g of HMB/day.

12.3.1.1 Adverse Events

Adverse event questionnaires were given during the studies and consisted of 32 questions relating to adverse events in major bodily systems. The questionnaires asked the subjects if they had any adverse symptoms over the last 3 days. Supplementation of HMB resulted in no differences in the occurrence of these events when compared to placebo-supplemented subjects.

12.3.1.2 Blood Chemistry and Hematology

Extensive blood chemistry (approximately 30 parameters) and hematology (approximately 20 parameters) data were reported. Supplemental HMB had no negative effects on any of these serum parameters when compared with the placebo-supplemented subjects. Blood potassium was minimally (<2%) but significantly ($p < 0.01$) decreased in HMB-supplemented subjects. This may have been due to the difference in mineral intakes between the treatment groups, as the HMB-supplemented group had a daily intake of 400 mg of calcium, 135 mg of phosphorous, and 170 mg of potassium, whereas the placebo group was not balanced for these nutrients. Blood hematology parameters measured during the studies included white blood cells (WBCs), red blood cells (RBCs), hemoglobin, hematocrit, platelets, and WBC subclasses. The only effect of HMB supplementation on any of these parameters was a small ($p < 0.05$) 0.5% decrease in hematocrit; however, no significant difference was noted in initial or ending values for hematocrit for the HMB- and placebo-supplemented groups.

12.3.1.3 Blood Lipids

Blood lipid profiles were measured during the studies and consisted of total cholesterol, high-density lipoprotein cholesterol (HDL), very low-density lipoprotein cholesterol (VLDL), low-density lipoprotein cholesterol (LDL), and triglycerides. In HMB-supplemented subjects, HDL cholesterol showed no change, while in the placebo-supplemented subjects, a 4% increase in HDL cholesterol was seen ($p < 0.04$). Of particular interest is that supplemental HMB significantly ($p < 0.03$) lowered total cholesterol by 3.7% in all subjects and by 5.8% in subjects with cholesterol levels over 200 mg/dl. The decrease in total cholesterol with HMB supplementation was mainly the result of a significant decrease in LDL cholesterol of 5.7% in all subjects ($p < 0.05$) and an even greater decrease of 7.3% ($p < 0.01$) in the high cholesterol subjects with starting cholesterol levels of >200 mg/dl.

12.3.1.4   Blood Pressure

Resting blood pressures were also measured in seven of the nine studies. Supplementation with HMB resulted in a significant decrease in systolic blood pressure of 4.4 mmHg. In a subset of subjects with systolic blood pressures of >130 mmHg, the decrease was even greater. Diastolic blood pressure was unaffected by HMB supplementation.

12.3.1.5   Emotional Profile

Emotional changes were measured using the circumplex test of emotion.[57] This consists of a questionnaire of 48 words that describe various emotions and the subjects are instructed to rate each on a scale from 1 (very slightly or not at all) to 5 (extremely) based upon their degree of feeling for that emotion. When compared with the placebo-supplemented group, no negative changes in emotional profile were noted with HMB supplementation during the studies. Supplementation with HMB resulted in a decrease of about 10% in the "unactivated unpleasant affect," which is described by the words *tired*, *drowsy*, *sluggish*, *dull*, *bored*, and *droopy*, indicating HMB had a slight but positive effect on emotion.

12.3.2   Safety at Higher Dosages

Since the first study was published, two studies have investigated the use of higher dosages of HMB (6 g/day).[7,9] It was concluded that a higher dose of HMB does not appear to promote additional increases in one repetition maximum strength or fat-free mass.[7,9] Gallagher et al.[58] studied the effects of HMB consumption at 0, 38, or 76 mg HMB/kg of body weight/day for 8 weeks on hematology and hepatic and renal function. The dosages studied corresponded to dosages of approximately 0, 3, or 6 g of HMB/day for the average person, with the 6 g/day level being twice the normally recommended dosage. Thirty-seven healthy male volunteers 18 to 29 years of age took the HMB supplements while undergoing a resistance exercise program. No differences in liver function were seen between any of the treatment groups (0, 38, or 76 mg HMB/kg body weight/day). There were also no differences in hematology parameters between the treatment groups, except for an increase ($p < 0.05$) in basophils in the 38 mg of HMB/kg of body weight/day. However, this increase in basophils was not seen in either the 0 or 76 mg of HMB/kg of body weight/day supplemented groups. Additionally, no differences were seen in lipid profiles, blood urea nitrogen, or hemoglobin between the treatment groups. Renal function was assessed by urine pH and the presence of glucose, protein, and ketones. No treatment differences existed for any of the values, and all data were within normal limits. Similarly, Kreider et al.[7] also studied the effects of supplementing HMB at 0, 3, and 6 g/day and showed no adverse effects on hematological or metabolic profiles for the higher dose group as well as the 3 g/day dose group.

In conclusion, supplementation of 3 g of HMB/day for several weeks should be considered safe. Additionally, studies of adult males consuming up to 6 g of HMB/day for up to 8 weeks had no adverse effects on measures of hematology or hepatic and renal function. Health-related positive effects of consuming 3 g of HMB/day include decreasing LDL and total cholesterol, decreasing blood pressure, and feeling better (improved mood).

12.4 RECOMMENDATIONS

Based on the combined published data, HMB has several benefits, and applications can be recommended for a broad range of people, such as athletes, fitness enthusiasts, those with an active lifestyle, and individuals experiencing unwanted muscle loss. Recommendations are based on the fact that HMB supplementation clearly augments strength and fat-free mass gains from resistance training, minimizes muscle damage and soreness, and has been shown to improve endurance.

12.4.1 WELL-TRAINED ATHLETES

For a well-trained athlete who is accustomed to a high training volume, it is important to maintain a proper dosage of 38 mg of HMB/kg of body weight (2 to 5 g of HMB/day) to minimize the muscle damage that occurs when training intensity or duration changes. For maximal gains, the addition of creatine to the HMB dose should be considered.

12.4.2 CASUAL ATHLETE AND FITNESS ENTHUSIAST

A second group that would benefit from HMB supplementation is the fitness enthusiast or casual athlete who frequently changes his training routine through periods of low to moderate to high activity and often participates in strenuous single bouts of competitive activity, such as road races, softball games, golf tournaments, etc. Supplementation of 3 g of HMB/day should improve the gains experienced from either resistance or endurance training as well as help minimize the muscle damage that occurs during those single bouts of strenuous activity. Furthermore, HMB supplementation also provides an additive health benefit to exercise.

12.4.3 ACTIVE LIFESTYLE

People with an active lifestyle but who rarely participate in a set training regimen will benefit mainly from the health benefits of HMB supplementation, but older adults may also benefit by reduced muscle loss and potentially muscle gain. Furthermore, supplementation of 3 g of HMB/day a few weeks prior to and during planned times of strenuous activity (active vacation, golf outing, long hike, etc.) should minimize the muscle damage and soreness that is normally experienced following these activities. Lower doses of 1.5 to 2.0 g/day may be sufficient, as the physical demands of this group are rather low.

12.5 FUTURE RESEARCH

As recently summarized in a meta-analysis, HMB is one of the few supplements to clearly enhance strength and lean gains with resistance exercise.[13] Further research investigating the effect of HMB on resistance training is not likely based on the current body of evidence. However, research examining the effect of HMB on endurance is not as clear-cut. Only three studies on the use of HMB as an endurance supplement have been conducted. While these studies showed positive results on increasing VO_2 max and decreasing muscle damage, further studies of HMB use for long-distance cyclists, marathon runners, or other elite endurance athletes would provide increased evidence for HMB use by these athletes. Further work should focus on the effect of HMB on VO_2 max or lactic acid accumulation, which could indicate an increase in fatty acid oxidation, therefore benefiting the endurance athlete. Future studies should also concentrate on the muscle damage caused by these types of exercise and the recovery after the endurance event.

Another potential use for HMB is in preserving lean mass in persons losing weight. Many calorie-restrictive diets also limit the amount of protein intake. A combination of protein and calorie restriction causes loss of muscle as well as fat tissue during weight loss. Therefore, it could be hypothesized that HMB could be used to preserve lean muscle during the process of weight loss. Maintenance of muscle while losing body fat would better accomplish the goal of maintaining a permanent weight loss because maintaining more muscle would result in a greater resting metabolic rate. This in turn would help maintain body weight once the caloric restriction ended.

Although HMB has been shown to decrease muscle protein degradation[3] and CPK leakage from muscle cells,[6] the exact mechanism is still unknown. Evidence points to HMB having a direct effect on stabilizing muscle cell membranes; however, thus far this is only a hypothesis. While the literature clearly shows that HMB carbon is incorporated into cholesterol,[31,32] suggesting that through this mechanism HMB supplies more cholesterol for cell membrane synthesis, actual experiments showing that HMB carbon is incorporated into cell membranes have yet to be reported. Additionally, HMB has been shown to decrease muscle protein breakdown.[3] In an animal model to examine protein degradation, it appears HMB may have an effect on decreasing protease activity.[46] Therefore, HMB could have a primary effect on the genes expressing proteases or the proteases themselves, or the decrease in protein degradation may be secondary to minimizing cellular membrane damage.

12.6 SUMMARY

HMB is one of only a few ergogenic aids that have unequivocal science backing the augmentation of strength and fat-free mass gains associated with resistance training. In general, HMB doubled the effects of resistance training on strength and fat-free mass gains. Furthermore, HMB is an ergogenic aid that has a positive effect on the cardiovascular disease risk profile through lowering blood pressure and cholesterol. HMB also has a strong database of safety showing no harmful effects and, in general, improving emotional profiles. HMB supplementation may also have value in improving endurance and minimizing muscle damage, as well as preventing unwanted muscle loss. In conclusion, there is strong evidence that 3 g of HMB/day can magnify both the strength and lean gains as well as the health benefits of exercise.

REFERENCES

1. Nair KS, Schwartz RG, Welle S. Leucine as a regulator of whole body and skeletal muscle protein metabolism in humans. *Am J Physiol* 1992; 263:E928–E934.
2. Frexes-Steed M, Lacy DB, Collins J, Abumrad NN. Role of leucine and other amino acids in regulating protein metabolism *in vivo. Am J Physiol (Endocrinol Metab)* 1992; 262:E925–E935.
3. Nissen S, Sharp R, Ray M, Rathmacher JA, Rice J, Fuller JC, Jr., Connelly AS, Abumrad N. The effect of the leucine metabolite β-hydroxy-β-methylbutyrate on muscle metabolism during resistance-exercise training. *J Appl Physiol* 1996; 81:2095–2104.
4. Nissen SL, Abumrad NN. Nutritional role of the leucine metabolite β-hydroxy-β-methylbutyrate (HMB). *J Nutr Biochem* 1997; 8:300–311.
5. Vukovich MD, Dreifort GD. Effect of beta-hydroxy-beta-methylbutyrate on the onset of blood lactate accumulation and VO_2 peak in endurance-trained cyclists. *J Strength Cond Res* 2001; 15:491–497.
6. Knitter AE, Panton L, Rathmacher JA, Petersen A, Sharp R. Effects of β-hydroxy-β-methylbutyrate on muscle damage following a prolonged run. *J Appl Physiol* 2000; 89:1340–1344.
7. Kreider RB, Ferreira M, Wilson M, Almada AL. Effects of calcium beta-hydroxy-beta-methylbutyrate (HMB) supplementation during resistance-training on markers of catabolism, body composition and strength. *Int J Sports Med* 1999; 20:503–509.
8. Panton LB, Rathmacher JA, Baier S, Nissen S. Nutritional supplementation of the leucine metabolite β-hydroxy-β-methylbutyrate (HMB) during resistance training. *Nutrition* 2000; 16:734–739.
9. Gallagher PM, Carrithers JA, Godard MP, Schulze KE, Trappe SW. β-Hydroxy-β-methylbutyrate ingestion. Part I. Effects on strength and fat free mass. *Med Sci Sports Exerc* 2000; 32:2109–2115.
10. Vukovich MD, Stubbs NB, Bohlken RM. Body composition in 70-year old adults responds to dietary β-hydroxy-β-methylbutyrate (HMB) similar to that of young adults. *J Nutr* 2001; 131:2049–2052.
11. Jówko E, Ostaszewski P, Jank M, Sacharuk J, Zieniewicz A, Wilczak, J, Nissen S. Creatine and β-hydroxy-β-methylbutyrate (HMB) additively increases lean body mass and muscle strength during a weight training program. *Nutrition* 2001; 17:558–566.
12. Slater G, Jenkins D, Logan P, Lee H, Vukovich MD, Rathmacher JA, Hahn A. β-Hydroxy-β-methylbutyrate (HMB) supplementation does not affect changes in strength or body composition during resistance training in trained men. *Int J Sport Nutr Exerc Metab* 2001; 11:384–396.
13. Nissen SL, Sharp RL. Effect of dietary supplements on lean mass and strength gains with resistance exercise: a meta-analysis. *J Appl Physiol* 2003; 94:651–659.
14. Eubanks May P, Barber A, Hourihane A, D'Olimpio JT, Abumrad NN. Reversal of cancer-related wasting using oral supplementation with a combination of β-hydroxy-β-methylbutyrate, arginine, and glutamine. *Am J Surg* 2002; 183:471–479.

15. Clark RH, Feleke G, Din M, Yasmin T, Singh G, Khan F, Rathmacher J. Nutritional treatment for acquired immunodeficiency virus-associated wasting using β-hydroxy-β-methylbutyrate, glutamine and arginine: a randomized, double-blind, placebo-controlled study. *J Parenter Enter Nutr* 2000; 24:133–139.
16. Levenhagen DK, Vaughan SR, Niedernhofer E, Carr C, Flakoll PJ. Dietary supplementation of arginine, lysine and β-hydroxy-β-methylbutyrate (HMB) to blunt loss of muscle, strength and functionality in elderly females. *FASEB J* 2001; 15:A277 (abstract).
17. Sabourin PJ, Bieber LL. Formation of β-hydroxyisovalerate from α-ketoisocaproate by a soluble preparation from rat liver. *Dev Biochem* 1981; 18:149–154.
18. Wagenmakers AJM, Salden HJM, Veerkamp JH. The metabolic fate of branched chain amino acids and 2-oxo acids in rat muscle homogenates and diaphragms. *Int J Biochem* 1985; 17:957–965.
19. Krebs HA, Lund P. Aspects of the regulation of the metabolism of branched-chain amino acids. *Adv Enzyme Regul* 1977; 15:375–394.
20. Sabourin PJ, Bieber LL. Subcellular distribution and partial characterization of an α-ketoisocaproate oxidase of rat liver: formation of β-hydroxyisovaleric acid. *Arch Biochem Biophys* 1981; 206:132–144.
21. Sabourin PJ, Bieber LL. Formation of β-hydroxyisovalerate from α-ketoisocaproate by a soluble preparation from rat liver. In *Metabolism and Clinical Implications of Branched Chain Amino and Ketoacids*, Walser M, Williamson JR, Eds. Elsevier North Holland, New York, 1981, pp. 149–154.
22. Sabourin PJ, Bieber LL. Purification and characterization of an alpha-ketoisocaproate oxygenase of rat liver. *J Biol Chem* 1982; 257:7460–7467.
23. Sabourin PJ, Bieber LL. The mechanism of α-ketoisocaproate oxygenase. Formation of β-hydroxyisovalerate from α-ketoisocaproate. *J Biol Chem* 1982; 257:7468–7471.
24. Sabourin PJ, Bieber LL. Formation of β-hydroxyisovalerate by an α-ketoisocaproate oxygenase in human liver. *Metabolism* 1983; 32:160–164.
25. Lee MH, Zhang ZH, MacKinnon CH, Baldwin JE, Crouch NP. The C-terminal of rat 4-hydroxyphenylpyruvate dioxygenase is indispensable for enzyme activity. *FEBS Lett* 1996; 393:269–272.
26. Mock DM, Henrich CL, Carnell N, Mock NI. Indicators of marginal biotin deficiency and repletion in humans: validation of 3-hydroxyisovaleric acid excretion and a leucine challenge. *Am J Clin Nutr* 2002; 76:1061–1068.
27. Mock DM, Mock NI, Weintraub S. Abnormal organic aciduria in biotin deficiency: the rat is similiar to the human. *J Lab Clin Med* 1988; 112(2):240–247.
28. Van Koevering M, Nissen S. Oxidation of leucine and α-ketoisocaproate to β-hydroxy-β-methylbutyrate *in vivo*. *Am J Physiol (Endocrinol Metab)* 1992; 262:E27–E31.
29. Vukovich MD, Slater G, Macchi MB, Turner MJ, Fallon K, Boston T, Rathmacher J. β-Hydroxy-β-methylbutyrate (HMB) kinetics and the influence of glucose ingestion in humans. *J Nutr Biochem* 2001; 12:631–639.
30. Nissen SL, Abumrad NN. Nutritional role of the leucine metabolite β-hydroxy-β-methylbutyrate (HMB). *J Nutr Biochem* 1997; 8:300–311.
31. Bloch K, Clark LC, Haray I. Utilization of branched chain acids in cholesterol synthesis. *J Biol Chem* 1954; 211:687–699.
32. Adamson LF, Greenberg DM. The significance of certain carboxylic acids as intermediates in the biosynthesis of cholesterol. *Biochim Biophys Acta* 1957; 23:472–479.

33. Gey KF, Pletsher A, Isler O, Ruegg R, Wursch J. Influence of iosoprenoid C5 and C6 compounds on the incorporation of acetate in cholesterol. *Helv Chim Acta* 1957; 40:2354–2368.

34. Zhang Z, Rathmacher J, Coates C, Nissen S. Occurrence of β-hydroxy-β-methyl butyrate in foods and feeds. *FASEB J* 1994; 8:A464 (abstract).

35. Zhang Z. Distribution of β-Hydroxy-β-Methylbutyrate in Plant and Animal Tissues. M.S. thesis, Iowa State University, Ames, 1994.

36. Zhang Z, Talleyrand V, Rathmacher J, Nissen S. Change in plasma β-hydroxy-β-methylbutyrate (HMB) by feeding leucine, alpha-ketoisocaporate (KIC) and isovaleric acid (IVA) to pigs. *FASEB J* 1993; 7:A392 (abstract).

37. Zachwieja JJ, Smith SR, Nissen SL, Rathmacher JA. Beta-hydroxy-beta-methylbutyrate (HMB) is produced *in vivo* in humans from leucine. *FASEB J* 2000; 14: A747 (abstract).

38. Gakhokidze AM. Condensation of ketones with esters of organic acids. I. Condensation of acetone with esters of formic, acetic and propionic acids. *J Gen Chem* (Russian) 1947; 17:1327–1331.

39. Gresham TL, Jansen JE, Shaver FW, Beears WL. Beta-propiolactone. XIV. Beta-isovalerolactone. *J Am Chem Soc* 1954; 76:486–488.

40. Coffman DD, Cramer R, Mochel WE. Synthesis by free-radical reactions. V. A new synthesis of carboxylic acids. *J Am Chem Soc* 1958; 80:2882–2887.

41. Searles S, Ives EK, Nukina S. Base-catalyzed cleavage of 1,3-diols. *J Organ Chem* 1959; 24:1770–1775.

42. Watanabe S, Suga K, Fujita T, Fujiyoshi K. The direct synthesis of beta-hydroxyacids by lithium naphthalene and acetic acid. *Isr J Chem* 1970; 8:731–736.

43. Chen HW. Role of cholesterol metabolism in cell growth. *Fed Proc* 1984; 43:126–130.

44. Dabrowski MP, Peel WE, Thomson AE. Plasma membrane cholesterol regulates human lymphocyte cytotoxic function. *Eur J Immunol* 1980; 10:821–827.

45. Ostaszewski P, Kostiuk S, Balasinska B, Jank M, Papet I, Glomot F. The leucine metabolite 3-hydroxy-3-methylbutyrate (HMB) modifies protein turnover in muscles of the laboratory rats and domestic chicken *in vitro*. *J Anim Physiol Anim Nutr* (Swiss) 2000; 84:1–8.

46. Jank M, Ostaszewski P, Rosochacki S, Wilczak J, Balasinska B. Effect of 3-hydroxy-3-methylbutyrate (HMB) on muscle cathepsins and calpain activities during the postdexamethasone recovery period in young rats. *Polish J Vet Sci* 2001; 3:213–218.

47. Panton L, Rathmacher J, Fuller J, Gammon J, Cannon L, Stettler S, Nissen S. The effect of β-hydroxy-β-methylbutyrate and resistance training on strength and functional ability in elderly men and women. *Med Sci Sports Exerc* 1998; 30:S194 (abstract).

48. Fujioka S, Matsuzawa Y, Tokunaga K, Tarui S. Contribution of intra-abdominal fat accumulation to the impairment of glucose and lipid metabolism in human obesity. *Metabolism* 1987; 36:54–59.

49. Ernst ND, Obarzanek E, Clark MB, Briefel RR, Brown CD, Donato K. Cardiovascular health risks related to overweight. *J Am Diet Assoc* 1997; 97(Suppl):S47–S51.

50. O'Connor DM, Crowe MJ. Effects of β-hydroxy-β-methylbutyrate and creatine monohydrate supplementation on the aerobic and anaerobic capacity of highly trained athletes. *J Sports Med Phys Fitness* 2003; 43:64–68.

51. Byrd P, Mehta P, DeVita P, Dyck D, Hickner R. Changes in muscle soreness and strength following downhill running: effects of creatine, HMB and Betagen supplementation. *Med Sci Sports Exerc* 1999; 31:S263 (abstract).

52. Williams J, Abumrad N, Barbul A. Effect of a specialized amino acid mixture on human collagen deposition. *Ann Surg* 2002; 236:369–375 (abstract).
53. Kirk SJ, Hurson M, Regan MC, Holt DR, Wasserkrug HL, Barbul A. Arginine stimulates wound healing and immune function in elderly human beings. *Surgery* 1993; 114:155–159.
54. Karinch AM, Pan M, Lin CM, Strange R, Souba WW. Glutamine metabolism in sepsis and infection. *J Nutr* 2001; 131(Suppl):2535S–2538S.
55. Field CJ, Johnson I, Pratt VC. Glutamine and arginine: immunonutrients for improved health. *Med Sci Sports Exerc* 2000; 32(Suppl):S377–S388.
56. Nissen S, Panton L, Sharp RL, Vukovich M, Trappe SW, Fuller JC, Jr. β-Hydroxy-β-methylbutyrate (HMB) supplementation in humans is safe and may decrease cardiovascular risk factors. *J Nutr* 2000; 130:1937–1945.
57. Russell JA. A circumplex model of affect. *J Pers Soc Psychol* 1980; 39:1161–1178.
58. Gallagher PM, Carrithers JA, Godard MP, Schutze KE, Trappe SW. β-hydroxy-β-methylbutyrate ingestion. Part II. Effects on hematology, hepatic, and renal function. *Med Sci Sports Exerc* 2000; 32:2116–2119.

13 Branched-Chain Amino Acids

Michael Gleeson

CONTENTS

13.1 INTRODUCTION

The three branched-chain amino acids (BCAAs), leucine, isoleucine, and valine, are not synthesized in the body, and therefore are classified as essential amino acids that must be supplied in the diet.[1] They are required for protein synthesis and neurotransmitter synthesis. The basic structure of all amino acids consists of an amine ($-NH_2$) group and a carboxyl ($-COOH$) group attached to a single carbon atom: also present is an organic side chain, and it is the structures of these side chains that give the different amino acids their characteristic structures. The structures of the BCAAs are shown in Figure 13.1, and they are so called because they each possess a short, branched hydrocarbon chain as the side group attached to the alpha carbon of the amino acid molecule. They are the only essential amino acids

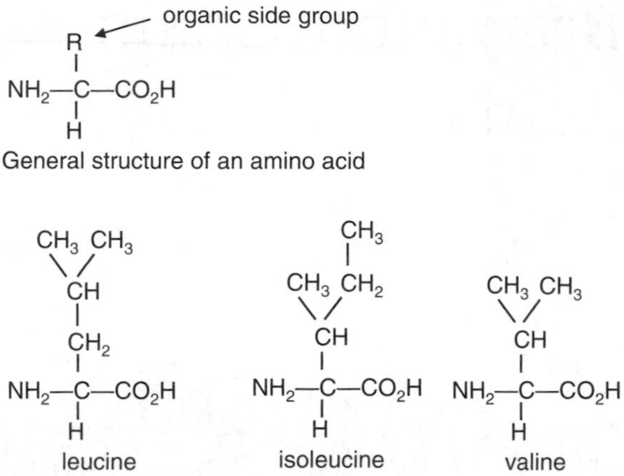

FIGURE 13.1 The general structure of amino acids and the structures of the branched-chain amino acids: leucine, isoleucine, and valine.

that are oxidized to a significant extent during exercise, and they must therefore be replenished by the diet. In the late 1970s, BCAAs were suggested to be the third fuel for skeletal muscle after carbohydrate and fat, and BCAAs are sometimes supplied to athletes in energy drinks to provide extra fuel. Claims have also been made that BCAA supplementation can reduce net protein breakdown in muscle during exercise, reduce fatigue, enhance performance via effects on the brain, and speed up the repair of muscle following exercise-induced muscle damage.

However, the majority of studies, using various exercise and treatment designs and several forms of administration of BCAAs (infusion, oral, and with and without carbohydrates), have failed to find a performance-enhancing effect. Leucine does appear to provide a stimulatory signal for muscle protein synthesis and thus has an anticatabolic effect during and after exercise in humans, but there is only very limited scientific evidence to support the claim that BCAA supplements may accelerate the repair of muscle damage or reduce muscle soreness after exercise. Acute intakes of BCAA supplements of up to about 30 g/day seem to be well tolerated and without ill effect, though the suggested reasons for taking such supplements have not received much support from well-controlled scientific studies.

13.2 METABOLIC FUNCTIONS OF BCAAs

13.2.1 A FUEL FOR EXERCISE

Muscle has a limited capacity to oxidize amino acids, and mammalian skeletal muscle has been shown to be capable of oxidizing only six of the amino acids: alanine, aspartate, glutamate, leucine, isoleucine, and valine.[2] Of these, the BCAAs may be quantitatively the most significant, and it is known that BCAA oxidation is promoted by exercise.[3] The BCAAs can act as precursors of the tricarboxylic acid cycle (Krebs cycle) intermediates following removal of their amino group by reversible transamination, as illustrated in Figure 13.2. Transamination is followed by

(a)

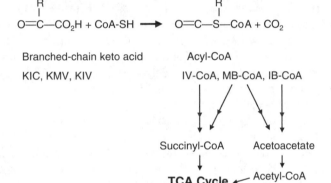

Branched-chain aminotransferase

$$NH_2—\underset{\underset{H}{|}}{\overset{\overset{R}{|}}{C}}—CO_2H + \text{α-ketoglutarate} \longleftrightarrow O{=}\overset{\overset{R}{|}}{C}—CO_2H + \text{glutamate}$$

amino acid   keto acid

LEU, ILE, VAL   KIC, KMV, KIV

(b)

Branched-chain keto acid dehydrogenase

$$O{=}\overset{\overset{R}{|}}{C}—CO_2H + \text{CoA-SH} \longrightarrow O{=}\overset{\overset{R}{|}}{C}—S—CoA + CO_2$$

Branched-chain keto acid   Acyl-CoA

KIC, KMV, KIV   IV-CoA, MB-CoA, IB-CoA

Succinyl-CoA   Acetoacetate

TCA Cycle ← Acetyl-CoA

FIGURE 13.2 The role of BCAAs in energy metabolism. Following removal of their amino group by reversible transamination (a) and the irreversible decarboxylation of the resulting branched-chain α-keto acids to form coenzyme A (CoA) compounds (b), BCAAs act as precursors of acetyl CoA and tricarboxylic acid cycle intermediates. CoA-SH, reduced form of CoA; IB-CoA, isobutyryl-CoA; ILE, isoleucine; IV-CoA, isovaleryl-CoA; KIC, α-ketoiso-caproate; KIV, α-ketoisovalerate; KMV, α-keto-β-methylvalerate; LEU, leucine; MB-CoA, α-methylbutyryl-CoA; NADH$_2$, reduced nicotinamide adenine dinucleotide; VAL, valine.

irreversible oxidative decarboxylation of the branched-chain α-keto acid transami-nation products, the branched-chain α-keto acids.[4] The oxidative decarboxylation step of BCAA catabolism is common to all three BCAAs and is the rate-limiting step in their oxidation. The activity of the branched-chain α-keto acid dehydrogenase complex is controlled by covalent modification. Phosphorylation of subunits of the complex by a branched-chain kinase causes inactivation when there is a need to conserve BCAAs for protein synthesis, and dephosphorylation of the complex by a branched-chain phosphatase causes activation when BCAAs are present in excess. Elevated levels of α-ketoisocaproate (formed by the transamination of leucine) have a potent inhibitory effect on the activity of the branched-chain kinase, thus activating the branched-chain α-keto acid dehydrogenase complex and elevating catabolism of all three BCAAs.[3,4] The keto acids of isoleucine and valine (α-keto-β-methylval-erate and α-ketoisovalerate, respectively) have a similar but far less potent effect.

Thus, increasing the availability of leucine alone could result in a potentially harmful BCAA imbalance by inducing a relative deficiency of isoleucine and valine.[3] Reduced capacity to oxidize BCAAs, as in the hereditary disorder maple syrup urine disease, results in excess BCAAs in the blood and profound neurological dysfunction and brain damage.[4]

The BCAA catabolic enzymes are distributed widely in body tissues and, with the exception of nervous tissue, all reactions occur in the mitochondria of the cell. Oxidation of the BCAAs by muscle results in the problem of disposal of the amino groups, and some of these will be transferred to pyruvate in a transamination reaction, with the formation of alanine, which will be transported via the circulation to the liver for entry into the urea cycle. In resting muscle, amino acid oxidation does not account for more than about 10% of total adenosine triphosphate (ATP) turnover, and the fractional contribution decreases during exercise as the rate of oxidation of other fuels (i.e., carbohydrate and fat) increases.[2] Where the availability of other fuels is limited, as in states of glycogen depletion, the contribution of amino acid oxidation to energy provision will again become more important. There are large increases in the oxidation rates of BCAAs during exercise; for example, the rate of oxidation of leucine may increase up to fivefold during strenuous exercise.[7] The mechanism responsible for this is attributed to the activation of the branched-chain α-keto acid dehydrogenase complex.

Although early studies suggested that BCAAs can act as a fuel during exercise in addition to carbohydrate and fat, later it was shown that the activities of the enzymes involved in the oxidation of BCAAs are too low to allow a major contribution of BCAAs to energy expenditure in humans.[5,6] Detailed studies with a ^{13}C-labeled BCAA (^{13}C-leucine) showed that the oxidation of BCAAs only increases two to fivefold during submaximal exercise, whereas the oxidation of carbohydrate and fat increases 10- to 20-fold.[7,8] Also, carbohydrate ingestion during exercise can prevent the increase in BCAA oxidation (Figure 13.3).[9] BCAAs, therefore, do not seem to play a major role as a fuel during exercise, and from this point of view, the supplementation of BCAAs during exercise is unnecessary.[10]

13.2.2 Effects on Protein Turnover

The claims that BCAAs reduce protein breakdown were initially based on early *in vitro* studies, which showed that adding BCAAs to an incubation or perfusion medium stimulated tissue protein synthesis and inhibited protein degradation. A few *in vivo* studies in healthy individuals[11–13] failed to confirm the positive effect on protein balance that had been observed *in vitro*. However, several studies in recent years have inferred an anabolic effect of leucine or the BCAAs on muscle protein breakdown and a stimulatory effect on muscle protein synthesis. Very recent work suggests that leucine itself, not its metabolites, acts as a signal to stimulate protein synthesis and acts via a pathway involving activation of the protein kinase mTOR (the mammalian target of rapamycin), which controls cellular functions in response to amino acids and growth factors.[14] During exercise, muscle protein synthesis decreases together with a net increase in protein degradation and stimulation of BCAA oxidation, resulting in falls in the intramuscular and plasma leucine concentrations. After exercise, recovery of

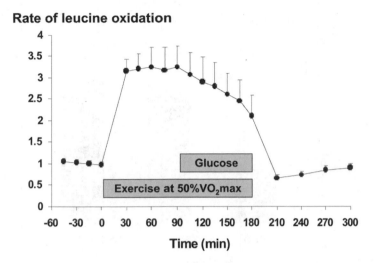

Rate of leucine oxidation

FIGURE 13.3 Carbohydrate ingestion during exercise can prevent the increase in BCAA oxidation as determined by the oxidation of infused ^{13}C-labeled leucine. (Data from Davies, C.T.M. et al., *J. Physiol.*, 332, 41P–42P, 1982.)

muscle protein synthesis requires dietary protein or BCAA to increase tissue levels of leucine in order to activate the mTOR signaling pathway.[15] Leucine's effect on mTOR is synergistic with insulin via the phosphoinositol 3-kinase signaling pathway. Together, insulin and leucine promote net skeletal muscle protein accretion. Insulin's main effects are to increase muscle amino acid uptake and inhibit protein degradation, whereas leucine's main effect is to promote protein synthesis. Recently it has been reported that co-ingestion of protein and leucine with carbohydrate stimulates muscle protein synthesis and optimizes whole-body protein balance compared to the intake of carbohydrate only after a 45-min bout of resistance exercise (Figure 13.4).[16] Thus, evidence is accumulating that supports the commercial claims that orally ingested BCAAs have an anticatabolic effect during and after exercise.[4]

13.2.3 PRECURSOR OF SEROTONIN AND ROLE IN CENTRAL FATIGUE

The central fatigue hypothesis, illustrated in Figure 13.5a, was proposed by Eric Newsholme and colleagues in 1987[17] as an important mechanism contributing to the development of fatigue during prolonged exercise. This hypothesis predicts that during exercise, free fatty acids (FFAs) are mobilized from adipose tissue and transported via the blood to the muscles to serve as fuel. Because the rate of mobilization is greater than the rate of uptake by the muscle, the blood FFA concentration increases. Both FFAs and the amino acid tryptophan bind to albumin and compete for the same binding sites. Tryptophan is prevented from binding to albumin by the increasing FFA concentration, and therefore, the free tryptophan (fTRP) concentration and the fTRP:BCAA ratio in the blood rise. Furthermore, the plasma concentration of BCAAs falls during prolonged exercise as circulating BCAAs are taken up by the contracting muscles for oxidative metabolism at a higher rate than

Fractional synthetic rate (%/h)

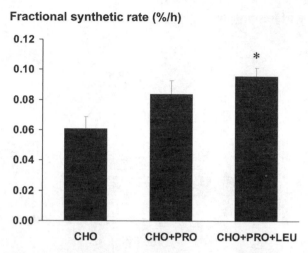

FIGURE 13.4 Fractional synthetic rate (FSR) of mixed muscle protein in the recovery phase during trials in which carbohydrate only (CHO), carbohydrate with protein (CHO + PRO), and carbohydrate with protein and leucine (CHO + PRO + LEU) were consumed by men following a 45-min bout of resistance exercise. Co-ingestion of protein and leucine with carbohydrate stimulated muscle protein synthesis (and optimized whole-body protein balance) compared to the intake of carbohydrate only after the resistance exercise bout. Values are means ± SE. *, $p < 0.05$ significantly different from CHO. (From Koopman, R. et al., *Am. J. Physiol. Endocrinol. Metab.*, 288, 645–653, 2005. Used with permission from the American Physiological Society.)

the rate at which the plasma BCAA pool is replenished through breakdown of whole-body proteins. The decline in plasma BCAA concentration during exercise will result in a further increase in the fTRP:BCAA ratio. Experimental studies in humans have confirmed that these events occur. The central fatigue hypothesis predicts that the increase in fTRP:BCAA ratio results in an increased fTRP transport across the blood–brain barrier because BCAA and fTRP compete for carrier-mediated entry into the central nervous system by the large neutral amino acid (LNAA) transporter.[18,19] Once taken up, the conversion of tryptophan to serotonin (5-hydroxy-tryptamine, or 5-HT) occurs and leads to a local increase of this neurotransmitter.[19] Serotonin has been shown to depress motor neuron excitability, influence autonomic and endocrine function, and suppress appetite in both animal and human studies. Furthermore, serotonin plays a role in the onset of sleep and is a determinant of mood and aggression. Therefore, the increase in serotoninergic activity might subsequently lead to the development of central fatigue, forcing athletes to stop exercise or reduce the exercise intensity. Of course, the assumption that increased fTRP uptake leads to increased serotonin synthesis and activity of serotoninergic pathways (i.e., increased synaptic serotonin release) is a rather large leap of faith.

The central fatigue hypothesis also predicts that ingestion of BCAAs will raise the plasma BCAA concentration, and hence reduce transport of fTRP into the brain. Subsequent reduced formation of serotonin may alleviate sensations of fatigue (Figure 13.5b) and, in turn, improve endurance exercise performance.

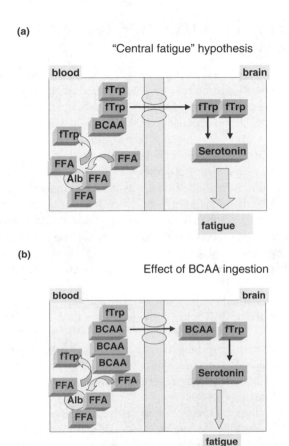

(a)

"Central fatigue" hypothesis

(b)

Effect of BCAA ingestion

FIGURE 13.5 Central fatigue hypothesis. (a) The central fatigue hypothesis proposes that during exercise free fatty acids (FFAs) are mobilized from adipose tissue and transported via the blood to the muscles to serve as fuel. Because the rate of mobilization is greater than the rate of uptake by the muscle, the circulating FFA concentration increases. Both FFA and the free amino acid tryptophan (fTRP) bind to albumin (ALB) and compete for the same binding sites. fTRP is displaced from binding to albumin by the increasing FFA concentration and, therefore, the fTRP concentration and the fTRP:BCAA ratio in the blood rise. Experimental studies in humans have confirmed that these events occur. The central fatigue hypothesis predicts that the increase in this ratio results in an increased fTRP transport across the blood–brain barrier because BCAAs and fTRP compete for carrier-mediated entry into the central nervous system by the large neutral amino acid (LNAA) transporter. Once taken up, the conversion of fTRP to serotonin (5-hydroxytryptamine, or 5-HT) occurs and leads to a local increase of this neurotransmitter. It has been well established that serotonin plays a role in the onset of sleep, and that it is a determinant of mood and aggression. It was therefore hypothesized that the increase in serotoninergic activity subsequently leads to central fatigue, forcing athletes to stop exercise or reduce exercise intensity. (b) The involvement of plasma fTRP and BCAAs in the central fatigue hypothesis also predicts that ingestion of BCAAs will raise the plasma BCAA concentration, and hence reduce transport of fTRP into the brain. Subsequent reduced formation of serotonin may alleviate sensations of fatigue, and hence improve endurance exercise performance.

13.3   EFFECTS OF BCAA INGESTION ON EXERCISE PERFORMANCE

The effect of BCAA ingestion on physical performance was investigated for the first time in a field test by Blomstrand et al.[20] One hundred and ninety-three male subjects were studied during a marathon in Stockholm. The subjects were randomly divided into an experimental group receiving BCAA in plain water and a placebo group receiving flavored water. The subjects also had free access to carbohydrate-containing drinks. No difference was observed in the marathon time of the two groups. However, when the original subject group was divided into fast and slower runners, a significant reduction in marathon time was observed in subjects given BCAAs in the slower runners only. This study has since been criticized for its design and statistical analysis. For example, fluid and carbohydrate ingestion were not controlled during the race, subjects receiving BCAAs were not matched to controls in terms of previous performance, and the retrospective division of subjects into groups relating to their performance times in the race has been criticized as statistically invalid.

A study that examined the effect of BCAA ingestion during exercise in the heat (ambient temperature of 34°C) has provided some further evidence in support of these early findings.[21] A 14% increase in the capacity to perform relatively low intensity exercise (40% of maximal oxygen uptake, VO_2max) was reported following BCAA supplementation, compared with placebo (Figure 13.6). No difference in peripheral markers of fatigue was reported between the BCAA and placebo treatments, and the BCAA supplementation (which began 1 h before the start of exercise) resulted in a two to threefold reduction in the plasma ratio of fTRP to BCAAs. The capacity to perform prolonged exercise is reduced at high ambient temperatures, and this premature fatigue is not adequately explained by peripheral mechanisms. Indeed, there is now some convincing evidence that central fatigue plays an important role in limiting exercise capacity in the heat.[22] However, two recent studies that have examined the effects of BCAA supplementation (approximately 20 g of BCAAs consumed before and during exercise) on cycling exercise capacity in the heat at two different exercise intensities (60% VO_2max at 35°C and 50% VO_2max at 30°C) failed to find any effect on exercise capacity or ratings of perceived exertion.[23,24]

Indeed, the majority of studies, using various exercise and treatment designs and several forms of administration of BCAA (infusion, oral, and with and without carbohydrates), have failed to find a performance-enhancing effect.[25–29] Van Hall et al.[27] studied time trial performance in trained cyclists consuming carbohydrate (6% sucrose solution) during exercise with and without BCAAs. A high (18 g/l) and a low (6 g/l) dose of BCAAs were given, but no differences were seen in time trial performance (Figure 13.7). One limitation of most of the studies that have investigated possible performance-enhancing effects of ingested BCAAs is that they have lacked sufficient statistical power to identify small but useful enhancements of performance.

If the central fatigue hypothesis is correct and the ingestion of BCAAs reduces the exercise-induced increase of brain fTRP uptake and thereby delays fatigue, the opposite must also be true; that is, ingestion of tryptophan before exercise should reduce the time to exhaustion. A few studies have included supplemental tryptophan

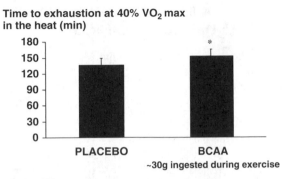

FIGURE 13.6 Time to exhaustion during cycling at 40% VO_2max in the heat with or without ingestion of ~30 g of BCAA. *, $p < 0.05$ significantly different from placebo. (Data from Mittleman, K.D. et al., *Med. Sci. Sports Exerc.*, 30, 83–91, 1998.)

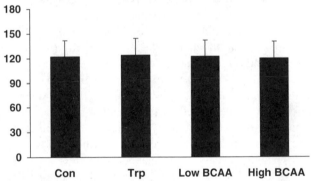

FIGURE 13.7 Time to exhaustion during cycling at 75 to 80% VO_2max. No significant effect on exercise performance is seen with drinks containing tryptophan (3 g/l), a small dose of BCAAs (6 g/l), or a large dose of BCAAs (18 g/l) compared with the control drink. All drinks contained carbohydrate in the form of sucrose (60 g/l). (From van Hall, G.J. et al., *J. Physiol.*, 486, 789–794, 1995. With permission from Blackwell Publishing.)

in human subjects before or during exercise,[27,30] and from these studies (as illustrated in Figure 13.7) the conclusion must be drawn that tryptophan has no effects on exercise performance.

The effect of chronic administration of BCAAs on exercise performance has also been examined.[31] Following 2 weeks of BCAA supplementation (16 g/day), performance of a 40-km cycling time trial in temperate ambient conditions was improved by 12% compared with placebo. However, the data from this study are still not published as a full paper, precluding any definitive conclusions on those results. The influence of chronic BCAA supplementation on exercise performance warrants further investigation.

13.4 EFFECTS OF BCAA INGESTION ON RECOVERY FROM MUSCLE-DAMAGING EXERCISE

Because of the stimulation of muscle protein synthesis by leucine and the suppression of exercise-induced increases in protein breakdown by BCAAs, it has been suggested that BCAA supplements might accelerate the repair of muscle damage after exercise; however, at present, evidence for this is limited. For example, it has been reported that oral ingestion of BCAAs (12 g/day for 2 weeks and an additional 20-g dose both before and after the exercise bout) was associated with a smaller rise in serum creatine kinase (CK) activity (a marker of muscle fiber damage) for several days after 2 h of cycle ergometer exercise at 70% VO_2max, compared with a placebo group.[32] The drawback with this study is that cycling involves concentric muscle actions and so is not usually associated with muscle damage, and the rises in serum CK activity observed were considerably smaller than those observed with eccentric exercise modes. However, a similar effect was observed in a study in which subjects ingested 1.33 g of BCAAs (as part of a 3.6-g amino acid mixture) before and after an exercise test and two doses each day of the same mixture for 4 days after an eccentric exercise test.[33,34] In this study, 24 subjects performed two bouts of exercise of the elbow flexors (different arms) separated by 3 to 4 weeks with either amino acid or placebo supplementation in a double-blind crossover design. Peak plasma levels of CK, aldolase, and myoglobin were substantially (40 to 60%) and significantly lower for the amino acid than the placebo treatment. Furthermore, peak ratings of muscle soreness during palpation and extension (but not flexion) were significantly lower for the amino acid than the placebo treatment. However, there were no significant differences between the two treatments for changes in muscle function (assessed by maximal isometric voluntary force of contraction at an elbow angle of 90°) and range of motion. Another recently published study reported beneficial effects of BCAA supplementation on delayed-onset muscle soreness and muscle fatigue in the days following a squat exercise protocol in humans.[35] Additional, well-controlled studies are needed to confirm these preliminary findings and to determine if the observed effects are specifically due to the increased availability of leucine, all three BCAAs, or all nine essential amino acids. An alternative mechanism to altered protein turnover for the observed reduction in muscle soreness following damaging exercise could possibly be modification of brain neurotransmitters and pain perception with BCAA supplements. However, at present, this is just speculation.

13.5 EFFECTS OF BCAA INGESTION ON IMMUNE RESPONSES TO EXERCISE

Prolonged strenuous exercise is associated with a temporary immunodepression that affects macrophages, neutrophils, and lymphocytes.[36-38] The mechanisms involved are not fully established and appear to be multifactorial, including the actions of stress hormones (e.g., catecholamines and cortisol), inhibition of macrophage and T-cell cytokine production, altered heat shock protein expression, increased oxidative stress, and a fall in the plasma concentration of glutamine.[38,39] BCAAs are nitrogen donors for glutamine synthesis, and some studies have evaluated the effectiveness of BCAA supplements during exercise to maintain the plasma glutamine concentration and modify immune responses to exercise. One recent study showed that BCAA supplementation (6 g/day) for 2 to 4 weeks and a 3-g dose 30 min before a long-distance run or triathlon race prevented the 24% fall in the plasma glutamine concentration observed in the placebo group and also modified the immune response to exercise.[40] These authors reported that BCAA supplementation did not affect the lymphocyte proliferative response to mitogens before exercise, but did prevent the 40% fall in lymphocyte proliferation observed after exercise in the placebo group. Furthermore, blood mononuclear cells obtained from athletes in the placebo group after exercise presented a reduction in the production of several cytokines, including tumor necrosis factor-α (TNF-α), interferon-γ (IFN-γ), interleukin-1 (IL-1), and IL-4, compared with before exercise. BCAA supplementation restored the production of TNF-α and IL-1 and increased that of IFN-γ. However, athletes given BCAA supplements presented an even greater reduction in IL-4 production after exercise. There were, however, flaws in the experimental design and statistical analysis of the data in this study, and the results need to be confirmed in more controlled studies. Since several previous studies have indicated that glutamine supplementation during exercise does not prevent the exercise-induced fall in lymphocyte proliferation,[41,42] these findings must be viewed with some caution.

13.6 DIETARY AND SUPPLEMENTAL SOURCES OF BCAAS

The human adult daily maintenance requirement for total BCAA intake is estimated to be 68 to 144 mg/kg (10 to 22% of the maintenance protein requirement).[43] Among the athletic population, several groups of athletes can be identified that consume relatively large amounts of BCAAs. The BCAAs can be obtained from one of four possible sources: whole food proteins, protein supplements, solutions of protein hydrolysates, and free amino acids. The reasons why athletes can have quite high intakes of BCAAs include having high dietary protein intakes and consuming protein and amino acid supplements.

13.6.1 FROM DIETARY PROTEIN INTAKE

The BCAAs, leucine, isoleucine, and valine, represent 3 of the 20 amino acids that are used in the formation of proteins. Thus, on average, the BCAA content of food proteins is about 15% of the total amino acid content. If we take an average man with a sedentary lifestyle, his daily energy intake will be about 10 MJ/day, and let us say that 15% of this will come from protein. Thus, he consumes about 1500 kJ as protein, which is equivalent to about 63 g. Therefore, his intake of BCAAs is about 9.5 g. Contrast this with a Tour de France cyclist: the energy intake of these elite athletes has been measured as averaging around 25 MJ/day over a 2- to 3-week period.[44,45] The proportion of protein in the diet may be a little less, as much of the extra energy consumed is in the form of carbohydrates, but even so, the protein content of the diet is still about 12% of the total energy content. Thus, the elite cyclist consumes about 3000 kJ as protein, which is equivalent to 126 g of protein, which in turn represents about 19 g of BCAAs, or twice the amount of the sedentary individual. The requirement for protein may actually be higher in the endurance athlete because some amino acids, including the BCAAs, are oxidized in increased amounts during exercise compared with rest.[3,6–9] On the other hand, the efficiency of protein utilization appears to be increased with exercise training, and thus the dietary protein requirement may not be very different in athletes compared with less active or even sedentary individuals.[46,47]

13.6.2 FROM HIGH-PROTEIN DIETS AND PROTEIN SUPPLEMENTS

Debate has always raged over how much dietary protein is required for optimal athletic performance, partly because muscle contains a large proportion of the protein in a human body (about 40%). Muscle also accounts for 25 to 35% of all protein turnover in the body. Both the structural proteins that make up the myofibrils and the proteins that act as enzymes within a muscle cell can change as an adaptation to exercise training. Indeed, muscle mass, muscle protein content, and muscle protein composition change in response to training. Interest in protein consumption is very high among amateur and professional athletes. Therefore, the fact that meat, which contains high-quality protein, is a very popular protein source for athletes (especially strength athletes) is not surprising. This preference for meat probably dates back to ancient Greece, where athletes in preparation for the Olympic games consumed large quantities of meat.

A strong belief among many athletes is that a high protein intake or certain protein or amino acid supplements increase muscle mass and strength. Despite the long history of protein use in sports, debate continues over even simple questions, such as whether protein requirements are increased in athletes, and no uniform opinion exists as to what should be measured as an endpoint. A large intake of dietary protein is common practice in weight lifters and bodybuilders. Daily protein intakes as high as 3 g/kg of body mass (b.m.) are not uncommon in these sports, where the aim is to develop a large muscle mass.[1] For a 100-kg individual, this means a protein intake of 300 g/day, and therefore a daily BCAA intake of about 45 g (450 mg/kg of b.m.) is expected.

13.6.3 FROM PROTEIN HYDROLYSATES AND MIXTURES OF ESSENTIAL AMINO ACIDS

Protein hydrolysates are produced from purified protein sources (e.g., casein) by heating with acid or, more usually, by addition of proteolytic enzymes followed by purification procedures. Such hydrolysates contain peptides, of which up to about 40% may be dipeptides and tripeptides. Consumption of amino acids as dipeptides and tripeptides results in faster absorption into the bloodstream, compared with the ingestion of whole proteins or single amino acids. This is a desirable characteristic for athletes who wish to maximize amino acid delivery to the muscles, although whether this has a practical effect of improving muscle protein synthesis, accretion of muscle mass, or improved recovery from exercise has not yet been established.

Nevertheless, this possibility remains attractive to consumers, and there is some strong recent evidence that carbohydrates consumed together with protein hydroly-sates with added leucine and phenylalanine promote higher insulin secretion than can be achieved with carbohydrate intake alone.[48] The potential advantages of this effect are that it may (1) further promote muscle glucose uptake and stimulate muscle glycogen synthesis, and so both increase the stores of this important fuel prior to exercise and enhance its restoration in the recovery phase after exercise, and (2) stimulate muscle amino acid uptake and protein synthesis during recovery from exercise.

13.6.4 BCAA SUPPLEMENTS FROM DRINKS

Although this practice is not common, as few drinks containing significant amounts of BCAAs are commercially available, there are some studies that have suggested that BCAA intake during prolonged exercise may enhance endurance performance by delaying the onset of central fatigue. This suggestion, although not confirmed by many studies, appears to be enough to convince some athletes that ingesting BCAAs during prolonged exercise is worthwhile. BCAAs have only limited solubility in water, and their taste is bitter and rather unpleasant, which is likely to limit the amount consumed by athletes in the form of drinks.

13.7 TOXICITY AND HEALTH RISKS OF BCAAs

As mentioned previously, a reduced capacity to oxidize BCAAs, as in the hereditary disorder maple syrup urine disease, results in excess BCAAs in the blood and profound neurological dysfunction and brain damage. It is hypothesized that the symptoms of excess intake would mimic the neurological symptoms of hereditary diseases of BCAA metabolism.[4] However, the studies on BCAA supplementation that have been conducted on physically active humans indicate that a rather large dietary excess of the three BCAAs is well tolerated when consumed in diets con-taining surfeit amounts of protein. Ingestion of BCAAs in the diet up to 450 mg/kg of b.m./day, which is a little over three times the estimated average requirement, appears to cause no adverse effects in healthy adults. Furthermore, the ingestion of acute doses of BCAA supplements containing all three BCAAs appears to be well tolerated by adults in amounts up to 450 mg/kg of b.m., or around 30 g/day, and without ill effect. Although leucine is the most potent of the BCAAs in promoting protein synthesis, supplementation with leucine alone may cause BCAA imbalance via the activating effect of its keto acid (α-ketoisocaproate) on the branched-chain α-keto acid dehydrogenase complex.[4]

Despite the lack of strong evidence for the efficacy of BCAA supplements for improving exercise performance, athletes continue to use them. Intake of individual amino acids has no added nutritional value compared with the intake of proteins containing these amino acids, and normal food alternatives are available and are almost certainly cheaper than BCAA supplements. For example, a typical BCAA supplement sold in tablet form contains 100 mg of valine, 50 mg of isoleucine, and 100 mg of leucine. A chicken breast (100 g) contains approximately 470 mg of valine, 375 g of isoleucine, and 656 mg of leucine, the equivalent of about seven BCAA tablets. One quarter of a cup of peanuts (60 g) contains even more BCAA and is equivalent to 11 tablets.

13.8 SUMMARY

The requirement for BCAAs is higher in endurance athletes than in sedentary individuals because the BCAAs are oxidized in increased amounts during exercise compared with rest, and they must therefore be replenished by the diet. In the late 1970s, BCAAs were suggested to be the third fuel for skeletal muscle after carbohydrate and fat. However, the majority of later studies, using various exercise and treatment designs and several forms of administration of BCAA (infusion, oral, and with and without carbohydrates), have failed to find a performance-enhancing effect. Leucine appears to provide a stimulatory signal for muscle protein synthesis, and thus has an anticatabolic effect during and after exercise in humans. Studies on the effects of post-exercise nutrition (including BCAA ingestion) on adaptations to training are needed to establish if the physiological role of leucine in stimulating muscle protein synthesis following acute exercise translates into meaningful benefit (e.g., increasing hypertrophy and strength gains with resistance training). There is, at present, limited valid scientific evidence to support the claim that BCAA supplements may accelerate the repair of muscle damage after exercise, and additional research in this area is needed. Some athletes can have quite high intakes of BCAAs because of their high energy and protein intakes, and also because they consume protein supplements, solutions of protein hydrolysates, and free amino acids. Acute intakes of BCAA supplements of up to about 30 g/day seem to be without ill effect. However, the suggested reasons for taking such supplements have not received much support from well-controlled scientific studies.

REFERENCES

1. Jeukendrup, A.E. and Gleeson, M., *Sports Nutrition: An Introduction to Energy Production and Performance*, Human Kinetics, Champaign, IL, 2004.
2. Maughan, R.J. and Gleeson, M., *The Biochemical Basis of Sport Performance*, Oxford University Press, Oxford, 2004.
3. Shimomura, Y., Murakami, T., Nakai, N., Nagasaki, M., and Harris, R.A., Exercise promotes BCAA catabolism: effects of BCAA supplementation on skeletal muscle during exercise, *J. Nutr.*, 134, 1583S–1587S, 2004.
4. Hutson, S.M., Sweatt, A.J., and LaNoue, K.F., Branched-chain amino acid metabolism: implications for establishing safe intakes, *J. Nutr.*, 135, 1557S–1564S, 2005.
5. Wagenmakers, A.J.M., Brookes, J.H., Coakley, J.H., Reilly, T., and Edwards, R.H.T., Exercise-induced activation of branched-chain 2-oxo acid dehydrogenase in human muscle, *Eur. J. Appl. Physiol.*, 59, 159–167, 1989.
6. Wagenmakers, A.J.M., Beckers, E.J., Brouns, F., Kuipers, H., Soeters, P.B., van der Vusse, G.J., and Saris, W.H.M., Carbohydrate supplementation, glycogen depletion, and amino acid metabolism during exercise, *Am. J. Physiol.*, 260, E883–E890, 1991.

7. Wolfe, R.R., Goodenough, R.D., Wolfe, M.H., Royle, G.T., and Nadel, E.R., Isotopic analysis of leucine and urea metabolism in exercising humans, *J. Appl. Physiol.*, 52, 458–466, 1982.

8. Knapik, J., Meredith, C., Jones, B., Fielding, R., Young, V., and Evans, W., Leucine metabolism during fasting and exercise, *J. Appl. Physiol.*, 70, 43–47, 1991.

9. Davies, C.T.M., Halliday, D., Millward, D.J., Rennie, M.J., and Sutton, J.R., Glucose inhibits CO_2 production from leucine during whole-body exercise in man, *J. Physiol.*, 332, 41P–42P, 1982 (abstract).

10. Wagenmakers, A.J., Amino acid supplements to improve athletic performance, *Curr. Opin. Clin. Nutr. Metab. Care*, 2, 539–544, 1999.

11. Louard, R.J., Barrett, E.J., and Gelfand, R.A., Effect of infused branched-chain amino acids on muscle and whole-body amino acid metabolism in man, *Clin. Sci.*, 79, 457–466, 1990.

12. Frexes-Steed, M., Lacy, D.B., Collins, J., and Abumrad, N.N., Role of leucine and other amino acids in regulating protein metabolism *in vivo*, *Am. J. Physiol.*, 262, E925–E935, 1992.

13. Nair, K.S., Matthews, D.E., Welle, S.L., and Braiman, T., Effect of leucine on amino acid and glucose metabolism in humans, *Metabolism*, 41, 643–648, 1992.

14. Lynch, C.J., Halle, B., Fujii, H., Vary, T.C., Wallin, R., Damuni, Z., and Hutson, S.M., Potential role of leucine metabolism in the leucine-signaling pathway involving mTOR, *Am. J. Physiol.*, 285, E854–E863, 2003.

15. Norton, L.E. and Layman, D.K., Leucine regulates translation initiation of protein synthesis in skeletal muscle after exercise, *J. Nutr.*, 136, 533S–537S, 2006.

16. Koopman, R., Wagenmakers, A.J.M., Manders, R.J.F., Zorenc, A.H.G., Senden, J.M.G., Gorselink, M., Keizer, H.A., and van Loon, L.J.C., Combined ingestion of protein and free leucine with carbohydrate increases postexercise muscle protein synthesis *in vivo* in male subjects, *Am. J. Physiol. Endocrinol. Metab.*, 288, 645–653, 2005.

17. Newsholme, E.A., Acworth, I.N., and Blomstrand, E., Amino acids, brain neurotransmitters and a functional link between muscle and brain that is important in sustained exercise, in *Advances in Myochemistry*, Benzi, G., Ed., John Libby Eurotext, London, 1987, pp. 127–138.

18. Chaouloff, F., Kennett, G.A., Serrurrier, B., Merino, D., and Curzon, G., Amino acid analysis demonstrates that increased plasma free tryptophan causes the increase of brain tryptophan during exercise in the rat, *J. Neurochem.*, 46, 1647–1650, 1986.

19. Hargreaves, K.M. and Pardridge, W.M., Neutral amino acid transport at the human blood-brain barrier, *J. Biol. Chem.*, 263, 19392–19397, 1988.

20. Blomstrand, E., Hassmen, P., Ekblom, B., and Newsholme, E.A., Administration of branched-chain amino acids during sustained exercise: effects on performance and on plasma concentration of some amino acids, *Eur. J. Appl. Physiol.*, 63, 83–88, 1991.

21. Mittleman, K.D., Ricci, M.R., and Bailey, S.P., Branched-chain amino acids prolong exercise during heat stress in men and women, *Med. Sci. Sports Exerc.*, 30, 83–91, 1998.

22. Nielsen, B. and Nybo, L., Cerebral changes during exercise in the heat, *Sports Med.*, 33, 1–11, 2003.

23. Watson, P., Strachan, A.T., Shirreffs, S.M., and Maughan, R.J., Branched-chain amino acids and prolonged exercise capacity in a warm environment, *Proc. Nutr. Soc.*, 61, 109A, 2002 (abstract).

24. Watson, P., Shirreffs, S.M., and Maughan, R.J., Effect of acute branched-chain amino acid supplementation on prolonged exercise capacity in a warm environment, *Eur. J. Appl. Physiol.*, 93, 306–314, 2004.

25. Varnier, M., Sarto, P., Martines, D., Lora, L., Carmignoto, F., Leese, G.P., and Naccarato, R., Effect of infusing branched-chain amino acid during incremental exercise with reduced muscle glycogen content, *Eur. J. Appl. Physiol.*, 69, 26–31, 1994.

26. Blomstrand, E., Andersson, S., Hassmen, P., Ekblom, B., and Newsholme, E.A., Effect of branched-chain amino acid and carbohydrate supplementation on the exercise-induced change in plasma and muscle concentration of amino acids in human subjects, *Acta Physiol. Scand.*, 153, 87–96, 1995.

27. Van Hall, G.J., Raaymakers, S.H., Saris, W.H.M., and Wagenmakers, A.J.M., Ingestion of branched-chain amino acids and tryptophan during sustained exercise in man: failure to affect performance, *J. Physiol.*, 486, 789–794, 1995.

28. Madsen, K., MacLean, D.A., Kiens, B., and Christensen, D., Effects of glucose, glucose plus branched-chain amino acids, or placebo on bike performance over 100 km, *J. Appl. Physiol.*, 81, 2644–2650, 1996.

29. Blomstrand, E., Hassmen, P., Ek, S., Ekblom, B., and Newsholme, E.A., Influence of ingesting a solution of branched-chain amino acids on perceived exertion during exercise, *Acta Physiol. Scand.*, 159, 41–49, 1997.

30. Stensrud, T., Ingjer, F., Holm, H., and Strømme, S.B., L-Tryptophan supplementation does not improve running performance, *Int. J. Sports Med.*, 13, 481–485, 1992.

31. Hefler, S.K., Wideman, L., Gaesser, G.A., and Weltman, A., Branched-chain amino acid (BCAA) supplementation improves endurance performance in competitive cyclists, *Med. Sci. Sports Exerc.*, 27, S149, 1995 (abstract).

32. Coombes, J.S. and McNaughton, L.R., Effects of branched-chain amino acid supplementation on serum creatine kinase and lactate dehydrogenase after prolonged exercise, *J. Sports Med. Phys. Fitness*, 40, 240–246, 2000.

33. Nosaka, K., Muscle soreness and amino acids, *Training J.*, 289, 24–28, 2003.

34. Nosaka, K., Sacco, P., and Mawatari, K., Effects of amino acid supplementation on muscle soreness and damage, *Int. J. Sport Nutr. Exerc. Metab.*, 16, 620–635, 2006.

35. Shimomura, Y., Yamamoto, Y., Bajotto, G., Sato, J., Murakami, T., Shimomura, N., Kobayashi, H., and Mawatari, K., Nutraceutical effects of branched-chain amino acids on skeletal muscle, *J. Nutr.*, 136, 529S–532S, 2006.

36. Shephard, R.J., *Physical Activity, Training and the Immune Response*, Cooper, Carmel, IN, 1997.

37. Mackinnon, L.T., *Advances in Exercise and Immunology*, Human Kinetics, Champaign, IL, 1999.

38. Gleeson, M., Ed., *Immune Function in Sport and Exercise*, Elsevier, Edinburgh, 2005.

39. Pedersen, B.K. and Bruunsgaard, H., How physical exercise influences the establishment of infections, *Sports Med.*, 19, 393–400, 1995.

40. Bassit, R.A., Sawada, L.A., Bacurau, R.F., Navarro, F., Martins, E., Jr., Santos, R.V., Caperuto, E.C., Rogeri, P., and Costa Rosa, L.F., Branched-chain amino acid supplementation and the immune response of long-distance athletes, *Nutrition*, 18, 376–379, 2002.

41. Rohde, T., MacLean, D.A., and Pedersen, B.K., Effect of glutamine supplementation on changes in the immune system induced by repeated exercise, *Med. Sci. Sports Exerc.*, 30, 856–862, 1998.

42. Krzywkowski, K., Petersen, E.W., Ostrowski, K., Kristensen, J.H., Boza, J., and Pedersen, B.K., Effect of glutamine supplementation on exercise-induced changes in lymphocyte function, *Am. J. Physiol.*, 281, C1259–C1265, 2001.

43. Baker, D.H., Tolerance for branched-chain amino acids in experimental animals and humans, *J. Nutr.*, 135, 1585S–1590S, 2005.

44. Brouns, F., Saris, W.H.M., Stroecken, J., Beckers, E., Thijssen, R., Rehrer, N.J., and ten Hoor, F., Eating, drinking, and cycling. A controlled Tour de France simulation study, Part I, *Int. J. Sports Med.*, 10, S32–S40, 1989.

45. Saris, W.H.M., van Erp-Baart, M.A., Brouns, F., Westerterp, K.R., and ten Hoor, F., Study on food intake and energy expenditure during extreme sustained exercise: the Tour de France, *Int. J. Sports Med.*, 10, S26–S31, 1989.

46. Butterfield, G.E., Whole-body protein utilization in humans, *Med. Sci. Sports Exerc.*, 19 (Suppl.), S157–S165, 1987.

47. Tarnopolsky, M.A., Gibala, M., Jeukendrup, A.E., and Phillips, S.M., Nutritional needs of elite endurance athletes. Part II. Dietary protein and the potential role of caffeine and creatine, *Eur. J. Sport Sci.*, 5, 59–72, 2005.

48. Manninen, A.H., Protein hydrolysates in sports and exercise: a brief review, *J. Sports Sci. Med.*, 3, 60–63, 2004.

14 Glutamine

Satya S. Jonnalagadda

CONTENTS

14.1 INTRODUCTION

Glutamine was first isolated in 1883 from beet juice. Glutamine is one of the most abundant free amino acids in the human body (muscle and plasma), comprising approximately 50% of the free amino acid pool in the blood and skeletal muscle.[1,2] Glutamine is considered a nonessential amino acid (dispensable) since it can be produced in the body from other amino acids, namely, glutamic acid, in the liver and skeletal muscle. The skeletal muscle is the most active tissue for glutamine synthesis, storage, and release, thus playing a critical role in the maintenance of plasma glutamine concentrations. However, under certain physiological conditions

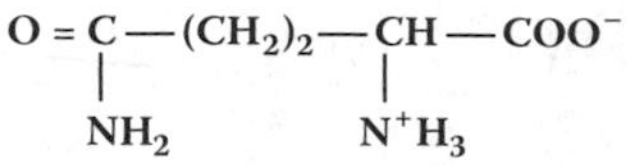

$$O = C - (CH_2)_2 - CH - COO^-$$
$$\quad\; | \qquad\qquad\qquad | $$
$$\quad NH_2 \qquad\qquad N^+H_3$$

FIGURE 14.1 Chemical structure of glutamine.

(trauma, infection, stress), glutamine can become a conditionally essential amino acid (indispensable), and exogenous sources (diet and supplements) may be required to meet the needs of the body.

14.1.1 CHEMICAL STRUCTURE

Glutamine is a five-carbon compound with two nitrogen groups (Figure 14.1), is a relatively ubiquitous amino acid, and is unstable in the liquid phase. Glutamine is an amide derivative of the acid amino acid, glutamic acid (or glutamate). The conversion of glutamate to glutamine can occur in key tissues such as liver, brain, kidney, skeletal muscle, and intestine and is catalyzed by the enzyme glutamine synthase.[1,2]

Glutamine is a neutral polar amino acid, with an amine functional group, which is highly polar, and is capable of forming strong hydrogen bonds. This nature of the side chain enables glutamine to contribute to the stability of the protein molecule. The hydrogen bonding capacity of the amine group also enables interaction with water, making glutamine a highly hydrophilic amino acid.[1,2]

Glutamine is degraded to α-ketoglutarate, which is an important intermediate in several metabolic pathways, such as the citric acid cycle and the transamination process.[1,2] Glutamine can also be converted to glutamate by the enzyme glutaminase, and thus plays an important role in the transamination process, in the synthesis of several key proteins, as precursors of other nonessential amino acids, and in the synthesis of excitatory neurotransmitters. Figure 14.2 summarizes the metabolism of glutamine.

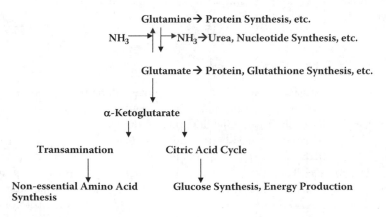

FIGURE 14.2 Brief overview of glutamine metabolism.

TABLE 14.1
Physiological Functions of Glutamine

- Nitrogen carrier
  - Interorgan transporter
- Metabolic intermediate
  - Energy source
    - Oxidation to lactate (partial) or carbon dioxide (full)
  - Main energy substrate for:
    - Immune system
    - Gastrointestinal system
  - Respiratory substrate
    - Enterocytes
    - Lymphocytes
  - Regulator of protein synthesis
  - Regulator of peptide synthesis
  - Precursor of nonessential amino acid synthesis
  - Purine, pyrimidine, nucleotide synthesis (amine group)
  - Formation of glucosamine (amine group)
  - Fatty acid synthesis (acetyl group)
  - Gluconeogenesis (carbon skeleton)
- Glutathione metabolism
- Muscle-sparing effect
- Acid–base homeostasis

14.2 METABOLIC FUNCTIONS

Glutamine is essential for maintaining many homeostatic functions and for the optimal functioning of a number of body tissues, most importantly the gut and immune system. Glutamine is the most versatile amino acid and has several key regulatory functions in the body. It plays a central role in acid–base homeostasis, is a precursor for nucleic acids and nucleotide biosynthesis, is used in the synthesis of amino sugars, and participates in interorgan nitrogen transport. Glutamine is a key anapleuretic, energy-yielding substrate under conditions of hypoxia, anoxia, and dysoxia, and a key gluconeogenic metabolite under normal postabsorptive conditions.[3] Additionally, glutamine is an important component of the flavor- and taste-enhancing compound monosodium glutamate. Table 14.1 summarizes the metabolic functions of glutamine. However, under catabolic states, such as exhaustive exercise, infection, surgery, and trauma, skeletal glutamine reserves are depleted, making this amino acid a conditionally essential amino acid.

14.2.1 PROTEIN SYNTHESIS AND DEGRADATION

Glutamine plays a significant role in the synthesis of proteins and nonessential amino acids. Glutamine is referred to as competence factor since it stimulates protein synthesis.[4] It is an amino group donor in various biosynthetic reactions of purine, pyrimidine, and amino sugar syntheses. Glutamine also serves as a storage and transport form of ammonium and plays a significant role in the removal of excess ammonia by playing a critical part in the urea synthesis process. Glutamine is a regulator of urea synthesis since the enzyme carbomyl phosphate synthetase is allosterically activated by N-acetylglutamate for the utilization of the first nitrogen molecule in the urea synthesis. Glutamine utilization of the cells increases dramatically during hypercatabolic conditions such as trauma and sepsis to fulfill the energy demands and to provide nitrogen for the protein synthesis occurring during these states.[1,2]

Glutamine regulates muscle protein levels and has been shown to have antiproteolytic effects on noncontractile protein components in the rat model.[5] Decreasing intramuscluar glutamine concentrations has been shown to increase muscle catabolism.[5] Glutamine has also been observed to regulate the myosin heavy-chain synthesis seen in glucocorticoid-induced muscle atrophy.[5] Fatigue due to increased exercise can increase overall protein catabolism and lower plasma and muscle concentration of amino acids; glutamine has been observed to play a key role in restoring these amino acid concentrations.[5] Glutamine supplementation has been observed to stimulate an increase in muscle protein synthesis, especially immediately after exhaustive exercise.[6]

Glutamine also plays an important role in the regulation of acid–base balance by allowing the kidneys to excrete an acid load, thereby protecting the body against acidosis, and serves as the most important nitrogen shuttle, supplying nitrogen for metabolic purposes.[1,2] Glutamine is a precursor for the synthesis of nucleic acids. It also plays a role in the synthesis of glutathione, a tripeptide molecule synthesized from glycine, cysteine, and glutamate. Glutathione plays a role in the transport of certain amino acids and in the synthesis of leukotriene (which regulates the inflammation response), and it protects the cells from the harmful effects of free radicals.[7]

14.2.2 GLUCOSE REGULATION

Glutamine is as important as lactate in contributing to the net gluconeogenesis in the postabsorptive state, contributing to 20 to 25% of the whole-body glucose production. Glutamine gluconeogenesis contributes to approximately 5% of the systemic glucose appearance, and renal production of glucose from glutamine accounts for nearly 75% of all glucose derived from glutamine.[8] However, in trained cyclists, glutamine supplementation did not show any significant impact on the rate of glycogen resynthesis, i.e., muscle glycogen concentrations, despite a twofold increase in plasma glutamine concentrations,[9] suggesting that the impact of glutamine supplementation on glycogen synthesis post-exercise needs to be further evaluated.

14.2.3 IMMUNE REGULATION

Leukocytes comprise a heterogeneous mix of cells circulating between the lymphoid tissues and organs and the blood and lymph, and play a very important role in maintaining a functional immune response system.[10] Some of the main leukocytes are neutrophils, which comprise 60 to 70% of circulating leukocytes, lymphocytes (T-, B-, and natural killer cells), which comprise 20 to 35% of circulating leukocytes, and monocytes, which comprise 15% of circulating leukocytes.[10] Additionally, glycoproteins such as immunoglobulins (Ig) and antibodies produced by B-cells are also found in the serum and other body secretions and play an important role in the immune response.

A moderate level of exercise has been suggested to enhance immunity and lower the risk of sickness among active individuals.[4,11] On the other hand, heavy training has been suggested to suppress the immune system of athletes.[4] Natural killer cell activity, which protects against viruses and tumor cells, has been observed to be higher among athletes than nonathletes.[11] However, depending on the severity of the training, neutrophil activity, which is the body's defense against bacteria and viruses, has been observed to be depressed.[11] Lagranha et al.[12] observed oral glutamine supplementation to partially prevent exercise-induced apoptosis in neutrophils by possibly preserving mitochondrial function in sexually immature and mature rats. In healthy men performing 2 h of cycle ergometry, Hiscock et al.[13] observed that supplementation with glutamine during and 2 h after exercise induced an 18-fold increase in plasma IL-6 concentrations. However, the impact on these changes, in the immune cell responses, on the risk of infection of athletes is inconclusive. Although plasma glutamine concentrations are kept constant during and after acute, strenuous exercise, glutamine supplementation does not appear to abolish the post-exercise decrease in *in vitro* cellular immunity, including low lymphocyte number, impaired lymphocyte proliferation, and impaired natural killer and lymphokine-activated killer cell activity, implying that the glutamine hypothesis may explain immunodepression related to stressful conditions such as trauma and burns, but not exercise-induced immunodepression.[14] Given the impact of an altered immune system on an athlete's performance and the role of certain nutrients in development and maintenance of the immune system, attention has focused on the use of specific nutrients in the prevention of infections among athletes, one such nutrient being glutamine.

Glutamine is considered an immunonutrient and is used in medical foods for hypercatabolic situations, including burns, cancer, infection, surgery, transplants, and trauma.[15,16] Additionally, stressors such as prolonged exercise and overtraining can cause a reduction in skeletal muscle and plasma glutamine concentrations. Muscle glutamine levels have been observed to decrease in a dose-dependent manner based on the degree of stress. Glutamine is also referred to as an anticatabolic nutrient.[15,16] Glutamine has been shown to strengthen the immunity under conditions of major trauma, especially in the gastrointestinal tract.[15,16] It is also needed for wound healing given its role in the regulation of protein synthesis. Glutamine serves as a fuel for enterocytes, colonocytes, lymphocytes, and proliferating cells. It has been observed to be important for lymphocyte proliferation and generation of lymphokine-activated killer cell activity *in vitro*. However, Rohde et al.[17,18] did not observe any benefit of glutamine supplementation following prolonged intense exercise on suppressing the decline in lymphokine-activated killer cell activity. Lymphocyte proliferation and synthesis of interleukin 1 by macrophages and interleukin 2 by lymphocytes have been observed to decrease with glutamine deficiency.

Acute effects of aerobic and anaerobic exercise on the immune system may include increase in leukocyte counts in peripheral circulation with transient immunosuppression in the ability of lymphocytes to respond to immune challenges. The duration and intensity of exercise can also impact the immune response. Exhaustive prolonged exercise can decrease muscle glutamine levels, which is typically magnified after athletic injury. Castell et al.[19] observed that glutamine supplementation (5 g in 330 ml of water) immediately after and 2 h after a marathon decreased the incidence of upper respiratory tract infections up to 7 days following the race. Likewise, Bassit et al.[20] observed that branched-chain amino acid supplements (6 g/day for 15 days), which are precursors for glutamine, prior to a triathlon or 30-km run prevented a 40% decline in the nitrogen-stimulated lymphocyte proliferation observed in the control group post-exercise. Additionally, the branched-chain amino acid supplementation prevented the post-exercise fall in plasma glutamine concentrations and was also associated with an increase in interleukin 2 and interferon production, suggesting a potential role for these amino acids in the regulation of the immune system. High-intensity exercises have been suggested to suppress neutrophil functions, which play a major role in nonspecific host defense and constitute 50 to 60% of the blood leukocyte pool. Walsh et al.[21] observed that glutamine supplementation during exercise and recovery helped maintain plasma glutamine concentrations and prevented the reduction in plasma glutamine levels. However, glutamine supplementation did not have any effect on the post-exercise changes in leukocytosis or whole-blood neutrophil degranulation following prolonged exercise activity. Furthermore, glutamine as a precursor of glutamate plays a major role in cellular synthesis of glutathione in lymphocytes, which plays a role in the redox system of the cell by protecting the cells against the harmful effects of oxidants (free radicals) produced during the various metabolic processes.[7]

In athletes, a consequence of overtraining, i.e., excessive training over a prolonged period, is immunosuppression, resulting in a higher incidence of infections, slower wound healing, fatigue, impaired immune function, and decreased exercise performance. Overtraining has been associated with a decrease in plasma glutamine concentrations.[22–24] Plasma glutamine concentrations have been observed to decrease acutely after intense exercise and during periods of intense training. During periods of stress, glutamine metabolism is increased to promote cell division, antibody production, and protein synthesis. Elite Olympic athletes who had lasting fatigue after intense training periods had 33% lower plasma glutamine levels than those who had no long lasting fatigue; however, the impact on athletic performance was minimal.[25] Additionally, athletes with plasma glutamine levels less than 450 μmol/l were more susceptible to infections, further suggesting that glutamine may have an impact on the synthesis of immune cells.[25]

14.2.4 Energy Supply

Glutamine provides nitrogen and carbon molecules for synthesis of macromolecules and production of energy.[1,2] Glutamine is a direct respiratory fuel for enterocytes and mucosal epithelial cells of the small intestine. Glutamine is also utilized as an energy source by lymphocytes, macrophages, and replication cells of the stomach, large intestine, spleen, and pancreas. Plasma glutamine concentrations have been observed to decrease after exhaustive exercise, which has been attributed to increased utilization of glutamine in the liver for gluconeogenesis and urea formation and an increased rate of glutamine utilization by the kidneys and immune system.[26,27]

14.3 BODY STORES AND REGULATION

Glutamine accounts for more than half of the total intramuscular free amino acid pool, making it one of the most abundant and versatile amino acids in the plasma and skeletal muscle.[28] Glutamine is predominantly synthesized and stored in the skeletal muscle by the action of the enzyme glutamine synthetase. Adipose tissue, lungs, liver, and brain are also sites of synthesis of glutamine.

14.3.1 SKELETAL MUSCLE

In the skeletal muscle glutamine is needed to maintain protein levels, immune system function, and glucose–glycogen metabolism, all of which can be very significant for an active individual such as an athlete.[28] Much of the glutamine is stored in skeletal muscle, and athletes who overuse these muscles may deplete their glutamine stores and increase their susceptibility to infection or slow their rate of recovery from injuries. In the postabsorptive state, skeletal muscle glutamine is a major contributor (48%) to the amino acid nitrogen released into the circulation.[29] Furthermore, 4 h after a mixed meal, skeletal glutamine accounts for 71% of the amino acid released and 82% of the nitrogen released from the muscle.[29] Plasma glutamine concentrations decreased 10 to 25% after moderate- to high-intensity exercise (50 to 80% VO_2max), which could be due to an increase in muscle protein synthesis during recovery.[29] Glutamine may also be a stimulator of post-exercise glycogen synthesis in the muscle, probably due to the direct conversion of glutamine (carbon skeleton) to glycogen or glutamine-induced cell swelling, which stimulates glycogen synthesis.[30] However, addition of protein to carbohydrate supplements post-exercise has not been consistently observed to increase glycogen synthesis beyond that produced with carbohydrate only.[30,31] A high correlation exists between muscle glutamate concentrations and muscle glutathione concentrations, suggesting that glutamate plays a determining role in the glutathione synthesis process, and thus oxidation pathway.[32] During exercise, glutamate plays a critical role in energy provision because it participates in the tricarboxylic acid cycle and the purine nucleotide cycles critical for protein synthesis. Kargotich et al.[33] observed high-intensity exercise in well-trained swimmers to result in a significant reduction in plasma glutamine during the post-exercise period, suggesting that glutamine could be a marker of overtraining.

14.3.2 LIVER AND KIDNEY

Glutamine in the liver and kidney is catabolized to glutamate and ammonia with the help of the enzyme glutaminase.[1,2] In the absorptive state or during periods of alkalosis, liver glutaminase activity increases ammonia production for the urea cycle.[1,2] Under the acidotic state, use of glutamine in the urea cycle decreases, and instead, glutamine is released from the liver and transported to the kidneys, where it is catabolized by the renal tubular enzyme glutaminase to produce ammonium and glutamate.[1,2] This glutamate may be catabolized by the enzyme glutamate dehydrogenase to produce α-ketoglutarate, which can be used for energy production via the citric acid cycle or nonessential amino acid synthesis via the transamination process, and ammonium.[1,2]

Iwashita et al.[34] observed that glutamine supplementation to exercising dogs stimulated whole-body glucose production during and after exercise above a normal exercise response by 24%. Hepatic uptake of glutamine and alanine was higher with glutamine supplementation during exercise, and hepatic glucose output was increased sevenfold during exercise with glutamine supplementation. Glutamine supplementation was observed to increase glucose utilization by 16% after exercise, suggesting that glutamine availability can modulate glucose homeostatis during and after exercise. Renal glutaminase activity and ammonium excretion increase with acidosis and decrease with alkalosis.[1,2] Thus, given the ubiquitous synthesis of glutamine in the cells and its ability to diffuse in and out of cells, it serves as a major transporter of nitrogen.

14.4 DIETARY INTAKE

14.4.1 FOOD SOURCES

Dietary sources rich in glutamine include all foods that are rich in protein, particularly milk protein and meats. Three ounces (85 g) of meat, chicken, or fish contains 3 to 4 g of glutamine. Plant foods such as spinach, parsley, and cabbage are also sources of glutamine. Table 14.2 provides some examples of food sources of

TABLE 14.2
Food Sources of Glutamine

Food	Amount (g) per 100 g of Cooked, Edible Portion[a]
Whole egg, large, raw	1.68
Turkey breast	2.79
Whole-wheat bread	2.96
Salmon	3.30
Tuna	3.81
Wheat germ	3.99
Beef T-bone steak	4.18
Pork chops	4.29
Chicken breast	4.64

[a] As glutamic acid.

From USDA National Nutrient Database for Standard Reference, available at http://www.nal.usda.gov/fnic/cgi-bin/nut_search.pl, accessed June 7, 2006.

TABLE 14.3
Summary of Available Glutamine Supplements[a]

Brand	Number of Servings	Grams Per Serving	Price Per Gram	Price
ABB Gluta-Force, 1.1 lb	100	5	$0.05	$27.49
All American Pharmaceutical Liquid Glutamine, 16 fl oz	32	—	$0.90	$28.95
Bioplex L-Glutamine, 1000 g	100	10	$0.03	$32.99
EAS L-Glutamine, 400 g	80	5	$0.05	$18.55
Fitness Technologies Pure Glutamine, 2000 g	400	5	$0.03	$69.95
Nature's Best L-Glutamine, 600 g	120	4.6	$0.05	$29.99
Optimum Glutamine Powder, 1000 g	222	4.5	$0.04	$40.98
Twinlab Glutamine Fuel, 120 capsules	60	1.5	$0.21	$18.45

[a] Not a comprehensive list.

glutamine and amount per 100 g. Under normal conditions, diet, in addition to what is produced by the body, can meet the glutamine needs of an individual. However, under certain physiological conditions such as injuries, surgery, infections, and extreme stress, body glutamine stores can be depleted and supplemental glutamine may be required.

14.4.2 SUPPLEMENTAL SOURCES

Glutamine is a popular supplement consumed by active individuals. Glutamine supplements are available as L-glutamine either as an individual amino acid supplement or as part of a protein supplement. These supplements are available in powder, capsule, tablet, or liquid form, with most claiming to enhance muscular recovery from intense workouts, with the recommended intake being post-workout or with meals. An Internet search (Google search engine, June 7, 2006) using the term *glutamine supplements* produced 2,040,000 hits. Table 14.3 provides some examples of currently available glutamine supplements. Like all dietary supplements, caution should be used when taking glutamine supplements, and these supplements should be taken under the supervision of a health care provider. Individuals with kidney and liver disease should not take glutamine supplements given the central role of these organs in glutamine metabolism. Glutamine supplements should be taken several hours before or after a meal to prevent interaction with amino acids in the regular diet of the individual.

14.4.3 DIGESTION AND ABSORPTION

The proteolytic enzymes produced by the pancreas and the brush border facilitate the release of glutamine from dietary protein. Glutamine is absorbed efficiently in the human jejunum and is transported across the intestinal brush border by both a sodium-dependent and a sodium-independent system. Following protein digestion and absorption across the brush border and basolateral membranes, glutamine is primarily used by the enterocytes, is the main energy source for these cells, and exhibits tropic effects on the gastrointestinal mucosal cells. The gastrointestinal tract utilizes approximately 40% of the glutamine entering the system. Given the dependence of the enterocytes on glutamine, a deficiency of this amino acid can decrease gut function due to a loss of protection against bacterial or endotoxin translocation from the gut lumen into the portal circulation.[1,2]

14.5 NUTRITIONAL STATUS ASSESSMENT

Plasma glutamine concentrations can be evaluated to determine an individual's glutamine status. Among high-performance athletes (speed skating, swimming, skiing) under a variety of training conditions, Smith and Norris[35] observed plasma glutamine concentrations to range from 402 to 741 μmol/l. Under conditions of rest, the average plasma glutamine concentration in these athletes was 585 μmol/l, while under heavy training conditions, a significant reduction to 522 μmol/l was observed. Additionally, under conditions of overtraining, plasma glutamine concentrations decreased to 488 μmol/l. Therefore, it has been proposed that glutamine concentrations decrease when the work volume exceeds the athlete's tolerance level; however, low glutamine levels are not necessarily indicative of the training status of an athlete. Hiscock and Mackinnon[22] also observed differences in resting plasma glutamine concentrations based on the athlete's sport, with cyclists having the highest concentration (1395 μM/l), runners and swimmers having intermediate levels (691 and 632 μM/l, respectively), and power lifters having the lowest levels (556 μM/l), suggesting that the physical and metabolic demands of a sport may influence an athlete's glutamine status. However, it is unclear if this is due to the effect of the sport or a combination of the sport and dietary practices of these athletes. Furthermore, dietary protein intake, when expressed as gram per kilogram of body weight, was observed to be negatively associated with plasma glutamine concentrations, which may be attributed to the role of glutamine in maintaining acid–base balance, with high protein diets increasing the acid load and thereby increasing glutamine needs by the kidneys.

In addition to exercise, an individual's dietary intake can also have an influence on his plasma glutamine concentrations. Blanchard et al.[28] observed high-carbohydrate (70%) diets to increase plasma glutamine concentrations compared to low-carbohydrate (45%) (i.e., high-protein) diets in endurance-trained men completing exercise trials. However, muscle glutamine concentrations did not differ between the two groups, and no association was observed between plasma glutamine concentrations and changes in muscle glycogen concentrations. This suggests that the effect of carbohydrate intake on plasma glutamine is not influenced by the muscle glycogen stores. Likewise, Gleeson et al.[29] observed low-carbohydrate diet (7%) to be associated with a reduction in plasma glutamine concentrations during recovery compared to a high-carbohydrate diet (75%). Low-carbohydrate and high-protein intakes have been suggested to result in lowering plasma glutamine levels due to a disruption in the acid–base balance, stimulating the kidneys to increase the uptake of glutamine to buffer the hydrogen ion concentration and restore normal pH.

Additionally, glutamine may serve as a precursor for gluconeogenesis, with low carbohydrate intakes, further reducing plasma glutamine concentrations. Branched-chain amino acid supplementation was also observed to maintain plasma glutamine concentrations among triathletes compared to placebo, which resulted in a 23% reduction after the triathlon.[20] This ability of branched-chain amino acids to maintain glutamine concentrations is attributed to their influence of glutamate metabolism in the skeletal muscle with the subsequent release of NH_3, which is used in the production of glutamine. Therefore, when assessing an individual's glutamine status, it is important to assess both his dietary intake and exercise patterns.

14.6 ERGOGENIC EFFECTS

14.6.1 ENDURANCE ACTIVITIES

The speculation that glutamine supplementation can enhance performance during endurance activities is largely based on the acute immune system suppression observed during strenuous exercise. Since glutamine is utilized as a fuel source for immune system cells, the assumption is that supplementary glutamine will attenuate the mobilization of glutamine from the skeletal muscle. Prolonged endurance exercise, such as marathon running, may reduce plasma glutamine concentration. Plasma glutamine concentrations seem to significantly decrease in overtrained athletes compared to control, nonovertrained athletes.[36] Physical stress such as illness or increased physical activity can induce hypercatabolic states, thereby decreasing the body's endogenous rate of glutamine synthesis, making it a conditionally essential amino acid. Early studies suggested that glutamine may be beneficial to endurance athletes because of its impact on muscle glycogen synthesis, by serving as a substrate for gluconeogenesis in the liver, thereby decreasing amino acid release from muscle during extended exercise and decreasing muscle protein degradation. Mourtzakis and Graham[37] observed that during prolonged exercise, carbohydrate oxidation peaked at 30 min of exercise and decreased for the remainder of the exercise bout, while pyruvate production was greatest at 1 h of exercise and was closely linked to glutamate concentrations, which was the predominant amino acid taken up during exercise and recovery. Alanine and glutamate were associated with pyruvate metabolism and comprised ~68% of the total amino acids released during exercise and recovery, thus implying that a reduced supply of these amino acids can limit endurance exercise performance.

Glutamine supplementation has also been shown to decrease incidence of infection secondary to overtraining and to improve the response of cells of the immune system, thereby enabling athletes to maintain training at a greater frequency and intensity.[11] However, other studies have not found any beneficial effects of glutamine supplementation in athletes.[17,18,31]

Strenuous exercise can cause significant immunosuppression along with a reduction in plasma glutamine levels. Following intense exercise of greater than 1 h, lymphocyte count, natural killer cell activity, and lymphokine-activated killer cell activity were observed to decline.[4,11] Additionally, the lymphocyte proliferative response to T-cell mitogens decreased during exercise. Concomitant decline in plasma glutamine concentrations may play a role in impaired immune function after sustained physical activity. It has been shown that glutaminase activity is increased during immunologic challenges, which in rapidly dividing cells is a source of nitrogen and carbon, which can serve as precursors for macromolecules and energy.[38] Thus, under life stresses and disease states, several dispensable amino acids can become conditionally essential because their utilization within the body exceeds their endogenous production.

While oral or parenteral glutamine supplementation has helped maintain muscular glutamine concentrations, improve nitrogen balance, and increase protein synthesis,[39] the benefits for athletes are not well established. Castell et al.[19] investigated the effects of consumption of glutamine-containing drinks immediately after heavy exercise and 2 h after exhaustive exercise in middle-distance, marathon, and ultramarathon runners and in elite rowers during training and competition. The glutamine-supplemented group reported a reduced instance of infections compared to the placebo group. Castell et al.[40] later observed that glutamine supplementation did not appear to have an effect on immune function (as assessed by lymphocyte distribution) following completion of the Brussels marathon. Similarly, Rohde et al.[17,18] examined the impact of glutamine supplementation on exercise-induced immune change after 30, 45, and 60 min at 75% VO_2max. Arterial glutamine concentration decreased by 20% after the last exercise bout in the placebo trial, whereas the glutamine concentration was maintained at a level above rest at all times in the glutamine-supplemented group (900 mg/kg body weight). However, these differences between the two groups were not significant. The concentration of leukocytes increased during and after each exercise bout, which was attributed to an increase in neutrophils, lymphocytes, and monocytes (during) and neutrophils and monocytes (after); however, no differences were observed between the placebo and glutamine groups. Thus, the post-exercise immune changes did not appear to be caused by decreased plasma glutamine concentrations.[17,18] Kargotich et al.[41] observed glutamine responses to strenuous interval exercise before and after 6 weeks of endurance training. Prior to training, glutamine concentrations progressively decreased (16 to 18%) post-exercise. However, with training glutamine concentrations increased by 14%, suggesting that training-induced changes in glutamine may be able to prevent the decline in glutamine levels following strenuous exercise below a threshold where immune function might be acutely compromised. These results further suggest that oral glutamine supplements may prevent the post-exercise reduction in plasma glutamine concentrations without influencing the immune system, but the ergogenic benefits of glutamine supplementation need further examination.

14.6.2 NONENDURANCE ACTIVITIES

Antonio and Street[42] propose that the ergogenic benefits of glutamine observed in certain groups of athletes and not in others may be due to its protective role against protein degradation, potentially enhancing recovery following resistance training sessions; however, this is yet to be determined among athletes participating in such sports. Since strength and resistance training result in glycogen depletion and increased protein turnover, Antonio and Street[42] have suggested that glutamine supplementation may be beneficial for these athletes. However, the data on non-endurance activities and glutamine supplementation are scarce. Antonio et al.[43] observed that pre-exercise glutamine supplementation (0.3 g/kg body weight) in men performing weight-lifting exercise did not result in any changes in maximal repetitions performed in the leg press or bench press, suggesting that short-term ingestion of glutamine does not enhance weight-lifting performance in resistance-trained men. The supposition that glutamine may act as a buffering agent for repeated bouts of high-intensity activities originates from the potential ability to maintain the acid–base balance in the body. However, Haub et al.[44] in a study of the effects of glutamine or placebo supplementation (0.03 kg/kg) did not observe any beneficial effects of the supplementation on five repeated bouts of cycling at 100% VO_2max peak (four bouts lasting 60 sec and the fifth bout continued to fatigue). The results indicated that acute ingestion of L-glutamine did not enhance buffering potential or performance or delay the onset of fatigue during high-intensity exercise in these athletes.

In another study, Candow et al.[45] examined the effect of oral glutamine supplementation combined with a weight resistance program on 1 rep maximum leg press and bench press, peak knee extension torque, on lean tissue and muscle protein degradation. Subjects were supplemented with glutamine (0.9 g/kg lean body mass/day) or placebo for 6 weeks of training. Although increases in strength (31% for squat and 14% for bench press), torque (6%), lean tissue mass (6%) and 3-methylhistidine (41%) were observed in the glutamine-supplemented group, similar increases were observed in the placebo group. The researchers concluded that glutamine supplementation resulted in no significant effect on muscle performance, body composition, or muscle protein degradation during resistance training. Similarly, van Hall et al.[31] also did not observe any beneficial effects of oral glutamine supplementation on glycogen resynthesis following intense interval exercise. Antonio et al.[46] also investigated glutamine supplementation and its effects on weight-lifting performance. Resistance-trained individuals (n = 6) performed weight-lifting exercises in a double-blind, placebo-controlled, crossover design supplemented with glutamine or glycine (0.3 g/kg; average intake, 23 g) mixed with calorie-free fruit juice or placebo. One-hour postingestion of the supplement, subjects performed exercises to muscular failure. Acute ingestion of glutamine did not enhance weight-lifting performance, and no differences were observed in the average number of maximal repetitions performed in the leg or bench press exercises, suggesting that short-term ingestion of glutamine (1 h before the event) may not have any ergogenic benefits for individuals participating in resistance type activities. The effects of long-term ingestion of glutamine are yet to be determined.

This lack of an effect of glutamine supplementation during resistance training may be due to the utilization of glutamine by other tissues before it reaches the peripheral circulation and skeletal muscle. Glutamine serves as a gluconeogenic precursor when muscle glycogen is depleted by approximately 90%; however, resistance training typically produces approximately 40% depletion in muscle glycogen, which may not be severe enough to benefit from glutamine supplementation.[46] Serving as an energy source of the immune cells is another proposed ergogenic effect of glutamine.[19,40] Exhaustive endurance exercise has been shown to suppress the immune system in some athletes; however, heavy resistance exercise has not been observed to have any significant impact on the immune system,[47,48] suggesting that some of the ergogenic benefits of glutamine may be dependent on the type of exercise performed. In a recent review by Ohtani et al.,[49] chronic supplementation with a mixture of amino acids, including branched-chain amino acids, arginine, and glutamine, was observed to result in a quicker recovery from muscle fatigue, following eccentric exercise training. At the highest doses of the amino acid supplementation (6.6 g/day) for 1 month, blood oxygen-carrying capacity was increased, while muscle damage was observed to decrease, thus resulting in improved training efficiency.

14.7   DRUG–NUTRIENT INTERACTIONS

Interactions of glutamine supplements with other nutrients and dietary supplements are not known.[50] Since glutamine is metabolized to glutamate, which can act as an excitatory neurotransmitter, the potential for antagonizing the anticonvulsant effects of certain epilepsy medications exists.[50] Furthermore, since glutamine is metabolized to ammonia, it can potentially antagonize the antiammonia effects of lactulose.[50] Although the aforementioned interactions are theoretically possible, no known adverse effects have been reported with glutamine supplementation. Glutamine supplements, especially the powders, should not be added to hot beverages because heat can destroy the amino acid. Individuals with kidney or liver disease should not take glutamine supplements. It has been suggested that glutamine may increase the effectiveness and reduce the side effects of chemotherapy treatments, therefore making it essential that individuals check with their health care providers before using supplements.

14.8   SAFETY AND TOXICITY

Intake of up to 40 g/day of glutamine supplements did not result in any significant adverse effects other than mild gastrointestinal discomfort in some individuals.[50] Such high intakes can be achieved only through supplement usage, and as such, these doses should be divided into two to four throughout the data to result in an increase in total body stores without resulting in significant competition for absorption with the other amino acids.

14.9   SUMMARY

Glutamine has established important physiological functions under both normal and hypercatabolic states. Glutamine has a central role to play in maintaining a healthy immune system and the energy levels of key cells. Adequate dietary protein intake can ensure that these functions of glutamine are fulfilled in the normal healthy individual, with hypercatabolic states requiring additional supplemental sources of glutamine. The immune-enhancing effects and the antiproteolytic effects of glutamine have implications for athletes involved in intense training activities.

However, the ergogenic benefits and the immune-enhancing effects of glutamine supplementation for the active individual are yet to be realized. Long-term studies examining the effect of glutamine supplementation on protein synthesis, body composition, prevention of infections, and increase in muscle glycogen stores are necessary before glutamine supplements can be advocated for athletes.

REFERENCES

1. Groff, J.L., Gropper, S.S., Protein, in *Advanced Nutrition and Human Metabolism*, Groff, J.L., Gropper, S.S., Eds., Wadsworth Thomson Learning, Belmont, CA, 1999, chap. 6.
2. Abcower, S.F., Souba, W.W., Glutamine and arginine, in *Modern Nutrition in Health and Disease*, Shils, M.E., Olson, J.A., Shike, M., Ross, A.C., Eds., Lippincott Williams and Wilkins, Media, PA, 1999, chap. 35.
3. Bailey, D.M., Castell, L.M., Newsholme, E.A., Davies, B., Continuous and intermittent exposure to the hypoxia of altitude: implications for glutamine metabolism and exercise performance, *Br J Sports Med*, 34, 210, 2000.
4. Cynober, L.A., Do we have unrealistic expectations of the potential of immunonutrition? *Can J Appl Physiol*, 26, S36, 2001.
5. Hargreaves, M., Snow, R., Amino acids and endurance exercise, *Int J Sports Nutr Exerc Metab*, 11, 133, 2002.
6. Rogero, M.M., Tirapegui, J., Pedrosa, R.G., de Castro, I.A., de Oliveira Pires, I.S., Effect of alanyl-glutamine supplementation on plasma and tissue glutamine concentrations in rats submitted to exhaustive exercise, *Nutrition*, 22, 564, 2006.
7. Chang, W.K., Yang, K.D., Shaio, M.F., Lymphocyte proliferation modulated by glutamine: involved in the endogenous redox reaction, *Clin Exp Immunol*, 117, 482, 1999.
8. Gerich, J., Meyer, C., Hormonal control of renal and systemic glutamine metabolism, *J Nutr*, 130, 995S, 2000.
9. van Hall, G., Saris, W.H.M., Wagenmakers, A.J.M., Effect of carbohydrate supplementation on plasma glutamine during prolonged exercise and recovery, *Int J Sports Med*, 19, 82, 1998.
10. Mackinnon, L.T., Chronic exercise training effects on immune function, *Med Sci Sports Exerc*, 32, S369, 2000.
11. Nieman, D.C., Exercise immunology: nutritional countermeasures, *Can J Appl Physiol*, 26, S45, 2001.
12. Lagranha, C.J., Senna, S.M., de Lima, T.M., Silva, E.P., Doi, S.Q., Curi, R., Pithon-Curi, T.C., Beneficial effect of glutamine on exercise-induced apoptosis of rat neutrophils, *Med Sci Sports Exerc*, 36, 210, 2004.
13. Hiscock, N., Petersen, E.W., Krzywkowski, K., Boza, J., Halkjaer-Kristensen, J., and Pedersen, B.K., Glutamine supplementation further enhances exercise-induced plasma IL-6, *J Appl Physiol*, 95, 145, 2003.
14. Hiscock, N. and Pedersen, B.K., Exercise-induced immunodepression—plasma glutamine is not the link, *J Appl Physiol*, 93, 813, 2002.
15. Gleeson, M., Bishop, N.C., Modification of immune responses to exercise by carbohydrate, glutamine and anti-oxidant supplements, *Immunol Cell Biol*, 78, 554, 2000.
16. Field, C.J., Johnson, I., Pratt, V.C., Glutamine and arginine: immunonutrients for improved health, *Med Sci Sports Exerc*, 32, S377, 2000.

17. Rohde, T., Asp, S., MacLean, D.A., Pedersen, B.K., Competitive sustained exercise in humans, lymphokine activated killer cell activity, and glutamine: an intervention study, *Eur J Appl Physiol*, 78, 448, 1998.

18. Rohde, T., MacLean, D.A., Pedersen, B.K., Effect of glutamine supplementation on changes in the immune system induced by repeated exercise, *Med Sci Sports Exerc*, 30, 856, 1998.

19. Castell, L.M., Poortmans, J.R., Newsholme, E.A., Does glutamine have a role in reducing infections in athletes? *Eur J Appl Physiol*, 73, 488, 1996.

20. Bassit, R.A., Sawada, L.A., Bacurau, R.F.P., Navarro, R., Costa Rosa, L.F.B.P., The effect of BCAA supplementation upon the immune response of triathletes, *Med Sci Sports Exerc*, 32, 1214, 2000.

21. Walsh, N.P., Blannin, A.K., Bishop, N.C., Robson, P.J., Gleeson, M., Effect of oral glutamine supplementation on human neutrophil lipopolysaccharide-stimulated degranulation following prolonged exercise, *Int J Sport Nutr Exerc Metab*, 10, 39, 2000.

22. Hiscock, N., Mackinnon, L.T., A comparison of plasma glutamine concentration on athletes from different sports, *Med Sci Sports Exerc*, 30, 1693, 1998.

23. Petibios, C., Cazorla, G., Poortmans, J.R., Deleris, G., Biochemical aspects of over-training in endurance sports, *Sports Med*, 32, 867, 2002.

24. Walsh, N.P., Blannin, A.K., Clark, A.M., Cook, L., Robson, P.J., Gleeson, M., The effects of high-intensity intermittent exercise on the plasma concentrations of glutamine and organic acids, *Eur J Appl Physiol*, 77, 434, 1998.

25. Kingsbury, K.J., Kay, L., Hjelm, M., Contrasting plasma free amino acid patterns in elite athletes: association with fatigue and infection, *Br J Sports Med*, 32, 25, 1998.

26. Newsholme, E.A., Biochemical mechanisms to explain immunosuppression in well-trained and overtrained athletes, *Int J Sports Med*, 15 (Suppl. 3), S142, 1994.

27. Newsholme, P., Why is L-glutamine metabolism important to cells of the immune system in health, postinjury, surgery or infection? *J Nutr,* 131, 2515S, 2001.

28. Blanchard, M.A., Jordan, G., Desbrow, B., Mackinnon, L.T., Jenkins, D.G., The influence of diet and exercise on muscle and plasma glutamine concentrations, *Med Sci Sports Exerc*, 33, 69, 2001.

29. Gleeson, M., Blannin, A.K., Walsh, N.P., Bishop, N.C., Clark, A.M., Effect of low- and high-carbohydrate diets on the plasma glutamine circulating leukocyte responses to exercise, *Int J Sport Nutr*, 8, 49, 1998.

30. Bowtell, J.L., Gelly, K., Jackman, M.L., Patel, A., Simeoni, M., Rennie, M.J., Effect of oral glutamine on whole body carbohydrate storage during recovery from exhaustive exercise, *J Appl Physiol*, 86, 1770, 1999.

31. van Hall, G., Saris, W.H.M., van de Schoor, P.A.I., Wagenmakers, A.J.M., The effect of free glutamine and peptide ingestion on the rate of muscle glycogen resynthesis in man, *Int J Sports Med*, 21, 25, 2000.

32. Rutten, E.P., Engelen, M.P., Schols, A.M., and Deutz, N.E., Skeletal muscle glutamate metabolism in health and disease: state of the art, *Curr Opin Clin Nutr Metab Care* 8, 41, 2005.

33. Kargotich, S., Rowbottom, D., Keast, D., Goodman, C., Dawson, B., and Morton, A.R., Plasma glutamine changes after high-intensity exercise in elite male swimmers, *Res Sports Med*, 13, 7, 2005.

34. Iwashita, S., Williams, P., Jabbour, K., Ueda, T., Kobayashi, H., Baier, S., and Flakoll, P.J., Impact of glutamine supplementation on glucose homeostasis during and after exercise, *J Appl Physiol*, 99, 1858, 2005.

35. Smith, D.J., Norris, S.R., Changes in glutamine and glutamate concentrations for tracking training tolerance, *Med Sci Sports Exerc*, 32, 684, 2000.
36. Williams, M.H., *Nutrition for Health, Fitness and Sport*, 5th ed., WCB/McGraw Hill, Dubuque, IA, 1999.
37. Mourtzakis, M., Graham, T.E., Glutamate ingestion and its effects at rest and during exercise in humans, *J Appl Physiol*, 93, 1251, 2002.
38. Wilmore, D.W., Rombeau, J.L., Role of mitochondrial glutaminase in rat renal glutamine metabolism, *J Nutr*, 131, 2491S, 2001.
39. Lacey, J.M., Wilmore, D.W., Is glutamine a conditionally essential amino acid? *Nutr Rev*, 48, 297, 1990.
40. Castell, L.M., Poortmans, J.R., Leclercq, R., Brasseur, M., Duchateau, J., Newsholme, E.A., Some aspects of the acute phase response after a marathon race, and the effects of glutamine supplementation, *Eur J Appl Physiol*, 75, 47, 1997.
41. Kargotich, S., Goodman, C., Dawson, B., Morton, A.R., Keast, D., and Joske, D.J., Plasma glutamine responses to high-intensity exercise before and after endurance training, *Res Sports Med*, 13, 287, 2005.
42. Antonio, J., Street, C., Glutamine: a potentially useful supplement for athletes, *Can J Appl Physiol*, 24, 1, 1999.
43. Antonio, J., Sanders, M.S., Kalman, D., Woodgate, D., and Street, C., The effects of high-dose glutamine ingestion on weightlifting performance, *J Strength Cond Res*, 16, 157, 2002.
44. Haub, M.D., Potteiger, J.A., Nau, K.L., Webster, M.J., Zebas, C.J., Acute L-glutamine ingestion does not improve maximal effort exercise, *J Sports Med Phys Fitness*, 38, 240, 1998.
45. Candow, D.G., Chilibeck, P.D., Burke, D.G., Davison, K.S., Smith Palmer, T., Effect of glutamine supplementation combined with resistance training in young adults, *Eur J Appl Physiol*, 86, 142, 2001.
46. Antonio, J., Sanders, M.S., Kalman, D., Woodgate, D., Street, C., The effects of high-dose glutamine ingestion on weightlifting performance, *J Strength Cond Res*, 16, 157, 2002.
47. Rall, L.C., Eoubenoff, R., Cannon, J.G., Abad, L.W., Dinarello, C.A., Meydani, S.N., Effects of progressive resistance training on immune system response in aging and chronic inflammation, *Med Sci Sports Exerc*, 28, 1356, 1996.
48. Flynn, M.G., Fahlman, M., Braun, W.A., Lambert, C.P., Bouillon, L.E., Bronson, P.G., Armstrong, C.W., Effects of resistance training on selected indexes of immune function in elderly women, *J Appl Physiol*, 86, 1905, 1999.
49. Ohtani, M., Sugita, M., Maruyama, K., Amino acid mixture improves training efficiency in athletes, *J Nutr*, 136, 538S, 2006.
50. Jellin, J.M., Gregory, P.J., Batz, F., Hichens, K., *Pharmacist's Letter/Prescriber's Letter Natural Medicines Comprehensive Database*, 4th ed., Therapeutic Research Faculty, Stockton, CA, 2002, p. 607.

15 Other Individual Amino Acids

Neal F. Spruce and C. Alan Titchenal

CONTENTS

15.1 INTRODUCTION

Many scientific publications have explored the roles of protein in the support of exercise performance and adaptation to the stresses of training. Along with this focus on the role of protein in general, many studies have been conducted about the functions and effects on performance of supplementation with specific amino acids (AAs). Perhaps more questions were raised than were answered by the many studies on the subject of AAs in sports published during the 20th century, and such research continues actively into the 21st century. Most of the research has been conducted on the branched-chain amino acids (BCAAs), glutamine, and ARG. Several of the other AAs are being studied for potential functions that may support sports performance. Also, since many AAs have complementary functions, AA mixtures are being actively studied for their potential to enhance exercise performance and adaptation to exercise stress.

15.2 AA CHEMICAL STRUCTURES AND CLASSIFICATION

15.2.1 CHEMICAL STRUCTURES

The structure of AAs consists of a central carbon atom that is bound to an amino group ($-NH_2$), an acid group ($-COOH$), and a side chain (R group) with the following basic structure:

$$H_2N-CH-COOH$$
$$|$$
$$R$$

The R group is what gives each AA its identity and determines its specific potential functions in the body. At the pH of body fluids, free AAs exist as dipolar ions (zwitterions) in the following basic form:

$$H_3N^+-CH-COO^-$$
$$|$$
$$R$$

The basic zwitterion form has no net electrical charge because the polar charges cancel each other out. However, some AAs have charged R groups that give them a net positive or negative charge. With the exception of glycine (R group = H), AAs can exist as D or L stereoisomers. The human body only uses L-AAs for protein synthesis (PS). The AA names used in this chapter refer to the L forms unless otherwise indicated. Figure 15.1 provides three additional illustrations of the general structure of most AAs.

15.2.2 CLASSIFICATION OF AAs BY CHEMICAL STRUCTURE

Various systems have been proposed to classify AAs by their chemical structures according to similar components in their R groups, net electrical charges in solution, and polarity in water at physiological pH. An example of amino classification used by Garrett et al.[1] based on polarity and electrical charge is illustrated in Figure 15.2 through Figure 15.5.

Nonpolar AAs (Figure 15.2) include those with alkyl chain R groups (alanine, valine, leucine, and isoleucine), as well as proline, methionine, and two aromatic AAs (phenylalanine and tryptophan). Nonpolar AAs are generally considered hydrophobic.

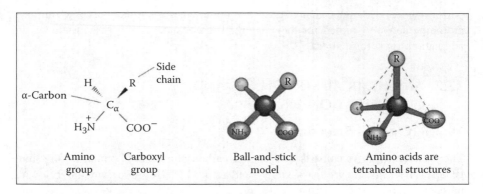

FIGURE 15.1 Anatomy of an AA. Except for proline and its derivatives, all of the amino acids commonly found in proteins possess this type of structure. Illustration, Irving Geis; Garrett RH, Grisham CM, *Biochemistry*, 3rd ed, Belmont, CA: Thomson Brooks/Cole, 2005. Rights owned by Howard Hughes Medical Institute. Not to be reproduced without permission.

Polar, uncharged AAs (Figure 15.3) except for glycine contain R groups that can form hydrogen bonds with water, making these generally more soluble in water than the nonpolar AAs.[1]

In the two acidic AAs (Figure 15.4), the R groups each contain a carboxyl group. Such negatively charged AAs play a unique role in proteins requiring metal binding sites for structural and functional purposes.

The two basic AAs (Figure 15.5) have R groups with a net positive charge and a neutral pH. ARG and lysine side chains participate in electrostatic interactions in proteins.

15.2.3 CLASSIFICATION OF AAs BY ESSENTIALITY

The human body is capable of producing some AAs via transfer of an amino group from one AA to the α-keto acid of another AA. If an AA can be produced this way in the body, it is considered to be nonessential or dispensable. The essential or indispensable AAs listed in Table 15.1 cannot be produced via such transamination reactions in humans, and therefore must be consumed in adequate amounts from foods or supplements.

15.3 COMMERCIAL PURIFICATION AND SYNTHESIS OF AAs

The isolation of protein from natural sources began as early as 1747 when Beccari reported on the isolation of gluten from wheat flour.[2] However, the discovery of specific AAs started in 1806 with the isolation of asparagine from asparagus shoots. By 1935, with the isolation of threonine, all of the AAs commonly found in natural proteins had been isolated. The industrial production of isolated AAs began in 1909 when L-glutamic acid was first extracted from a hydrolysate of

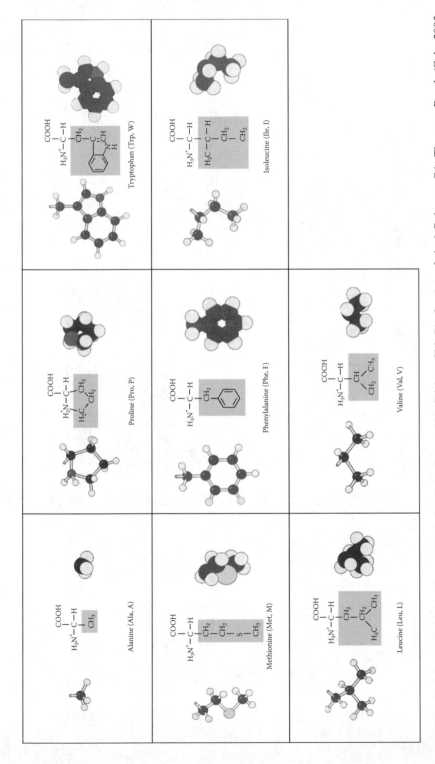

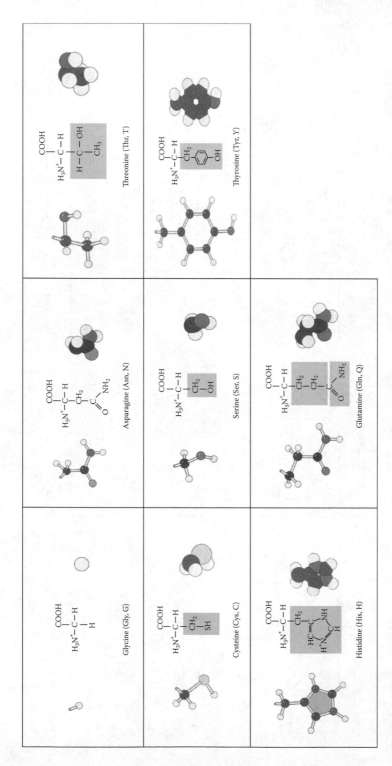

FIGURE 15.3 Polar, uncharged AAs. Illustration, Irving Geis; Garrett RH, Grisham CM, *Biochemistry*, 3rd ed, Belmont, CA: Thomson Brooks/Cole, 2005. Rights owned by Howard Hughes Medical Institute. Not to be reproduced without permission.

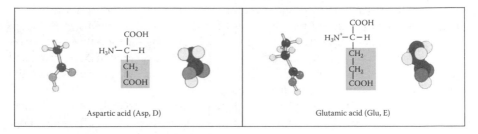

FIGURE 15.4 Two acidic AAs. Illustration, Irving Geis; Garrett RH, Grisham CM, *Biochemistry*, 3rd ed, Belmont, CA: Thomson Brooks/Cole, 2005. Rights owned by Howard Hughes Medical Institute. Not to be reproduced without permission.

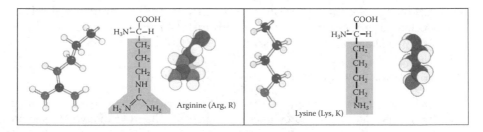

FIGURE 15.5 Basic AAs. Illustration, Irving Geis; Garrett RH, Grisham CM, *Biochemistry*, 3rd ed, Belmont, CA: Thomson Brooks/Cole, 2005. Rights owned by Howard Hughes Medical Institute. Not to be reproduced without permission.

TABLE 15.1
Classification of Essentiality

Essential		Nonessential		Semi-Essential[a]
Isoleucine	Threonine	Alanine	Glutamine	ARG
Leucine	Tryptophan	Asparagine	Glycine	Histidine
Lysine	Valine	Aspartic acid	Proline	
Methionine		Cysteine	Serine	
Phenylalanine		Glutamic acid	Tyrosine	

[a] Due to their rate of synthesis within the body, ARG and histidine are considered semi-essential AAs. It appears that these AAs cannot be synthesized by the body at a rate that will support growth (especially in children).

From Spruce, N., *Apex Fitness Group Certification Manual*, 4th ed., p. 15. Reprinted with permission of Apex Fitness Group, Camarillo, CA, 2003.

wheat gluten. This marked the beginning of marketing the sodium salt of L-glutamic acid (monosodium glutamate) for use as a flavor enhancer in Japan. Initially, the major commercial use for isolated AAs was for food flavoring. After 1950, as lower-cost production methods were developed, isolated AAs were used in a variety of new ways such as in pharmaceuticals, animal feeds, and the nutritional enhancement of human foods.[3]

A variety of methods have been developed to produce isolated AAs. For industrial production, the method used is determined primarily by cost efficiency. Four methods are utilized and reviewed briefly in the following subsections.[3]

15.3.1 EXTRACTION METHOD

Natural protein sources are hydrolyzed (typically by hydrochloric acid), and the resulting free AAs are subsequently isolated by taking advantage of the unique chemical properties of each one. This process often starts with separation of acidic, neutral, and basic AAs, and is followed by further separation with ion exchange resins or precipitants to produce purified L-AAs.

15.3.2 FERMENTATION METHOD

This technique takes advantage of specific microorganisms that synthesize large amounts of specific AAs when cultured on media containing carbohydrate and an inorganic source of nitrogen. Selective breeding over the years has resulted in cultures that produce specific AAs with great efficiency. Commercial fermentation commonly takes place in tanks with a capacity of 50,000 to 300,000 l. Upon completion of the fermentation process, a variety of separation and purification techniques are used to produce pure crystalline L-AAs. This is currently the major method used for industrial production.

15.3.3 ENZYMATIC METHOD

This method takes advantage of specific enzymes that convert chemical precursors for specific target AAs into the actual AA. This may involve the use of microorganisms that contain the necessary enzymes, or it may utilize solutions of partially purified enzymes. If the precursor compound is available at low cost, this can be a very efficient method for the production of purified L-AAs.

15.3.4 CHEMICAL SYNTHESIS METHOD

Numerous laboratory techniques have been developed to produce specific AAs through chemical reactions among organic and inorganic chemicals. These methods have become important when it has been difficult to produce a specific AA by the other methods. However, these techniques generally result in the DL form of an AA, necessitating optical separation of the L-AA form.

15.4   BODY RESERVES OF AAs

15.4.1   DYNAMIC STATE OF BODY PROTEIN

Proteins and other molecules derived from AAs in cells are catabolized sooner or later and must be replaced as needed to maintain cell function. Maintaining this balance requires a relatively constant supply of AAs, often referred to as the AA pool of free AAs available for synthesis of proteins or other nitrogenous compounds. The total AA pool in the human body includes AAs circulating in blood plasma and AAs found within cells. Under most conditions, the average person's AA pool contains about 150 g. Normally, the relative amounts of each AA in this pool stay fairly constant.[4]

The AA pool derives AAs both from the breakdown of body proteins and from the intestinal absorption of AAs derived from the digestion of dietary protein. The supply of AAs from the breakdown of body protein is referred to as endogenous AAs (derived from sources within the body), as opposed to exogenous AAs, derived directly from dietary protein or other ingested AAs.

The constant dynamic balance between protein degradation and PS is called *protein turnover*. Under normal homeostatic conditions in adult humans, the rates of PS and protein degradation are similar. During growth or the accumulation of muscle mass in adults, the rate of PS exceeds the rate of degradation, resulting in a net increase in the body protein content.

Normal PS requires an adequate amount of each AA to be available in cells. Since some AAs are needed in larger amounts than others, the pattern of AAs (relative proportions) in the AA pool is important. AAs present in excess of the amount needed for synthesis are typically utilized for energy by oxidation to carbon dioxide and water, with the nitrogen component disposed of primarily as urea in the urine.

The preferred AA pattern in cells is also partially maintained by converting one AA into another. This is possible only for the 11 dispensable AAs among the 20 AAs used in PS. The other nine AAs are considered to be indispensable or essential AAs that cannot be formed from another AA (or cannot be formed rapidly enough to meet needs) and must be supplied in adequate amounts from the diet. As long as there is enough total AA available, dispensable (nonessential) AAs can be formed from other AAs in adequate amounts to meet the needs of PS in cells.

15.4.2   IMPORTANCE OF BODY PROTEIN MASS IN HOMEOSTASIS

The human body has the capacity to store carbohydrate in the form of muscle and liver glycogen, and to store fat as triglycerides in adipose and muscle tissue. However, there is no comparable storage pool for protein. Yet, under conditions of energy or protein deficit, proteins that serve a variety of functions must be catabolized.[5] When needed, the body can utilize skeletal muscle protein as a somewhat dispensable protein and energy reserve. With an inadequate supply of protein, AAs can be mobilized from muscle protein catabolism and used to synthesize proteins more essential to survival than skeletal muscle. Similarly, with an inadequate supply of carbohydrate, AAs from protein catabolism are used as substrate for gluconeogenesis to maintain an adequate supply of blood glucose.

The maintenance of skeletal muscle and other body proteins is under regulatory control by the interplay of various hormones and the availability of a variety of AAs.[6] Whereas a transient sacrifice of body protein can benefit essential body functions dependent upon a steady supply of AAs, prolonged net loss of body protein eventually can compromise essential functions. The dispensability of skeletal protein has its limits, and a significant loss can soon impair work performance[6] and other body functions. Consequently, body protein (especially skeletal muscle protein) can function to some extent as an AA reserve to meet a variety of functions throughout the body. One of these functions is the skeletal muscle maintenance of plasma glutamine levels to meet the needs of various cells, such as those of the gastrointestinal and immune systems (see Chapter 14).

Individuals with greater skeletal muscle mass have a greater dispensable protein reserve, which may enhance the duration of an individual's ability to maintain homeostasis in various body functions during times of dietary protein deficit. For example, Castaneda et al. found that a low-protein diet (0.45 g/kg body weight) fed to elderly women caused a loss of body protein that impaired muscle function and immune response.[7] Conversely, an excessively high-protein intake can result in an adaptation to high intake such that the body will experience a rapid loss of protein if the diet is abruptly changed to a lower, but normally adequate, protein intake.[8]

15.5 GENERAL METABOLISM OF AAs

AAs are subjected to a variety of metabolic fates in the body, as shown in Figure 15.6.[9] These fates (functions) can be summarized in three basic categories:

1. Synthesis of body proteins
2. Catabolism for energy production
3. Synthesis of other nitrogen-containing compounds (creatine, carnitine, etc.)

15.5.1 SYNTHESIS OF BODY PROTEINS

Exogenous (from food or supplements) and endogenous (from body protein turnover) AAs form the AA pool that serves the body's needs for the synthesis of proteins such as:

- Enzymes that combine with other molecules in the cells to catalyze chemical reactions that take place in the body
- Immunoproteins that are involved in identifying and destroying foreign antigens
- Transport proteins that transport other substances throughout the body
- Peptide hormones that control many bodily functions, usually by regulating the synthesis or activity of enzymes
- Structural proteins, including skin, hair, nails, and muscle

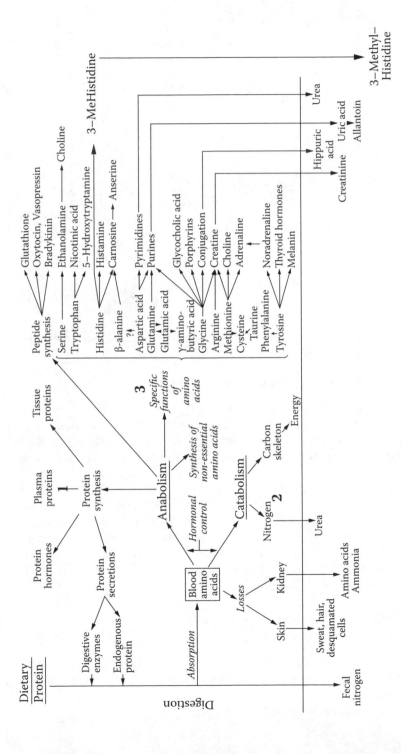

FIGURE 15.6 General features of mammalian protein metabolism. From Shils ME, Young VR, *Modern Nutrition in Health and Disease*, 7th ed., Philadelphia: Lea & Febiger, 1988. Permission granted by Wolters Kluwer Health.

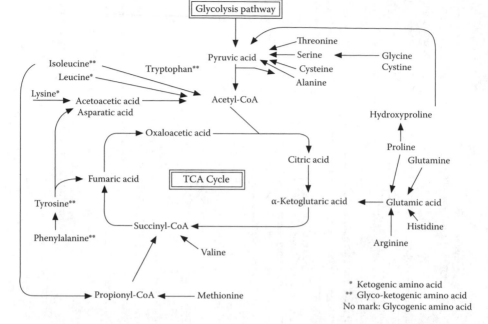

FIGURE 15.7 Metabolic pathway of AAs. Reprinted with permission from *Ajinomoto's Amino Acid Handbook*, Japan: Ajinomoto, 2004.

15.5.2 CATABOLISM OF AAS FOR ENERGY PRODUCTION

AAs absorbed from the gastrointestinal tract along with those released within the body via body protein turnover can be used as a source of energy. The various AAs can be converted to either glycolytic or tricarboxylic acid (TCA) cycle intermediates and enter the respective pathway for energy production. Endogenous proteins undergo a continuous process of turnover (breakdown and synthesis). Approximately 85% of the AAs are reutilized for biosynthesis of proteins, with the remaining 12 to15% oxidized as energy.[3] As shown in Figure 15.7, glycogenic (glucogenic) AAs can be converted to glucose. Some AAs can only be converted to acetyl-CoA. Consequently, they cannot be converted to glucose and can only be used for energy production or conversion to fatty acids or ketones. They are therefore commonly labeled ketogenic AAs. AAs capable of forming both glucose precursors and acetyl-CoA are sometimes called glyco-ketogenic.

15.5.3 SYNTHESIS OF OTHER NITROGEN-CONTAINING COMPOUNDS

Some free AAs are used for the synthesis of other nitrogen-containing compounds, such as creatine, carnitine, and epinephrine. A full discussion of this topic is beyond the scope of this chapter. Table 15.2 shows examples of some specific functions of AAs and various compounds derived from them.[10]

TABLE 15.2
Functions of AAs Other Than for PS and Energy Production

AA	Function
Alanine	Glucogenic precursor; N-carrier from peripheral tissues to liver for N-excretion
Aspartate	Urea biosynthesis; glucogenic precursor; pyrimidine precursor
Cysteine	Precursor of taurine (used in bile acid conjugation and for other functions); reducing agent; also part of glutathione (important in the defense of oxygen radicals)
Glutamate	Intermediate in AA interconversions; precursor of proline, ornithine, ARG, polyamines, neurotransmitters γ-aminobutyric acid (GABA); NH_3 source
Glutamine	Amino group donor to many non-AA reactions; N-carrier (crosses membranes easier than glutamate), NH_3 source
Glycine	Precursor in purine biosynthesis and for glutathione and creatine; neurotransmitter
Histidine	Precursor of histamine; donates to 1-C pool
Lysine	For cross-linking proteins (as in collagen); precursor of carnitine biosynthesis (used in fatty acid transport)
Methionine	Methyl group donor for many synthetic processes; cysteine precursor
Phenylalanine	Precursor of tyrosine; via tyrosine, precursor of catecholamines, DOPA, melanin, thyroxine
Serine	Constituent of phospholipids; precursor of sphingolipids; precursor of ethanolamine and choline
Tryptophan	Precursor of serotonin; precursor of nicotinamide (B-vitamin)
Tyrosine	See *phenylalanine*

Adapted from Linder, M.C., *Nutritional Biochemistry and Metabolism*, 2nd ed., Elsevier, New York, 1991, p. 93. With permission of Elsevier.

15.6 METABOLISM OF SPECIFIC AAs

15.6.1 ALANINE

A nonessential AA, alanine is produced in large amounts within skeletal muscle during exercise. Much of the amino nitrogen released from BCAA metabolism in muscle is utilized to produce alanine via transamination of pyruvate. During states of stress such as aerobic exercise, there is a net flux of alanine from muscle tissue into the blood for transfer of nitrogen from skeletal muscle to the liver. In the liver, alanine is deaminated back to pyruvate and ammonia. Pyruvate can enter liver gluconeogenesis for the production of glucose, and the fate of ammonia is mainly in the formation of urea for excretion via the kidneys. This process, often called the glucose–alanine cycle, allows the skeletal muscles to eliminate ammonia via a gluconeogenic precursor that the liver can return to the circulation as glucose to support continued muscular contractions.[11] To keep up with glucose demand in times of physiological stress such as exercise, alanine can become vital in helping to maintain blood glucose via gluconeogenesis in the liver. Ultimately, this helps maintain glucose delivery to muscle and to decrease skeletal muscle catabolism.[8] Alanine production in skeletal muscle is linear with exercise intensity.[8] Alanine and glutamine combined account for approximately 68% of the AAs released from skeletal muscle during exercise and rest.[12] Pitkanen et al. showed that alanine levels in muscle tissue decreased 30% at rest after resistance training[13] and increased approximately 27% in plasma.[14] A loss of alanine and other AAs from muscle during intense exercise, or due to a prolonged energy deficit, represents a temporary state of net muscle protein catabolism.[15]

As to its involvement in sports, alanine has generally not been studied or used alone as an ergogenic substance. However, its role in energy metabolism and cell swelling (cellular hydration) has led to its incorporation in different dietary supplement mixtures for athletes attempting to maximize PS, minimize skeletal muscle protein catabolism, or improve performance (see Section 15.7.3).

15.6.2 ARGININE

ARG is a conditionally essential dibasic AA, synthesized in the kidney from gut-derived citrulline.[16,17]

The typical American diet contains ~3 to 6 g/day of ARG, mainly from plant sources. Healthy adults can synthesize it in sufficient quantities. However, during periods of rapid growth or injury, the demand for ARG may not be met by such synthesis, and it is thereby placed in the conditionally essential AA category.

ARG is involved in the transport, storage, and excretion of nitrogen; in polyamine synthesis (important for cell division); and as a substrate for nitric oxide (NO) and creatine biosynthesis.[16] Arginine (ARG) is also used clinically as a test for growth hormone deficiency (GHD).[18] All of these factors have made ARG a popular candidate for study as an ergogenic aid. With regard to sports applications, the following areas are of interest:

- Research about ARG and GH
- ARG supplementation and NO production
- ARG, exercise, and performance
- Other sport concepts and applications

15.6.2.1 Research on ARG and Growth Hormone (GH)

Eto et al. tested the effects of ARG-glutamate salt (AGs) ingestion on exercise-induced hormonal changes in highly trained cyclists, aged 18 to 22 years. There was no effect on resting plasma GH, insulin, or cortisol levels. However, ingestion of AGs dramatically diminished the elevation of cortisol and hGH during and after exercise. The results, related to the AGs and exercise-induced hormonal changes, led the authors to state the possibility that AGs supplementation may alter energy metabolism during exercise.[19] Additional studies related to hormones and ARG supplementation are reviewed with AA blends and GH release in Section 15.7.3.2.

15.6.2.2 ARG Supplementation and Nitric Oxide (NO) Production

In a double-blind study, Schaefer et al., using intravenous L-ARG hydrochloride salt, found that the ARG load significantly decreased peak plasma ammonia and lactate during exercise, suggesting that the increase in NO production was the mechanism.[20]

McConell et al. found ARG infusion to significantly increase skeletal muscle glucose clearance, believing that ARG's ability to increase NO production may have been responsible.[21]

For more details on both studies, and rationale for NO in exercise, see AA blends (Section 15.7) and NO sections (Section 15.7.2.4 and Section 15.7.3.4).

15.6.2.3   ARG, Exercise, and Performance

ARG is also an important constituent of the urea cycle, which converts ammonia to urea, a harmless waste product. In early studies, ARG infusions were found to reduce ammonia levels in animals and humans. Intravenous doses of ARG at 1 to 4 g lowered induced high-ammonia levels.[22,23] In theory, ARG may be able to lower elevated ammonia levels as a result of high-intensity exercise, delaying fatigue. This condition has been investigated:

- Stevens et al. using ARG combined with glycine (glycine, ARG, α-ketoisocaproic acid (GAKIC)) significantly improved performance during anaerobic isokinetic exercise in 13 male subjects (average age, 21 years) (see Section 15.6.5).[24] Additionally, Buford and Koch found that the same formula improved performance of repeated cycling sprints (see Section 15.6.5 for additional details on both studies).[25]

- Colombani et al. incorporated a double-blind crossover design to study the general metabolic impact of ARG aspartate supplementation in 14 endurance-trained athletes, using 15 g of ARG aspartate or placebo for 14 days before a marathon run. The authors found no obvious metabolic benefit, including no differences in the respiratory exchange ratio, cortisol, insulin, ammonia, or lactate levels related to the supplementation of ARG aspartate.[26]

- Abel et al., using 5.7 g of ARG and 8.7 g of aspartate, investigated the effects of supplementation on selected performance, metabolic, and endocrine parameters in 30 male endurance-trained athletes during a 4-week trial. They found no differences in endurance performance (VO_2 peak, time to exhaustion), endocrine (concentrations of hGH, glucagon, cortisol, testosterone), and metabolic (lactate levels, ferritin, urea) parameters after ARG aspartate supplementation, compared to the placebo group.[27] At this dose, ARG aspartate appears to be ineffective as an ergogenic aid. (For more information on aspartates, see Section 15.6.4).

- A 1988 study examined the effects of ARG and ornithine (ORN) supplementation on the body composition of 18 untrained males in a resistance training program. After 5 weeks, the 10 supplemented subjects lost a significantly greater amount of fat (−0.85% vs. −0.20%) and body mass (−1.3 kg vs. −0.81 kg) than the placebo group.[28] This outcome has never been reproduced in a more comprehensive trial.

15.6.2.4   Other Sport Concepts/Applications

ARG is a precursor for creatine synthesis. In a 1976 study, ARG with glycine in equimolar amounts increased the rate of creatine biosynthesis.[29] Based on the availability and success of creatine supplementation, there appears to be no sport application for the use of supplemental ARG as a substrate for creatine synthesis.

15.6.3   LYSINE

L-Lysine is an indispensable dibasic AA (L-2,6-diaminohexanoic acid) required for human growth and for maintaining nitrogen balance in adults. Lysine cannot be synthesized by the body, and therefore must be supplied through diet.[30] Lysine and threonine are the only essential AAs whose amino groups do not contribute to the total body amino pool because they do not participate in transamination reactions.[31]

Metabolites of lysine catabolism enter the TCA cycle only at the acetyl-CoA site, and therefore cannot serve as substrates for glucose synthesis. Consequently, lysine functions strictly as a ketogenic AA.[31]

Lysine, like most other AAs, is a building block of body proteins. Among the indispensable AAs, lysine is present in the greatest amounts, at 93.0 and 38 mmol/dl in tissues and serum, respectively (see Table 15.3). Carnitine, a compound responsible for transport of long-chain fatty acids into the mitochondria for oxidation, is synthesized in the liver and kidneys from lysine and methionine.[32] Lysine is also required for collagen synthesis and may be central to bone health.[33,34] Lysine's effects

---

TABLE 15.3
AA Concentrations in Serum and Muscle (mmol/dl)

AA	Serum	Muscle
Dispensable		
Alanine	32.6	110
Glutamate	12.0	826
Glutamine	65.2	1038
Glycine	33.6	62
Indispensable		
Lysine	38.0	93.0
Threonine	20.3	33.0
Phenylalanine	6.9	5.9
Leucine	16.6	11.2
Valine	18.8	14.7
Isoleucine	10.8	6.8

From Morgan, H.E. et al., *J. Biol. Chem.*, 246, 2152, 1971.

---

on bone growth also may be related to its ability to enhance calcium absorption and renal conservation, as well as to its participation in the cross-linking process of bone collagen formation.[35–37] Additionally, lysine competes with the AA ARG for tissue uptake, which provides some of the basis for its clinical applications in the treatment and prevention of recurrent herpes simplex infections.[38]

The most common rationale in support of lysine supplementation in sport or fitness applications is in the raising of GH levels. According to the athletic culture theory, that effect should in turn enhance exercise-induced outcomes. The use of AAs for stimulating GH release dates back to the 1960s, when infusion of ARG was introduced as a potential diagnostic test for GH secretion.[39] Intravenous infusion of 183 mg of ARG per kilogram of body weight increased plasma GH 20-fold in females.[40] Infusion of other AAs in combination or singularly, including lysine, was also demonstrated to promote 8- to 22-fold increases in circulating GH levels.[41]

Lysine may exert its putative GH-releasing effects on the anterior pituitary by the production of one of its metabolites, pipecolic acid, which acts as an agonist for the gamma-aminobutyric acid (GABA) receptors and enhances the GABA influence on GH release.[42–45]

It may also have been assumed (perhaps falsely) that lysine's ability to enhance bone growth may be due to its effect on GH release. Both of these factors may have led to lysine's inclusion in AA preparations promoted as increasing GH.[35,36]

For the most part, lysine has not been studied or tested alone as an ergogenic substance.

As is true for all essential amino acids (EAAs), the body's need for lysine increases during periods of intensive exercise training, and therefore it is generally included in AA blends designed to maximize exercise-induced protein synthesis (see Section 15.7.3.5).

Lysine's action in the body may also be modified in the presence of ARG, because ARG's proposed mechanism of action in the body is to inhibit secretion of somatostatin, which is a GH inhibitor.[41] We therefore theorize lysine's action in combination with ARG to be an amplification of ARG's effects by attenuating NO production (which ARG supplementation enhances). NO production would otherwise inhibit the growth hormone-releasing hormone's (GHRH) effects on the pituitary release of GH.[37,46]

Finally, if lysine and ARG together truly raise GH levels in combination more than separately, it may simply be the additive effect of stimulating the anterior pituitary (AP) by two different mechanisms: (1) ARG inhibition of somatostatin[47] and (2) lysine stimulation of the GABA receptors.[42–45]

For more details on both studies and rationale for lysine and GH in exercise, see AA blends (Section 15.7) and GH sections (Section 15.7.2.2 and Section 15.7.3.2).

15.6.4 ASPARTIC ACID

The AA aspartic acid participates in several biochemical pathways, such as the tricarboxylic acid (TCA) and urea cycles.[48] It is involved in disposing excess metabolic nitrogen into the urea cycle, thus reducing elevated ammonia levels. Aspartic acid and oxalacetate are interchangeable by a transaminase reaction, which makes aspartic acid a glucogenic AA.

AA salts are hypothesized to be mineral transporters to subcellular sites. They thereby replenish electrolytes and aid in metabolism, including compartmentalization of energy production (e.g., sparing glycogen and increasing fatty acid utilization).[49] The transport of potassium and magnesium by aspartate salts has been used to treat asthma and heart conditions with varying degrees of success.[50-61] Potassium is the main cation of muscle and most other cells in the intracellular fluid. Potassium salts are widely used in medicine.[50-61] Magnesium is a component of intra- and extracellular fluids and is required for the activity of many enzymes, particularly those involved in oxidative phosphorylation (energy production).[62]

Animal studies report conflicting results using aspartate salts. Trudeau et al. used 1 g/kg body weight of a potassium-aspartate salt formula in rats during swimming and found that it did not support the hypothesis of sparing muscle or liver glycogen. A similar content of glycogen remained in the muscles and liver of control rats after a 60-min swim, or after swimming to exhaustion.[63] Marquezi et al. used 350 mM aspartate (ASP) and 400 mM asparagine (ASN) in rats and found that ASP + ASN supplementation might increase the contribution of oxidative metabolism in energy production and delay fatigue during exercise performed above the anaerobic threshold.[64] The supplemented rats exercised approximately 27 min longer and had lower lactate levels than the rats receiving the distilled water placebo.

The conflicting results may be related to differences in formulas, meaning the aspartate/asparagine combination may have positively influenced oxidative metabolism, whereas potassium aspartate had no effect at the given dose.

Potassium and magnesium are important minerals for the body involved in sports/fitness activities because they are essential for enzyme activity involved in energy production in subcellular locations, such as the electron transport chain. In addition, they are important in the stabilization of cellular membranes by normalizing intracellular levels of the two minerals.[49]

Aspartate salts act as a mineral delivery system to specific cell sites, and the aspartate component is involved in the detoxification of ammonia,[49,65-67] which can cause fatigue.

Aspartate also contributes to the TCA cycle via conversion to oxaloacetic acid.[65,66] During exercise, fatigue may be caused by: (1) depleting potassium and magnesium, (2) increasing ammonia, and (3) decreasing TCA cycle intermediates. If one of these three conditions is the limiting factor in performance, a potassium magnesium aspartate (PMA) supplement may delay fatigue until another factor causes it (such as lactate accumulation in muscle or central fatigue due to increased serotonin levels in the brain).

Aspartate is thought to reduce ammonia or increase the TCA cycle flux, and then deliver the potassium and magnesium to the subcellular locations to normalize intracellular concentrations.[49,65,66] These conditions could increase fatty acid oxidation, spare glycogen, and reduce ammonia-induced fatigue — and thus increase the time to exhaustion. However, there are no proven action mechanisms.

Human exercise studies have used 2 to 13 g of potassium and magnesium D or L aspartate. They employed exercise endurance (aerobic and anaerobic) testing protocols. Results have been mixed. Five studies found between a 14 and 50% increase in performance (increased time to exhaustion).[62,67–70] A more recent study found a decrease in blood lactate and blood ammonia levels compared to the placebo group.[67] In five other studies, aspartate salts produced no benefit.[71–75]

A deeper look into the study designs reveals the following: In four of six studies with trained subjects, there was no significant improvement in performance. In three of four studies with untrained subjects, there was a significant performance enhancement. In addition, higher dosages of 6 to 13 g were used in the studies finding benefits; 2 g per dose was ingested in four of the five studies reporting no effect, suggesting a dose–response. There also may have been differences between the D and L aspartate salts of potassium and magnesium on resynthesis of ATP, indicating the forms were critical.[76] D, L aspartate was used consistently in the positive studies.[62,65–70] Only one study showed no benefit when used in this form.[72]

This closer look at study designs and protocols suggests reasons why individuals may experience different effects when using supplementation. The dosage, form, and condition of athletes may have played a significant role in the results of the studies.

Lancha et al.[77] tested the effect of aspartate, ARG, and carnitine supplementation on metabolism of skeletal muscle during exercise. The group receiving the supplement was able to exercise 40% longer than the control group, and blood analysis determined a greater glycogen preservation and free fatty acid utilization.[77] These dramatic results would need to be confirmed by a better designed study that included a placebo group in order to be credited. See also Section 15.6.2.

Typical dosages, extrapolated from studies that suggest benefit and indicate safety, include 7 to 12 g per day of potassium and magnesium aspartate split over a 24-h period and administered acutely (5-day to 4-week periods). Chronic use for longer periods is not recommended. When ingested during intense training or before competition, performance may improve, especially with the novice to intermediate athlete.

15.6.5 GLYCINE

Glycine is a nonessential AA, but during periods of rapid growth glycine requirements increase. Creatine can be formed from glycine and ARG contributing to the creatine pool in skeletal muscle. Ingestion of glycine in combination with ARG has been shown to increase creatine synthesis.[78,79] Glycine's unique structure allows it to bind to various substances that are then excreted in bile or urine. Important pools for glycine in the body are the extracellular protein, collagen, and skeletal muscle. In fact, practically one third of the AAs found in collagen fibers are glycine. Pharmacological doses of intravenous glycine, in a dose-dependent manner, have been shown to significantly raise GH levels in humans.[80] Additionally, glycine is a significant contributor to cell volumization (see data on cell volume and glycine's role in Section 15.7.2.3), which is a major control point for protein metabolism. These properties of glycine have created some rationale for its investigation as a potential ergogenic agent.

Glycine alone has not been studied as a supplement for improving athletic outcomes.

In combination with ARG and α-ketoisocaproic acid, it has been shown to be a potential application in sport according to two studies:

- When 11.2 g (2.0 g of glycine, 6 g of ARG monohydrochloride, 3.2 g of α-ketoisocaproic acid dicalcium) were consumed in three equal aliquots over 45 min, muscle torque and work sustained during intense acute anaerobic exercise increased, as well as overall muscle performance by delaying muscle fatigue.[25]
- In the second study, lasting 23 days, Stevens et al. quantified the effects of the same formula of GAKIC used during high-intensity anaerobic isokinetic exercise.[24] The GAKIC subjects increased the mean resistance to fatigue (using a fatigue resistance index) up to 28% over controls consuming isocaloric amounts of sucrose. The overall increase in total muscle work sustained for at least 15 min, attributable to the supplement, was 10.5 ± 0.8% greater than in controls.

15.6.6 CYSTEINE

Cysteine is a principal source of sulfur in the diet, which is necessary for the production of coenzyme A and taurine. Cysteine is also utilized in PS, especially in the formation of hair and skin. It supports wound healing and stimulates white blood cell activity. The N-acetyl derivative of cysteine is N-acetyl cysteine (NAC), which is more stable and is the preferred form of cysteine for oral ingestion and infusion.[81] NAC has been shown to protect the liver from the effects of alcohol, acetaminophen, and cancer drugs.[82] NAC provides significant free radical protection and may be beneficial in reducing oxidative damage from exercise.[83]

At this time there are no published reports of the sole use of cysteine for the purpose of increasing sports or fitness performance. However, intravenous NAC has been shown to attenuate fatigue in male cyclists[84,85] and is commonly incorporated as an antioxidant into many commercially available products.

15.6.7 TYROSINE

Tyrosine, a nonessential AA, is created from the hydroxylation of phenylalanine. Catecholamine neurotransmitters such as dopamine, epinephrine, and norepinephrine are produced from it, and it is also a precursor of the hormones thyroxine and triiodothyronine. Fumarate, a TCA cycle intermediate, and acetoacetate are formed in the catabolism of tyrosine, making it both glucogenic and ketogenic.[86] Performance-related stress during intense military operations has been shown to be attenuated or reversed by exogenous tyrosine, apparently by increasing norepinephrine levels in the brain.[87–89]

Several studies indicate that tyrosine has little beneficial effect in sports applications:

- Struder et al. concluded that 20 g of tyrosine did not improve time to fatigue during physical performance.[90]
- Sutton et al. tested 150 mg/kg body weight of L-tyrosine on muscle strength and endurance and found no benefit compared with the placebo.[91]

- Chinevere et al. used 25 mg/kg body weight of L-tyrosine with nine competitive cyclists to test the AA effect on endurance and found no independent benefit from the tyrosine supplements.[92]

There is great interest in tyrosine supplementation for preventing environmental stresses (cold and heat) from impairing cognitive behavior.[93,94] It remains to be seen if tyrosine's ability to attenuate cognition-related stress (as noted during military operations) would translate to a benefit to athletes. Long-term use of large doses of tyrosine (>5 g) may have adverse health effects, based on its ability to alter sympathetic nervous system activity.[95]

15.6.8 GLUTAMIC ACID OR GLUTAMATE

Glutamic acid or glutamate is one of the most abundant AAs found in natural proteins (approximately 20%)[96] and a major excitatory transmitter within the brain. It mediates fast synaptic transmission and is active in approximately one third of all central nervous system (CNS) synapses.[97,98] It is also a precursor to gamma-aminobutyric acid (GABA), which is an inhibitory neurotransmitter important in brain metabolism. Glutamic acid readily participates in transamination reactions to produce other AAs and is converted to the TCA cycle intermediate α-ketoglutarate. The transport rate of glutamate from blood to brain in mature animals is much lower than that for neutral or basic AAs.[99]

The sodium salt form of glutamic acid is monosodium glutamate (MSG). The neurotoxic levels of MSG have been studied extensively in animal and human models. The available data indicate that, under normal conditions, mammals have the metabolic capacity to handle large oral doses of MSG. Glutamate salts have also been tested in exercise.

During the first 15 min of exercise, TCA intermediates increase 300%, while intramuscular glutamate decreases approximately 60%.[100] This decrease makes glutamate essential to several transamination reactions that affect the production of ammonia, alanine, glutamine, and TCA cycle intermediates during exercise.[101] Intensive exercise increases ammonia levels, a factor in fatigue, and can lead to a decrease in performance,[102] giving rise to the potential for glutamate salts to function as ergogenic aids.

Salt forms of glutamate (ARG-glutamate or MSG) have been used in exercise trials.

- Eto et al. noted a decrease in serum ammonia when cyclists were given 20 g of a glutamate-ARG salt prior to a 1-h bike ride at 80% VO_2 max.[103]
- Mourtzakis et al. administered 150 mg/kg body weight of MSG or placebo to seven male subjects. Results indicated increased alanine levels and decreased ammonia for the MSG group compared to the placebo group.[101]

Both studies appear to suggest that supplemental salt forms of glutamate may play a positive role in nitrogen and energy metabolism.

15.6.9 HISTIDINE

The end product of histidine catabolism is glutamate, making histidine one of the glucogenic AAs. Bacterial decarboxylation of histidine in the intestine gives rise to histamine. Similarly, histamine appears in many tissues through the decarboxylation of histidine, which in excess causes constriction or dilation of various blood vessels. The general symptoms are those of asthma and various allergic reactions. Histidine is generally considered to be an essential AA, although this has been a subject of debate. Kriengsinyos et al. investigated histidine's essentiality in healthy adult humans consuming a histidine-free diet for 48 days. They discovered a gradual decrease in protein turnover and a substantial decrease in plasma protein concentrations, including albumin, hemoglobin, and transferrin. So, although histidine deficiency may not affect nitrogen equilibrium, it can impact other important health parameters.[104] Histidine, like cysteine, also may have antioxidant properties.[105]

In regard to sports/fitness applications, histidine alone has not been studied as a supplement for improving athletic outcomes. Carnosine is related metabolically to histidine and histamine. It is a naturally occurring histidine-containing dipeptide present in muscle tissue. Being immunoprotective, carnosine has been shown to detoxify free radical species, protect cell membranes, and act as a buffer against lactic acid and hydrogen ions.[106] This is especially important in athletic events where lactic acid buildup (metabolic acidosis) can affect performance by causing fatigue.[107] Intracellular buffering agents such as phosphates and histidine-containing peptides may help delay fatigue by buffering hydrogen ions, reducing oxidative damage, and maintaining cell membrane integrity.[108–110]

Histidine appears to be one of the more toxic AAs. Unusually large doses (24 to 64 g/day) have been shown to have adverse effects.[111]

15.6.10 PROLINE

The nonessential AA proline is especially prevalent in connective tissue. Proline's structure contains a pyrrole ring such as that which forms the porphyrin component of hemoglobin and the cytochromes. Under extreme conditions, such as are found in severely traumatized patients or premature neonates, it has been suggested that proline may be a conditionally essential AA.[112–115]

During prolonged endurance events, serum proline is oxidized in skeletal muscle like the BC AAs. One study found that the increase in serum free fatty acids in post-exercise subjects, compared to those at rest, was correlated to the decrease in the concentrations of alanine and proline.[116] Therefore, although proline is considered to be dispensable, it may have an increased requirement under certain conditions.

In regard to sports/fitness applications, since proline levels decrease significantly during prolonged intense exercise, it may be prudent for energy-restricted athletes to maintain proline intake in line with their elevated needs for the essential AAs. Proline is often not included in specific AA blends designed to maximize exercise-induced protein synthesis (see data on AA blends in Section 15.7.3.5). It has not been tested alone as an ergogenic substance.

15.6.11 PHENYLALANINE

Phenylalanine (P) is an essential AA that participates in protein synthesis. It is converted to tyrosine via hydroxylation (see Section 15.6.7). Phenylalanine is both glucogenic and ketogenic.[4] Phenylketonuria (PKU) is a rare disease (generally diagnosed at birth) caused by an inborn error in the ability to metabolize P (lacking the enzyme phenylalanine hydroxylase). In affected people, if the diet is not controlled by severe restriction of P intake, PKU can lead to serious irreversible neurological disorders, such as mental retardation.

Sports drinks that contain a mixture of carbohydrate and free-form AAs, including P, can result in a greater insulin response than carbohydrate by itself.[117,118]

Phenylalanine has not been studied or tested alone as an ergogenic substance.

As is true for all essential AAs, the body's requirement for P increases during periods of intensive exercise training, and it is therefore generally included in AA blends designed to maximize exercise-induced PS (see data on AA blends in Section 15.7.3.5).

15.6.12 TRYPTOPHAN

Tryptophan (TRP) is a glucogenic and ketogenic essential AA that serves as a precursor for the synthesis of serotonin (5-hydroxytryptamine [5HT]) and melatonin. TRP's precursor potential has created interest in its use as a natural alternative to traditional antidepressants, used to treat unipolar depression and dysthymia.[119] Besides 5HT's involvement in mood, the chemical also helps to induce drowsiness and may play a role in CNS-related fatigue. Little is known about central fatigue in physical activity, but it has been suggested that changes in plasma AA concentrations (e.g., TRP and BCAA) during exercise may play a role by influencing the synthesis of neurotransmitters such as 5HT, which may in turn affect the perception of fatigue. It has also been proposed that the increase in nonesterified fatty acid (NEFA) mobilization that accompanies exercise, and the resulting rise in serum NEFA concentrations, indirectly promotes the entry of TRP into the brain, increasing the brain TRP pool. This process stimulates the synthesis and release of the neurotransmitter 5HT. Because increased 5HT release is associated with sleep and drowsiness, the notion is that such increases in 5HT promote central fatigue, and thereby impair athletic performance.[120-123] This is often referred to as the central fatigue hypothesis.[124]

BCAA competes with TRP for transport across the blood–brain barrier. Therefore, high doses of BCAA before and during exercise may slow TRP entry into the brain, decreasing the production of 5HT and therefore increasing time to exhaustion. This has been tested with equivocal results.[125-129]

In regard to sports/fitness applications, TRP has been studied as a possible performance-enhancing supplement.

- Segura and Ventura studied the effect of TRP supplementation on perceived pain and performance during strenuous physical activity (workload of 80% of VO$_2$ max to exhaustion). The authors showed that large doses (1.2 g) of TRP given to 12 runners improved endurance capacity by 49%, and surmised that the improvement may have been a result of a decrease in pain perception.[130]

- In a more comprehensively designed study, Stensrud et al. followed up the above trial with a randomized, double-blind placebo protocol using the same 1.2-g dosage. Forty-nine well-trained male runners, aged 18 to 44, ran to exhaustion (100% of VO$_2$ max). The authors found no improvement in time to fatigue.[131] The discrepancy between the results of the two studies may be attributed to the weaker design of the first trial, including the small number of subjects and the difference in run intensity.

As is the case for all essential AAs, TRP is generally included in AA blends designed to maximize exercise-induced PS (see AA blends information in Section 15.7.3.5).

Note: TRP was linked to eosinophilia-myalgia syndrome (EMS) during the late 1980s and early 1990s, leading the FDA to ban the sale of TRP products. It has since been generally accepted that the problem was not TRP itself, but a contaminated batch produced by a specific manufacturer.[132,133]

15.6.13 SERINE

A nonessential AA, serine participates in protein synthesis and is an important energy substrate during high-protein diets.[134] Serine contributes to the biosynthesis of purines and pyrimidines and, along with two fatty acids, is an important component of phosphatidylserine (PS). PS is a fat-like substance that may be important in determining neuronal membrane surface potential (the electrical potential at the membrane).[135] Animal studies have found that the use of PS can attenuate the neuronal effects of aging. Consequently, researchers have been testing the ability of PS supplementation to stave off age-related cognitive decline in humans.[135,136] PS has recently been studied for its anticatabolic effects. Administration of PS has been shown to blunt the cortisol response to exercise,[137,138] giving rise to its potential as an ergogenic aid. Theoretically, the anabolic response to exercise may be enhanced through the PS process of decreasing exercise-induced cortisol.

In regard to sports/fitness applications, serine has not been tested alone as an ergogenic substance, but PS has been studied for its effects on exercise-induced cortisol with a surprising outcome. Kingsley et al., in two recent studies using 750 mg/day of PS, found an improvement in exercise capacity in the supplemented group vs. the placebo group. Ironically, neither study found a reduction in the cortisol response from exercise at this dose.[139,140]

15.6.14 METHIONINE

Methionine (M) is a major source of sulfur in human diets and is an essential AA for normal growth and development. It is considered glucogenic, due to its conversion to pyruvic acid via succinyl CoA. It is a major methyl donor and is important in the metabolism of phospholipids. It is also prominent in methylation reactions and as a precursor for cysteine, which is the rate-limiting AA for glutathione synthesis. High levels of M are associated with hyperhomocysteinemia and endothelial dysfunction, which are risk factors for cardiovascular disease.[141] Deficiency of M produces hepatic steatosis similar to that seen with ethanol,[142] and supplementation with this lipotrope can prevent ethanol-induced fatty liver.[142]

Besides M's role in methyl group metabolism, and in serving as a substrate for PS, its other functions include participation in the synthesis of polyamines, catecholamines, nucleic acids, carnitine, and creatine.[143–145] Because of its many functions, M has a high intracellular turnover.[146,147] It may be the AA that is most rate limiting for the building of body proteins, including maintaining nitrogen balance and the effective reutilization of the other AAs.[148,149] Therefore, the requirement for M increases significantly during times of high protein turnover, such as is seen in burn and trauma patients.[150,151]

Intravenous doses of M have also been shown to increase GH,[41,152] but oral doses below pharmacological amounts have not been effective in raising GH levels in athletes.[153]

M has not been studied or tested alone as an ergogenic substance.

As is true for all essential AAs, the requirement for M increases during periods of intensive exercise training, and it is therefore generally included in AA blends designed to maximize exercise-induced protein synthesis (see AA blends information in Section 15.7.3.5).

Harden et al. tested an L-methionine combination (with B6, B12, folate, and magnesium) supplement for its effects on symptoms of upper respiratory tract infections and on performance in 21 ultramarathon runners before, during, and after exercise. They found no significant differences between the experimental and placebo groups. However, they did conclude that benefits may be found using a greater number of participants.[154]

Because homocysteinemia is linked with cardiovascular disease, long-term use of M supplements may be of concern.[95]

15.6.15 THREONINE

Threonine is an essential AA often low in vegetarian diets. Aminotransferases exist for all AAs except threonine and lysine. Its main routes of catabolism lead to both ketogenic and glucogenic metabolites.[10] The human requirement for threonine set by FAO/WHO/UNU at 7 mg/kg/day[155] has been challenged by more recent data suggesting a level more than twice this amount to maintain AA homeostasis[156,157] in healthy adults. The Institute of Medicine recently established a threonine RDA for adults at 27 mg/kg/day.[158]

Threonine has not been studied or tested alone as an ergogenic substance.

As is the case with all essential AAs, the requirement for threonine increases during periods of intensive exercise training, and it is therefore generally included in AA blends designed to maximize exercise-induced protein synthesis (see AA blends information in Section 15.7.3.5).

15.7 BLENDS OF AAs IN SPORTS (NOT INCLUDING BCAA AND GLUTAMINE)

15.7.1 INTRODUCTION

Due to their association with muscle PS, AAs attract the interest of athletes, and thus have a colorful history in the athletic community. Researchers and athletes have been well aware that specific combinations of AAs, especially high intakes or infusions of one or more of the AA, can lead to changes in behavior, hormone production, and rates of PS (specifically muscle).[159] This knowledge has led them in search of AA solutions to the "performance holy grail."

Various supplementation schemes have demonstrated safety and success in enhancing certain types of performance or increasing muscle size when compared to a nonsupplemented state.[160,161] Examples of such schemes are carbohydrate and creatine loading for specific athletes (endurance and strength, respectively). In healthy exercisers, under various conditions, AA supplementation, singular or in combinations, has been shown to positively alter the anabolic environment. Specific acute effects have included reducing muscle damage, increasing or indirectly decreasing specific related hormone levels (e.g., increased insulin and GH and decreased cortisol), increasing the rate of PS, and shortening time of recovery from intense exercise bouts. This has led many to the proverbial leap of faith that regular utilization of such acutely successful practices can enhance long-term training outcomes beyond that obtainable by following normal food intake patterns. Despite the preponderance of evidence in favor of various acute effects of AA supplementation, the answer to the question of ongoing benefits has been elusive.

This section attempts to correlate a wide variety of study results having to do with AA supplementation and sport, and thereby tease out some relevance to healthy athletes attempting to improve performance or increase muscle size. It also tries to develop some, albeit limited, practical recommendations based on current evidence. Additional data are continually becoming available, however, and this snapshot view is likely to need revision fairly soon.

Though it is currently difficult to support claims for long-term benefits from chronic AA supplementation in healthy, well-fed (nondieting) athletes, certain training conditions may warrant dietary supplementation with specific AAs or AA mixtures. The following sections present some of the purported scientific evidence in support of AA supplementation by athletes, discuss related studies in different populations (e.g., healthy, aging, exercising/sport, dieting, etc.), and attempt to present some potential practical applications for individual competitive exercisers.

15.7.2 SCIENTIFIC BASIS

15.7.2.1 Overview

The reason people take AA supplements is to increase muscle size or performance. The metabolic basis for increased muscle strength and size is stimulation of muscle PS to a rate that exceeds breakdown losses. Individual AA or mixtures of AA have been studied and applied in practice for their abilities to:

- Increase anabolic hormone levels, specifically GH[41,162]
- Contribute to cell swelling (volume)[163]
- Enhance NO production[164]
- Increase the rate of muscle PS[159]

The above actions can be modulated by intakes of AA, giving rise to some of the rationale for their use by athletes. The sections below address the scientific rationale and current evidence for each of these four categories as follows:

1. The use of various AAs to increase the natural release of GH from the pituitary gland in hopes of enhancing exercise-induced muscle development: A summary of current evidence indicates that the use of AA supplementation to stimulate GH release is unlikely to enhance exercise-induced results.
2. The use of AA blends to enhance cell swelling with the goal of producing a greater anabolic environment in muscle cells: Although cellular evidence exists for cell swelling to enhance PS, it is not known if this translates to a significant effect in muscle cells of athletes. Studies are reviewed on the AAs directly involved in cell volume regulation to illustrate the rationale for certain AA blends used in dietary supplements targeting athletes.
3. The use of NO boosters for the purpose of stimulating vasodilatation, with hopes of increasing blood flow to working muscles: Very little research related to healthy athletes exists for this category. A brief summary of current rationale and related data is presented.
4. The use of AA combinations by athletes for the purposes of (a) increasing the rate of muscle PS to hasten recovery following intense workouts and (b) increasing long-term muscle protein accretion (muscle hypertrophy): Volumes of literature exist on the effects of AAs on PS following exercise, especially during the post-exercise timeframe when the working muscles' sensitivity to incoming nutrients is at its greatest. The main focus is on the use of AA blends in PS.

15.7.2.2   AAs and GH Release

Many published reports have described how infusions or oral ingestion of various combinations of AAs can stimulate GH release. Some of these AAs, including ARG, lysine, ornithine, histidine, phenylalanine, glycine, and methionine, can induce large increases in circulating GH levels.[41,165] ARG and lysine have been the top contenders,[41,166–170] creating the basis for marketing AA blends to promote greater muscle or strength gains by increasing GH levels.

Injections of recombinant GH (rhGH) to raise GH levels in GH-deficient adults have well-known positive effects on lipid metabolism and changes in body composition.[171–174] Administration of supraphysiological doses to obese women and healthy elderly men has shown a similar outcome, albeit somewhat less dramatic.[175,176] However, as explained below, the results for athletes have been unimpressive.

15.7.2.2.1   rhGH Injections and Exercise

Recombinant GH injections in healthy strength training subjects produced no increase in strength compared to strength training alone.[177–181] It also did not improve endurance exercise capacity in healthy active young men and women.[182] A review of GH effects by Yarasheski suggests that any increase in fat free mass (FFM) from GH administration in healthy exercisers is primarily due to an increase in tissues other than skeletal muscle, and possibly fluids.[181] GH can influence metabolism by causing a shift in substrate oxidation. That shift has in turn been shown to increase basal metabolic rate (BMR) and total energy expenditure (TEE) in GH-deficient and healthy adults (possibly by stimulating uncoupling proteins causing futile cycling). That effect offers the rationale for elevating GH to decrease body fat.[183–185]

15.7.2.2.2   Summary

In summary, administering rhGH alone to healthy exercising subjects has offered no ergogenic benefit or increase in skeletal muscle hypertrophy over and above that attributable to training alone, but it may affect energy substrate utilization and TEE in ways that could positively influence body composition.[181,186] Table 15.4, adapted from Zachwieja and Yaresheski's review of studies using rhGH in older exercisers and nonexercisers, summarizes GH effects on body composition.[187]

This summary shows that even if AA supplementation could stimulate increases in GH levels in healthy exercisers, similar to daily injections of rhGH, the only outcome to expect is a shift in substrate utilization, and a mild increase in 24-h energy expenditure. Therefore, although the scientific rationale continues to be exploited by manufacturers of dietary supplements, no data at this time support the use of AAs to increase GH to improve exercise-induced performance or muscle hypertrophy outcomes. Also see Section 15.7.3 for study results and discussion.

15.7.2.3   AAs and Cell Volume

AA-induced cell swelling not only inhibits proteolysis, but also can simultaneously stimulate protein synthesis in liver cells.[188] Cell volume affects protein synthesis by an independent mechanism.[163] It has been shown that creatine and CHO loading can make significant contributions to muscle cell volume.[160,161] Also, mixtures of AA and other nutrients that have been shown to promote cell swelling are often added into dietary supplement formulas purported to increase muscle size or performance.

15.7.2.3.1   Role of Increased Cell Volume

Cells must avoid excessive swelling or shrinkage in order to survive. Most cell membranes are highly permeable to water and are too fragile to resist significant hydrostatic pressure gradients. Therefore, a change in cell volume is controlled by osmotically active substances that must be approximately equal in intra- and extracellular fluid, and which thereby establish osmotic equilibrium across the cell membrane.[189] This osmotic equilibrium is frequently altered by the transport of osmotically active substances, such as glucose, AAs, or electrolytes across the cell membrane.

Alterations in equilibrium may also result from cellular metabolism. Examples include degradation of glucose or AAs and formation or degradation of macromolecules such as protein or glycogen.[190] Because the dynamics of cellular

TABLE 15.4
Studies Investigating the Effects of rhGH Administration on Body Composition and Muscle Force in Older Men and Women

Study[a]	Initial Dosage (µ/kg/day)	Dosage Reduction	Subjects	Study Length	Exercise	Change in LBM	Change in Force	Side Effects
Marcus et al., 1990 (N = 18)	30–120	No	Men and women ≥ 60 years	7 days	No	NA	NA	None reported
Kaiser et al., 1991 (N = 5)	100	No	Men ≥ 60 years	3 weeks	No	NA	NA	None reported
Rudman et al., 1990 (N = 12)	30	Yes	Men ≥ 61 years	6 months	No	+8.8%	NA	None reported
Papadakis et al., 1996 (N = 26)	30	Yes	Men ≥ 69 years	6 months	No	+4.3%	No effect	Yes
Welle et al., 1996 (N = 5)	30	No	Men ≥ 60 years	3 months	No	+5.8%	+14% vs. placebo	Yes
Holloway et al., 1994 (N = 19)	43	No	Women ≥ 60 years	6 months	No	No change	NA	Yes
Thompson et al., 1995 (N = 5)	25	No	Women ≥ 65 years	4 weeks	No	+3.1%	NA	Yes
Zachwieja and Yarasheski, 1999 (N = 8)	24	Yes	Men ≥ 64 years	4 months	Yes	+8.4%	-3% vs. placebo	Yes
Taafe et al., 1994 (N = 10)	20	No	Men ≥ 65 years	10 weeks	Yes	+2.3%	No effect	Yes

[a] Marcus, R., Butterfield, G., Holloway, L., Gilliland, L., Baylink, D.J., Hintz, R.L., and Sherman, B.M., Effects of short term administration of recombinant human growth hormone to elderly people, *J. Clin. Endocrinol. Metab.*, 70, 519–527, 1990.

Kaiser, F.E., Silver, A.J., and Morley, J.E., The effect of recombinant human growth hormone on malnourished older individuals, *J. Am. Geriatr. Soc.*, 39, 235–240, 1991.

Rudman, D., Feller, A.G., Nagraj, H.S., Gergans, G.A., Lalitha, P.Y., Goldberg, A.F., Schlenker, R.A., Cohn, L., Rudman, I.W., and Mattson, D.E., Effects of human growth hormone in men over 60 years old, *N. Engl. J. Med.*, 323(1), 1–6, 1990.

Papadakis, M.A., Grady, D., Black, D., Tierney, M.J., Gooding, G.A., Schambelan, M., and Grunfeld, C., Growth hormone replacement in healthy older men improves body composition but not functional ability, *Ann. Intern. Med.*, 124(8), 708–716, 1996.

Welle, S., Thornton, C., Statt, M., and McHenry, B., Growth hormone increases muscle mass and strength but does not rejuvenate myofibrillar protein synthesis in healthy subjects over 60 years old, *J. Clin. Endocrinol. Metab.*, 81, 3239–3243, 1996.

Holloway, L., Butterfield, G., Hintz, R.L., Gesundheit, N., and Marcus, R., Effects of recombinant human growth hormone on metabolic indices, body composition, and bone turnover in healthy elderly women, *J. Clin. Endocrinol. Metab.*, 79, 470–479, 1994.

Thompson, J.L., Butterfield, G.E., Marcus, R., Hintz, R.L., Van Loan, M., Ghiron, L., and Hoffman, A.R., The effects of recombinant human insulin-like growth factor-I and growth hormone on body composition in elderly women, *J. Clin. Endocrinol. Metab.*, 80, 1845–1852, 1995.

Taaffe, D.R., Pruitt, L., Reim, J., Hintz, R.L., Butterfield, G., Hoffman, A.R., and Marcus, R., Effect of recombinant human growth hormone on the muscle strength response to resistance exercise in elderly men, *J. Clin. Endocrinol. Metab.*, 79, 1361–1366, 1994.

Zachwieja, J.J. and Yarasheski, K.E., Does growth hormone therapy in conjunction with resistance exercise increase muscle force production and muscle mass in men and women aged 60 years or older, *Phys. Ther.*, 19, 76–82, 1999.

Reprinted from Wolinsky, I. and Driskell, J.A., *Nutritional Ergogenic Aids*, CRC Press, Boca Raton, FL, 2004. With permission.

metabolism and extracellular osmolytes constantly disrupt osmotic equilibrium — thus threatening cell survival — cells have established cell volume regulatory mechanisms.[190] These regulatory mechanisms can be turned on and off during transport and metabolism by hormones and other mediators.

Cell swelling leads to the activation of K^+ and anion channels. Upon swelling, the K^+ channel is probably activated by an increase of intracellular calcium activity.[191] During swelling, electrolytes are released via these channels to achieve a regulatory volume decrease.

15.7.2.3.1.1   Role of Cell Shrinkage
Cell shrinkage leads to activation of a Na^+, K^+, and 2 Cl^- cotransporter, thus accumulating electrolytes, leading to a regulatory volume increase.[191] Alterations in cell volume modify the transport and metabolism of AAs, polyols (such as sorbitol and inositol), and methylamines (such as betaine and glycerophosphoryl-choline). Cell shrinkage stimulates the accumulation and formation of these substances (osmolytes), and cell swelling prompts their release. In addition, shrinkage activates the breakdown of protein to AAs and glycogen to its metabolites.[192] The resulting change in osmolarity contributes to cell volume regulation.[192]

15.7.2.3.1.2   Signals from Cell Volume
The intracellular signaling cascade is initiated in response to cell swelling, resembling responses triggered by growth factors.[193] This can explain why cell swelling acts like an anabolic signal with respect to protein and carbohydrate metabolism. Stress, trauma, hormones, or nutritional substrate availability can affect cellular hydration — which in turn affects protein anabolism and catabolism.[194] Thus, when muscle cell water content is high, PS is stimulated; when the water content is low, PS is inhibited and degradation increases.

15.7.2.3.1.3   Events in Cell Volume Decrease
Cell volume decrease occurs after exercise and other stresses, including normal life functions. During cell shrinkage — caused by oxidative and exercise stress,[195–197] glucagon activation,[198–202] and high urea concentration[203] — the following events take place:

- Decrease in glycogen synthesis[204–207]
- Decrease in glutamine uptake by inactivating transporters[208,209]
- Decrease in taurine efflux[210–217]
- Increase in the rate of release of glutamine and alanine from muscle[218]
- Increase in protein breakdown[198,200,202,219]

15.7.2.3.1.4   Events in Cell Volume Increase
Cell volume increase occurs as a regulatory or homeostatic response to volume decrease, but it must have the appropriate substrates to support an increase in cell volume and the associated anabolic response.

During cell swelling — caused by hormones, sugars, insulin, and a high concentration of certain AAs — the following events take place:

- Increase in glycogen synthesis[204–207]
- Increase in glutamine transporters, and therefore uptake[208,209]

- Decrease in rate of release of glutamine and alanine from muscle[218]
- Increase in taurine efflux by activating taurine transport pathways[220]
- At maximum swelling, inositol, betaine, and taurine efflux begin as the cell begins a regulatory decrease in cell volume[217,220,221]
- High cell volume activates the Cl channel, which begins the release of certain osmolytes (taurine, betaine, and inositol)
- Increase in lipogenesis by decreasing carnitine palmitoyl transferase[222-224]
- Decrease in protein breakdown and increase in synthesis[198,200,202,219]
- Stimulation of urea synthesis and ammonia formation from AAs[208]
- Decrease in glycogenolysis, glycolysis,[225-227] and glucose-6-phosphatase activity[206]
- Increase in alanine uptake[208,228-230]
- Increase in glycine oxidation[198]

15.7.2.3.2   Rationale for Cell Swelling AA Supplementation

15.7.2.3.2.1   Cell Volume Regulation

Cell volume regulators are not designed to keep volume constant. Thus, the small volume changes (hydration) act as a separate signal for cellular metabolism and gene expression. Hormones and AAs can trigger cell volume changes that send different cellular metabolism signals. Thus, hydration plays a physiological role in cell function.[194] In other words, hormones, oxidative stress, and nutrients can affect metabolism and gene expression by modifying cell volume. Cell volume may act as a second messenger of hormone action.

The increased concentration of AAs and potassium during cell shrinkage eventually leads to swelling, which triggers volume regulatory decrease (potassium efflux).[208,229,231] However, as long as the AA load is present, the cell swelling continues, because the potassium, taurine, and other osmolyte efflux keep the swelling from becoming excessive. Therefore, in the presence of certain organic osmolytes (such as specific AAs), the cell remains slightly swollen, thus transmitting the signals associated with high cellular hydration (such as PS). The degree of AA-induced cell swelling seems to be related largely to the steady state of the intra- or extracellular AA concentration gradient.[202,232]

15.7.2.3.2.2   Cell Volume Effects Potentially Related to the Athlete

As mentioned, cellular hydration is a major control point for protein metabolism.[202] Swelling stimulates synthesis,[188,190,233,234] and shrinkage enhances degradation.[198,200,202,219] Therefore, cell volume can mimic hormonal effects on protein metabolism, and if the nutrients involved in cell swelling can be applied at proper times and amounts, the goal would be to improve exercise-enhanced PS through this independent mechanism.

15.7.2.3.2.3   Nutrients in Cell Swelling

The primary chemical compounds involved in cell swelling and cell volume maintenance include L-glutamine,[208,209,235-238] creatine,[160] taurine,[217,220,221] glycine,[198,231,239] alanine,[208,228,229] betaine and inositol,[217,221] and glucose.[190,194]

15.7.2.3.2.4   Summary and Athletic Theory

In observing all the functions that take place during cell swelling, the most apparent finding is that cell swelling increases PS during recovery from trauma induced by exercise or other mechanisms. The mechanisms by which hydration exerts control over protein metabolism are unclear, but primary candidates are the cytoskeleton (cell stretching), regulatory proteins, and stretch-activated cation and anion channels.[240–243]   Various protein kinases and phophatases can also participate in the regulation of cell function by cell volume.[243,244–248] What is clear is that cell volume acts on PS independently from other influences such as exercise, creating demand for supplementation to produce a state of swelling. Athletes theorize that a steady supply of the nutrients that promote cell swelling (which often includes nitric oxide boosters) helps to produce and maintain this state as often or as long as possible. Therefore, they theoretically obtain the benefits associated with the growth signals occurring during the swelling process.

15.7.2.3.3   Conclusion

The goal of this section on cell volume is to shed light on why certain AAs appear in various supplements marketed to athletes. Much of the research demonstrating the cell-volumizing effects of these compounds (other than creatine and carbohydrates) has been conducted in preparations of liver cells and red blood cells. The studies conducted with muscle cells demonstrate similar general effects of increased cell volume, but compounds that promote cell swelling in liver cells may or may not promote swelling in muscle cells. Consequently, additional research is needed in order to help identify the substances and amounts (if any) that can enhance the maintenance of cell volume — specifically in muscle tissue — and potentially contribute to favorable exercise-induced outcomes.

15.7.2.4   AAs and NO Boosters

15.7.2.4.1   NO Action in the Body

L-ARG is the substrate for the production of endogenous nitric oxide (NO).[164] NO stimulates vasodilatation, which can result in increased blood flow. In a double-blind study, Schaefer et al.[20] measured cardiorespiratory parameters and the metabolic (lactate and ammonia) responses to maximal exercise after either an intravenous L-ARG hydrochloride salt or placebo load in eight subjects. There were no differences in cardiorespiratory parameters between the L-ARG and placebo groups. However, peak plasma ammonia and lactate were significantly decreased after the L-ARG loading. The authors found a significant inverse relationship between changes in lactate and citrulline concentrations with the L-ARG load. Since NO is produced in the body through the action of NO synthase (NOS) on the AA ARG, producing the by-product citrulline, this study appears to support the theory that L-ARG supplementation may enhance the body's NO production during exercise. The increase in NO production may have been the mechanism that caused the reduction in lactate and ammonia levels following exercise in the supplemented group.

15.7.2.4.2 ARG and NO in Exercise

In support of the above, L-ARG supplementation has been shown to increase the natural production of NO, and following intravenous infusions, L-ARG improved the exercise capacity in patients with vascular and arterial ailments.[249,250] In addition, NO production may affect glucose kinetics during exercise, as NOS inhibition has been demonstrated to lessen exercise-induced increases in muscle glucose uptake.[251,252] Recently, McConell et al.[21] infused 30 g of L-ARG in nine trained cyclists and found that although it had no effect on performance, the infused group showed a significant increase in skeletal muscle glucose clearance. The authors concluded that the greater NO production may have been responsible for the increase because plasma insulin levels were unaffected by the supplement.

Finally, if ARG alone has any effect on muscle PS, it is probably because of its effect on NO production. The action of consuming sufficient ARG to increase muscle blood flow via ARG's ability to increase NO production may not by itself contribute to enhancing exercise-induced PS. Theoretically, however, consumption of ARG with essential AAs immediately before training (so that the AAs are absorbed when muscle blood flow is elevated during exercise)[253] may cause the ARG-induced enhanced NO level to accelerate the uptake of EAA, and lead to an incremental contribution to protein balance/synthesis.

The functions described above establish the rationale for L-ARG being employed to increase NO production with the goal of improving oxygen and nutrient flow to the working muscles to increase performance and promote muscle repair, cell swelling, and removal of lactic acid. They have thereby brought about the release and marketing of at least a dozen products containing L-ARG, all touted as facilitating increase in muscle size. At this time two pilot studies have tested purported NO boosters in healthy exercisers with minor outcomes.[254,255] Also see Section 15.7.3 for study results and discussion.

15.7.2.5 AAs and Muscle Protein Balance (PB)

Resistance training stimulates an increase in the synthesis rate of muscle proteins[256–259] and an accompanying increase in the rate of breakdown.[256,258,260] Following exercise, PB is negative[256,258,260] until AAs are provided.[232,261,262] The feeding-induced stimulation of PS has been shown to be independent of insulin,[232,261–265] and probably due to the increased delivery of AAs to muscle.[266,267] In addition, the effects of feeding and exercise stimulation of PS are independent and additive. In other words, feeding and exercise induce PS by different mechanisms, and can thereby be delivered in close combination. PS can be maximized at that point in time, giving rise to the common practice of AA supplementation before and after exercise (see Figure 15.8a and b).

15.7.2.5.1 AA Inflow and Outflow

As mentioned earlier, exercise stimulates PS,[256] but it also causes protein breakdown during exercise and shortly afterward. AAs released from muscle during exercise therefore represent a net loss, at least temporarily. Without subsequent protein ingestion, the N balance of muscle will be negative. Bohe et al.[268] investigated the

(a)

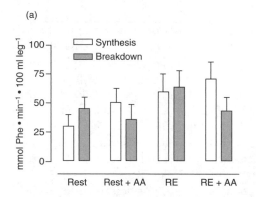

(b)

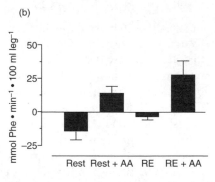

FIGURE 15.8 (a) Influence of AA consumption at rest, performance of RE, and AA consumption after RE on muscle protein synthesis and breakdown; (b) net protein balance (synthesis minus breakdown) under the same conditions. Values are means ± standard deviations. AA = amino acid; RE = resistance exercise. Reprinted with permission of Elsevier, from Phillips SM, Protein requirements and supplementation in strength sports, *Nutrition*, Jul-Aug:20(7-8):689-95, 2004.

relationship between AA inflow and leg PS using a balanced infusion of AAs. The increased inflow stimulated the inward transport of the AAs, and the authors found that a close relationship exists between the total intracellular rate of appearance of EAAs and muscle PS.

This tight relationship suggests that the rate of PS may be dictated by the intracellular availability of AAs (not intramuscular) and the sensing of the concentration of extracellular AAs, giving rise to a rationale for supplementation.

A point to consider is that when AA or protein is consumed, its appearance in the intracellular space of muscle cells depends on transport kinetics and initial clearance from the splanchnic bed, rendering a pattern of AAs in the intramuscular pool different from that in the original composition of the ingested proteins. The type of ingested protein (or combination of AAs) therefore determines the extent to which individual AAs will be increased in the intramuscular pool, suggesting a possible reason for isolating certain AAs for supplementation purposes.

The effects on infusion of AAs under rest and post-exercise conditions are shown in Figure 15.9. Inward transport proceeds at a greater rate following exercise than rest, which supports the concept of a higher inward transport of AAs leading to greater PS. That concept in turn suggests that the timing of AA ingestion in relation to an exercise bout will have at least an acute effect on muscle PS (see Figure 15.10).

Consequently, it appears that exercise and delivery of AA to muscle cells have additive effects on PS, since each contributes without the other, and when combined (intake soon after exercise), they cause PS to reach its highest point, as shown in Figure 15.11.[256,269,270]

AA intake can stimulate PS to some degree following each feeding session.[271–273] Bohe et al.[274] agree that the timing of ingestion can maximize PS at a given point in time, but they also demonstrated that at some level PS becomes unresponsive to a continuous increase in AA delivery. Tipton et al.[262] discovered no greater AA-

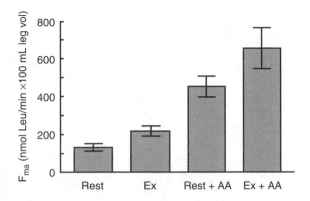

FIGURE 15.9 Effect of the infusion of a balanced mixture of AAs on the inward transport of leucine (F_{ma}). The infusion was done either at rest or in the first 3 h of recovery from a resistance workout (Ex). Leu = leucine. Reproduced with permission by the *American Journal of Clinical Nutrition*, Wolfe RR. Protein supplements and exercise. 2000 Aug;72(2Suppl):551S–7S. In review.

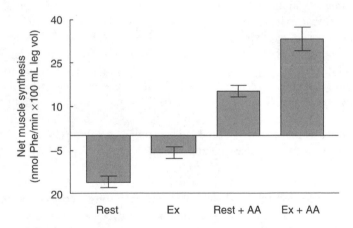

FIGURE 15.10 Effect of the infusion of a balance mixture of AAs on net muscle protein synthesis at rest and after resistance exercise (Ex). Reproduced with permission by the *American Journal of Clinical Nutrition*. Wolfe RR. Protein supplements and exercise. 2000 Aug;72(2Suppl):551S–7S. In review.

induced increase in muscle protein synthesis (MPS) in subjects given 40 g of EAA vs. 21 g of EAA, while Miller et al.[272] found that 6 g of EAA taken after exercise doubled the rate of PS compared to 3 g of EAA. Based on these observations, it appears that the maximal effect of EAA ingestion on PS exists between 6 and 21 g of ingested EAA. Of course, the amounts of AAs necessary to maximize the PS response to exercise likely vary based on body size and the total body workload, i.e., quantity and intensity of the exercise bout preceding ingestion.

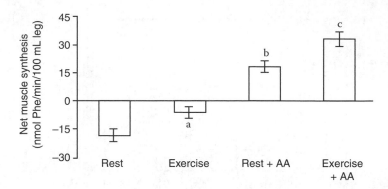

FIGURE 15.11 The influence of AAs on muscle protein net balance. Ordinate scale: net muscle balance, in nmol phenylalanine (PHE) min^{-1} 100 mL leg^{-1}. Values are means ± SEM. Reprinted with permission of the American Society for Nutrition; from Wolfe RR, Skeletal muscle protein metabolism and resistance exercise, *J. Nutr.*, 136, 526S, 2006.

15.7.2.5.2   Timing and Composition of AA Ingestion

It is well understood that when a supply of AA is provided to muscle after exercise, PS is greater than when the same quantity of AA is given at rest.[256,262,274] Thus, exercise opens the door to an enhanced utilization of AA by working muscles (Figure 15.11). The boundaries of this synergistic relationship are constantly being explored.

Based on work by Volpi et al.,[275] only the EAAs may be necessary to maximize PS following exercise. Ingesting 6 g of EAA after exercise had twice the effect on stimulating net protein balance as did 6 g of AAs made up of 3 g of NEAAs and 3 g of EAAs.[271] In addition, when 35 g of CHO was added to the 6 g of EAAs, the anabolic effect was less than that produced by the EAAs alone (Figure 15.12), which may be related to the increased insulin resulting in AA removal by the splanchnic bed.

However, when the same formula was given before exercise, it resulted in a greater stimulation of PS than any of the other aforementioned protocols.[253] A possible explanation for that outcome may be that because exercise increases blood flow to muscles, by having excess AA available at the onset of exercise, AA uptake could be greater than without immediate pre-exercise feeding. In addition, adding 35 g of CHO to the EAA intake (Figure 15.12) may have acted to spare protein by serving as an additional energy substrate and by increasing pre- and during exercise insulin levels, thereby blunting the effect of cortisol.[276,277] Taken together, these factors may have reduced the exercise-induced protein breakdown, allowing a greater net protein synthesis (NPS) to occur.

As noted above, Tipton et al.[253,261] found in acute studies that pre- and post-exercise ingestion of EAAs (6 g) and CHO (35 g) in healthy young subjects enhances PS over that found in connection with regular food feeding, which suggests that such a regular practice would enhance long-term results from resistance exercise training.

Esmark et al.[278] tested the timing of an oral protein supplement containing 10 g of protein and 7 g of CHO in supporting hypertrophy in elderly males with dramatic

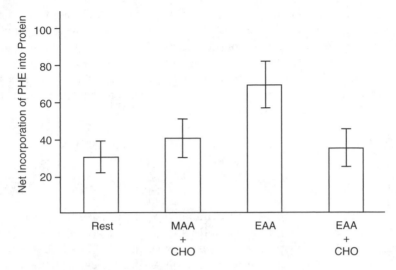

FIGURE 15.12 Response to 6g of EAA + 35g carbohydrate (CHO) following exercise. Area under the curve for net uptake (mg/leg) of phenylalanine over 1 h after ingestion of 6 g of different AAs by healthy human subjects. MAA, 6g mixed AAs (3g of essential AAs + 3g of nonessential AAs; MAA + CHO, 6g mixed AAs + 35g carbohydrate; EAA, 6g essential AAs; EAA + CHO, 6g essential AAs + 35g carbohydrate. Values are means ± SEM. Reprinted with permission of the American Society for Nutrition; from Wolfe RR, Skeletal muscle protein metabolism and resistance exercise, *J Nutr* 136, 527S, 2006.

results. During a 12-week, 3 days/week resistance training (RT) program, two groups took the supplement, but one delayed the ingestion for 2 h posttraining, as opposed to immediately posttraining (IPT) (both groups received no other food for the 2-h span). The delayed-intake group showed inferior strength gains and no hypertrophy, while the IPT group had a 25% increase in mean muscle fiber area.

   Results are surprising and must be primarily related to age because even in the absence of food intake RT has been shown to stimulate MPS for up to 48 h in younger adults.[257,258]

   Overall, the results suggest that older males are more resistant to the anabolic effects of AA feeding, including having a dramatically shorter metabolic window (i.e., the period of heightened nutrient sensitivity to the post-exercise effects of RT).

15.7.2.5.3 Summary
The rationale for AA supplementation is quite clear in the fact that their intake stimulates MPS independent of all other means. In addition, proper timing of ingestion and AA composition can dramatically amplify the anabolic response to regular exercise during each immediate post-workout period. The unresolved issue is whether these separate AA-induced increases in PS contribute to an incremental amount of nitrogen retention, translating into improved training outcomes, as opposed to ingesting intact proteins from traditional style meals. In other words, would the same result occur anyway over time?

All this begs the question whether — other than in aged, prolonged dieting, diseased, or other specific segments of the sport- and exercise-avoiding population — even if energy requirements and overall protein needs are met (which are generally accomplished by athletes not attempting to lower weight), there is an AA amount/blend regularly consumed immediately post-exercise that may enhance training outcomes for anyone, over and above that attributable to regular feeding patterns of three or four traditional food meals daily.

15.7.3 EFFICACY OF SUPPLEMENTING AA MIXTURES IN SPORT AND EXERCISE

15.7.3.1 Introduction

Exercise intensity, duration, frequency, training experience, and total energy intake can all presumably affect protein requirements,[279–281] with total energy intake having the greatest impact,[282,283] followed by training experience.[284–286] As with most dietary modulations, it appears that supplementing with AAs or protein beyond the Dietary Reference Intakes (DRIs) would yield its greatest effects on the inexperienced exerciser/weight lifter,[287] or for the experienced athlete, during periods of extreme unaccustomed work.[288] Both conditions would lead to relatively significant remodeling, but as muscle mass and workloads stabilize, supplementation of any kind may not be of much value,[279] as long as energy and basic protein requirements are met. In support of the concept of decreased protein requirements in habitual exercisers, Phillips et al.[258,289] suggest that there may be an improved intracellular reutilization of AAs during intense exercise, and that exercise itself improves protein retention (i.e., nitrogen economy). Energy intake probably has the greatest influence on the adjustment of protein needs, as has been clearly demonstrated many times.[290–296] Athletes lose mass during prolonged negative energy balance,[292,293] but by increasing protein (~27% of energy intake) most of the loss in lean body mass (LBM) may be avoided.[295]

Finally, all discussions regarding protein requirements for most athletes/exercisers may be moot, based on the typical routine protein intakes of this population, which far exceed most recommendations. Phillips[297] compiled the data from nine studies related to habitual protein intakes of resistance-trained athletes (Figure 15.13). The results indicate that the vast majority of athletes and exercisers are meeting protein requirements, except for those athletes who must endure extended periods of negative energy balance (e.g., bodybuilders preparing for competition or athletes working to achieve a specific weight class). Therefore, it is still questionable whether AA supplementation of any kind will enhance exercise-induced muscle hypertrophy if protein requirements are already regularly exceeded through dietary intake. Most positive evidence exists for athletes engaged in the early stages of heavy training, and for the elderly, as demonstrated by the dramatic results of Esmark et al.[278] Also, it appears that AA supplementation is beneficial during periods of inadequate protein intake or prolonged states of energy restriction. Consequently, there may be supportable rationale for AA supplementation for specific types of athletes and types of training programs. However, many athletes remain concerned that if

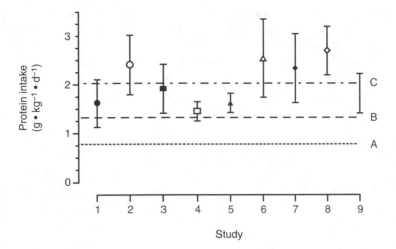

FIGURE 15.13 Reported habitual protein intakes in resistance-trained athletes in Studies 1[257], 2[362], 3[284], 4[281], 5[363], 6[364], 7[364], 8[279], 9[280]. Dietary reference protein intake (0.8 g/kg/d) is shown by line A, an estimated "safe" protein requirement (1.33 g/kg/d) is indicated by line B, and the mean reported protein intake (2.15 g/kg/d) is indicated by line C. Values are means ± standard deviations. From Phillips SM. Protein requirements and supplementation in strength sports. *Nutrition.* 2004 Jul-Aug;20(7-8):689-695.

they do not maximize their response (i.e., cover all their bases) to each MPS opportunity, they may compromise their exercise-induced results and not realize their maximum potential.

15.7.3.2 AAs and GH Release

Eto et al. investigated highly trained cyclists ages 18 to 22 ingesting 20 g of glutamate-ARG (AG) salt per day and found that although AG had no effect on resting plasma levels of hGH, the AG subjects had marked reduction in cortisol and hGH compared to the placebo group during and after exercise. Those results suggest that AG may modify energy metabolism during endurance exercise.

A study published by Hellman et al.[298] investigated an AA blend called Growlean 15® that contained 200 mg of L-glutamine, 200 mg of ornithine, 200 mg of L-ARG, 500 mg of glycine, 200 mg of lysine, 200 mg of tyrosine, and 600 mg of miscellaneous glandulars. The supplement was taken immediately before bed on an empty stomach and was touted to increase the body's natural production of GH. They found no differences between the placebo and experimental groups in plasma GH levels either before or after exercise challenge and no change in body composition. The amounts of AAs provided by the product were much lower than levels known to stimulate GH, which readily explains the lack of GH increase. As most other studies have discovered, the results of this study indicated that supplementing AAs will not raise GH beyond the level produced by exercise.

Fricker et al.[299] had found the same result in male and female strength athletes. Ingesting an AA mixture of 1.8 g of ARG, 1.2 g of ornithine, 0.48 g of methionine, and 0.12 mg of phenylalanine following an overnight fast, and before exercise (presumably to take advantage of a primed pituitary), did not raise GH levels beyond the exercise-induced increase.

Four well-controlled trials associated with exercise and fitness that investigated oral ingestion of AA blends are summarized in Table 15.5.[166–170] For comparison, the table also includes results of the studies by Isidori et al.[300] and Corpas et al.,[166] since they are so frequently cited in literature regarding AA supplementation and GH release. Isidori et al.'s research also appears in connection with the first noted sport-related use of specific AA combinations to boost GH. That research demonstrated a tenfold increase in plasma levels of GH at 90 min after oral ingestion of 1200 mg each of lysine and ARG in nonexercising subjects.[300] The prospect of athletes being able to enhance GH production with oral ingestion of relatively small doses of AAs was probably the spark that ignited the marketing and widespread use of these supplements as supposed secretagogues for GH release.

15.7.3.2.1 Discussion Including Other Factors Affecting GH Release

15.7.3.2.1.1 Age

Natural GH production declines with age,[301–308] and paradoxically, GH secretagogues appear to be more effective on normal subjects in younger age brackets.[166,168,300] Tanaka et al.,[309] using an AA infusion to stimulate GH release, demonstrated an inverse relationship between age and responsiveness to AA GH stimulus. Corpas et al.[166] reported that healthy male subjects over 60 years of age absorbed ARG as well as young men, but 3 g each of ARG and lysine, given twice daily, had no effect on GH or insulin-like growth factor-I (IGF-I) secretion.[166] This result was in stark contrast to Isidori's findings[300] that administration of 1200 mg of the same two AAs to 15- to 20-year-old males elicited up to a tenfold increase in GH. Suminski's subjects were 20 to 25 years of age, and in the absence of exercise, oral ingestion of 1200 mg each of ARG and lysine caused a 2.4-fold increase. Collectively, these three studies appear to support the theory of age-related decline in GH response to oral administration of an ARG/lysine mixture (Arg/Lys).[168]

15.7.3.2.1.2 Exercise

Exercise amount and intensity are strongly related to GH release.[310–317] Research incorporating high-intensity cycling and resistance training demonstrates up to a tenfold increase in GH concentration when blood is sampled immediately following exercise.[312,318]

The young bodybuilders used in Lambert's study exercised 5 to 10 h/week, maintained their normal diet (1.2 to 2.2 g of protein/day), and ingested the Arg/Lys supplement after an 8-h overnight fast (to take advantage of the anterior pituitary being naturally primed to secrete GH). Blood GH was measured in increments up to 180 min after ingestion. The mean increase of serum GH in the ARG and lysine group doubled that of the placebo group (Table 15.6). However, no firm conclusions should be drawn from these results because of the small group size (n = 7) and the dramatic variations among subjects.[167]

Exercise appears to have a significantly greater effect on GH release than ingestion of Arg/Lys. Consequently, exercise may overwhelm and obviate any simultaneous effects of supplementation.

Suminski et al.,[168] using 1500 mg of Arg/Lys, measured GH levels in subjects
before exercise and in a separate group without exercise. In the exercise group, they
measured GH levels before training and in 30- to 90-min intervals after exercise.
GH levels were measured in the nonexercise subjects at the same times. In the two
exercise groups (placebo and Arg/Lys), the GH levels were elevated equally (not
altered by supplementation) and exercise performances were not improved. In the
nonexercise groups (placebo and Arg/Lys), the GH level in the supplemented group
was 2.4 times higher than in the placebo group. These results suggest that AA
supplementation can raise GH in the absence of exercise, but there is no additive
effect to the GH stimulation resulting from exercise, at least when protein intake is
already adequate. The smaller increase in GH in the nonexercise group compared
to Isidori's results may be partly attributed to the age differences, since Suminski's
participants were 20 to 25 years old, whereas Isidori's 1982 study participants were
15 to 20 years old.[168,300] In addition, the dosages used by the exercisers may have
been too small because of the obligatory tissue uptake of AAs in response to exercise.
That tissue uptake diverts a significant portion of the Arg/Lys to muscle and the
splanchnic bed, and likely renders the remaining supplemental AAs ineffective in
stimulating the anterior pituitary.[256,319]

Lambert and Fogelholm also studied experienced weight lifters and found no
significant increases in GH release using 1.2 g each of Arg/Lys once daily, and 1 g
each of ARG, ornithine, and lysine twice daily. In contrast to the findings of Suminski
et al.,[168] they were unable to demonstrate an acute basal increase in GH in their
similar subjects — a result that might be attributed to differences in protein intake.

15.7.3.2.1.3   Dietary Protein

As discussed in the introduction to this section, exercisers typically have adequate
protein intake, and the timing of ingestion can play a role in enhancing the anabolic
environment following exercise.[262,279,320,321] The protein requirements for exercisers
may be twice those of sedentary counterparts.[322] This fact offers a possible explanation for results of the Lambert et al.[167] and Fogelhom et al.[169] studies, which
contradict results reported by Suminski relative to basal GH stimulation through
Arg/Lys supplementation. Lambert and Fogelholm's subjects ingested between 1.5
and 2.0 times the amount of protein during the trials as did Suminski's participants,
and diets high in protein, compared to "normal" balanced diets, are associated with
higher basal GH.[323] These results suggest that high-protein intake throughout the
day may exhaust the GH-releasing potential that Arg/Lys supplementation might
otherwise tap.

The only other study showing a significant increase in GH levels from Arg/Lys
oral supplementation was Isidori's. That study did not report protein intake, but the
subjects were nonexercisers, and we may assume they consumed the typical Italian
diet of the times, in which protein intake was probably not relatively high.[300]

Finally, in the absence of exercise (based on the effects of the cellular compartmentalization of circulating AAs from any source [see Section 15.7.2.5.1]), high

TABLE 15.5
Oral Ingestion of AA Blends

Reference	Number Treated/ Control	Age	Sex	Agent	Dose	Number of Doses	Oral/ IV	Duration	Time of Ingestion	GH Pretreatment	GH Posttreatment (Highest Average Reported)	IGF-I Base/ Peak	IGF Post-treatment	Diet (kcal/ protein)	Conclusion
Isidori et al.[360]	15	15–20	M	ARG + lysine	1.2 g of each	1	Oral	Single dose	Not given	15.4 ± 5 µg/l	108 ± 7.4 µg/l @ 90 min[a]	0.9–3.0 U/ml	3.0 U/ml	Not given	Young nonexercising males may have an acute response to Arg/Lys supplementation during fasting
	8	15–20	M	ARG	1.2 g	1	Oral	Single dose	Not given	7.3 ± 2.3 µg/l	13.5 ± 7.5 µg/l @ 30 min	ND[e]			
				Lysine	1.2 g	1	Oral	Single dose	Not given	4.8 ± 1.9 µg/l	15.8 ± 4.2 µg/l @ 120 min	ND[e]			
				ARG	2.4 g	1	Oral	Single dose	Not given	16.4 ± 4.1 µg/l	6.2 ± 4.1 µg/l @ 120 min				
Suminski et al.[168]	16	22–23	M	ARG+ lysine (C)	1.5 g of each	1	Oral	1 day	9:00 A.M.	2.78 µg/l	7.5 µg/l @ 90 min	Not given	Not given	1.12 ± 0.06	AAs were not additive to exercise
				Exercise + placebo (A)	0	1	Oral	1 day	9:00 A.M.	~3.0 µg/l	~26 µg/l[b]	Not given	Not given	1.11 ± 0.06	
				Exercise + ARG/LYS (B)	1.5 g each	1	Oral	1 day	9:00 A.M.	~2.0 µg/l	~22 µg/l[b]	Not given	Not given	1.14 ± 0.07	
				No Ex/No AA (D)	0	1	Oral	1 day	9:00 A.M.	~2.5 µg/l	~2.5 µg/l	Not given	Not given	1.11 ± 0.06	
Fogelholm et al.[169]	11	19–35	M	6 g ARG, lysine, ornithine, daily	6 g	2	Oral	6 days	1 P.M./9 P.M.	~5.5 µg/l	3.06 ± 1.2 µg/l (no change compared to placebo and pretreatment; $p < 0.55$)			3500 kcal/166 g (2.2 g/kg)	

Study	n	Age	Sex	Supplement	Dosage	No.	Route	Duration	Timing	Value	Value	Value	Value	Value
Fry et al.[170]	28		M	ARG, ornithine, lysine BCAAs	2.1 g argine, ornithine, lysine+2.1 g BCAA + 50 mg gln		Oral	7 days			No change compared to placebo			
Corpas et al.[166]	8/8	69 ± 5	M	ARG + lysine	1.5 g each 2 times/day for 3 days, then 3 g of each twice daily for 11 days	2	Oral	14 days	10 P.M. and 8 A.M.	2.7 ± 2.1 µg/l; 12 h mean; 1.0 ± 0.7 µg/l	2.7 ± 2.5 µg/l; 12 h mean; 1.2 ± 1.1 µg/l	142 ± 58 µg/l	147 ± 82 µg/l	Not given
Lambert et al.[167]	7	22–23	M	ARG + lysine	2.4 g total	1	Oral	5 1-day visits (1 week between each)	6:00 A.M. and after fasting	Placebo,~104 ± 57 ng min/ml[c,d]	283.7 ± 117.2 ng min/ml[d]			1.56 g/kg ± 0.13

a Statistically significant increase from pretreatment value.
b $p < 0.05$ compared to pretreatment.
c Placebo is the same as pretreatment since all subjects did a placebo trial in one of the five trials.
d Values in ng min/ml over 180 min.
e ND = No data.

TABLE 15.6
Integrated Concentrations of Serum Growth
Hormone (ng/min/ml⁻¹) for 180 minutes after
Ingestion of the Treatment or Infusion of rhGH

Subject	Placebo	A	B	C	rhGH
1	13.5	249.0	54.0	33.0	—
2	64.5	220.5	52.5	667.5	3605.9
3	441.5	357.0	709.5	1725.0	—
4	52.5	937.5	673.5	1597.5	644.3
5	21.0	42.0	30.0	415.5	800.9
6	85.5	144.0	723.0	49.5	654.3
7	51.0	36.0	39.0	36.0	325.5
Mean	104.2	283.7	325.9	646.3	1206.2[a]
± SE	57.0	117.2	133.1	277.2	511.3

Note: A = ARG/lysine; B = ornithine/tyrosine; C = Bovril®.

[a] $p < 0.05$; GH-RH vs. placebo; A, B, and C.

From Lambert, M.I. et al., *Int. J. Sport. Nutr.*, 3(3), 303, 1993. With permission.

circulating levels of AAs may mimic the effects of exercise that lead to an increase in GH production. Increasing the blood levels of AAs, a condition that takes place during and immediately after exercise,[256,258] may initially give a false signal of catabolism, which then triggers anabolism analogous to cell volumizing with different AAs.[194]

15.7.3.2.1.4   Time of Ingestion
Supplementation does not appear to amplify GH release during exercise, so ingesting Arg/Lys before training should not be of benefit to the GH response.[168–170] Pulsatile and continuous intravenous administration of GH have demonstrated similar effects on raising GH, with the latter having a greater effect on raising IGF-1 in GH-deficient subjects.[324,325] These results suggest that it may not be necessary to take advantage of the anterior pituitary (AP) when it is already primed for secretion. In all studies reviewed, with the exception of Fogelholm et al.'s,[169] the supplemental AAs were taken in fasting states (or at least postabsorptive), presumably to take advantage of a primed AP.[326,327]

Fogelholm et al.[169] fed 11 competitive male weight lifters an Arg/Lys/Orn mixture 1.5 h after an 11:30 A.M. meal and 3 h after a 6:00 P.M. meal, over a period of 4 days. They periodically measured serum GH levels and found no difference between the supplemented and placebo groups. Arg/Lys/Orn supplementation appears to have no additive effect to other stimuli affecting GH release.

15.7.3.2.1.5   Dosage

All dosages used in the trials mentioned previously were relatively small (Table 15.5) compared to infusions of AAs that show efficacy. These dosages were based on suggestions made by the product manufacturers.

15.7.3.2.2   Conclusions from Research

If AA supplementation or high-protein intakes stimulate GH secretion, the mechanisms involved may be the same as those for exercise.[194,256,258] When supplementation is combined with other stimuli like exercise, an additive capacity for GH release by the AP does not occur, especially in older individuals. In other words, for someone 25 or more years old who is already participating in moderate to intense exercise and consuming between 1.8 and 2.2 g/kg of protein throughout the day, with a portion consumed with carbohydrate shortly after exercise, additional GH response may not be possible by any means other than continuous injections of GH. Conversely, for someone under the age of 20 not exercising and consuming a low-protein diet, Arg/Lys supplementation may exert a potential for increasing GH levels.

All in all, AA supplementation to increase GH seems to be an exercise in futility under most normal conditions. Even GH injections have shown little to no effect on skeletal muscle hypertrophy or performance additive to the effects of training.[178–181]

15.7.3.3   AAs and Cell Volume

As of this writing, no human studies have been found on the use of AAs alone to increase cell volume and potentially related outcomes. For more on cell volume and sports, see Volek and Rawson's review on creatine supplementation in athletes[160] and Berneis et al.'s review on cell volume and whole-body protein and glucose kinetics.[163]

15.7.3.4   AAs and NO Boosters

There are no studies published to date using blends of orally ingested AAs for boosting NO with the goal of enhancing exercise-induced results. A form of ARG (ARG alpha-ketoglutarate, or AAKG) appears to be the only AA used in commercially available products claiming to boost NO production. A two-part unpublished study was conducted by Campbell et al.[254] to discover if 12 g/day of AAKG for 8 weeks had any significant effects on muscle mass and performance in 30- to 35-year-old weight-trained males.[255] Body composition results showed no differences between placebo and supplemented groups in fat free mass or body fat. No differences were found in total work or power between groups, but the supplemented group had a significantly greater 1RM bench press, sprint peak power, rate to fatigue, and hemoglobin level (hemoglobin was slightly increased in the AAKG group). These results were achieved without negatively impacting measured health markers such as blood pressure. As noted in Section 15.7.2.4, intravenous infusion of ARG improved exercise capacity, as would be expected in patients with vascular ailments,[249,250] but showed no performance improvement in trained cyclists.

15.7.3.5   AAs and PS

Many studies to date have demonstrated an acute increase in MPS following AA supplementation in association with exercise.[159,297,328] Consequently, the studies reviewed below are those that may address some of the open issues discussed in the introduction to this section (Section 15.7.3). The main question is whether the regular practice of ingesting appropriately formulated mixtures of AAs at proper times in relation to an exercise bout in healthy, normally fed (balanced diet and eating patterns) athletes will improve long-term results beyond those obtainable via dietary practices alone. A secondary question is whether specific types of athletes under specific training circumstances are more likely to benefit from a regular AA supplement program.

15.7.3.5.1   Diet

It is clear that total protein and EAA requirements increase during periods of prolonged negative energy balance. Consequently, AA supplementation may be logical and useful for athletes who regularly experience negative energy balance to meet various demands of their respective sports. However, assuming that using an AA supplement can positively affect PS, the question remains as to whether the results obtained from consuming the supplement can be incremental to those produced by ingesting adequate daily intact protein from typical foods consumed from a typical eating pattern (i.e., three of four traditional meals spaced throughout the day).

Paddon-Jones et al.[329] tested this by having seven subjects drink a beverage containing 15 g of EAAs combined with 30 g of carbohydrate (CHO) between meals consumed at 5-h intervals over a 16-h period, during constant infusion of labeled phenylalanine, to measure net phenylalanine balance and fractional synthetic rate of PS. The control and experimental groups consumed identical balanced meals that met energy needs. The study demonstrated that the EAA supplement produced a greater increase in fractional synthetic rate (FSR) of muscle proteins than did consumption of normal meals alone. Also, the EAA supplement did not interfere with normal metabolic responses to the meals. Based on previous work, the authors believe that acute improvement in FSR observed in this short study might translate into cumulative long-term results.[273,330]

15.7.3.5.2   AA Composition

Borsheim et al.[271] demonstrated that NEAAs are not needed to stimulate PS, in a study using an EAA composition that was to mimic the muscle AA profile (Table 15.7), with the objective of increasing the availability of the EAAs in proportion to their requirement for MPS. They also found a dose-dependent effect of EAA ingestion on MPS and a dose limit. No additional increase in MPS was realized by increasing the EAA dose beyond 21 g (under these study conditions). They observed equal MPS in response to intake of 40 g of AAs composed of 18 g of EAA and 22 g of NEAAs, compared to 40 g of all EAAs.[262] In addition, the Borsheim[271] study neatly demonstrated that AA ingestion following exercise stimulates PS independent of all other mechanisms (calories, insulin, exercise, etc.), and the authors calculated that approximately 26 g of muscle tissue (including muscle water content) was

TABLE 15.7
AA Composition of Drink

AA	% of Total AAs	Grams in EAA Drink
Histidine	10.9	0.6540
Isoleucine	10.1	0.6060
Leucine	18.6	1.1160
Lysine	15.5	0.9300
Methionine	3.1	0.1860
Phenylalanine	15.5	0.9300
Threonine	14.7	0.8820
Valine	11.5	0.6900
Total	99.9	5.994

Note: AA = amino acid; EAA = essential amino acids. Composition is based on a 70-kg person. Drink was given at 1 and 2 h after completion of exercise.

From Borsheim, E. et al., *Am. J. Physiol. Endocrinol. Metab.*, 283, E648–E657, 2002. Reprinted with permission of the American Physiological Society.

synthesized in response to the AA supplementation. Other studies have confirmed that under normal diet conditions, the EAAs are primarily responsible for the AA-induced stimulation of MPS.[275,273,329]

These results, and those of other recent related studies, show that the total amount of EAA supplementation that might be required to maximize MPS, at least for the average-sized human, seems to lie between 6 and 18 g, and should be consumed two or three times daily and close to the exercise period.[273,275,329,331]

15.7.3.5.3 Timing

AA ingestion and exercise increase net muscle protein balance[253,261,262] more acutely than exercise alone. However, it has also been suggested that there may be a diurnal physiological adjustment of the body protein pool such that this AA-induced elevation of net protein may be temporary. It may be counterbalanced at other times throughout the day, so that there is no longer-term net increase.

In a well-controlled study that maintained normal/adequate eating patterns, Tipton et al.[273] dosed seven subjects with 15 g of EAAs immediately before and 1 h after resistance exercise. Results of the study demonstrated that an increase in net muscle protein balance, as previously shown to take place within 3 h of AA ingestion and exercise,[232,262] was representative of changes in net muscle protein balance for a full 24-h period. Therefore, it was responsible for an incremental contribution to muscle protein.[273] In other words, the acute response to exercise and EAA ingestion was not temporary, but did in fact persist to maintain a positive muscle protein balance over the 24-h period, when compared to the resting nonsupplemented state.

15.7.3.5.4   Elderly

Nutritional supplementation with meal replacement formulas (balanced protein, fat, and CHO) used to increase the protein intake of elderly subjects has failed to increase NPS.[332–334] However, Volpi et al.,[335,336] using a balanced mixture of AAs administered by infusion or oral routes, observed a significant increase in PS in healthy elderly subjects.

The authors have subsequently surmised that MPS is resistant to the anabolic qualities of insulin driven by mixed meals in the elderly.[337–339] They clearly demonstrated that AA supplementation alone can overcome at least some of the age-related reduced stimulation (e.g., movement) or diminished sensitivity to normal anabolic factors,[338,339] suggesting a potential justification for long-term use of AA supplementation as a nutritional strategy for sarcopenia.

In contrast to the earlier studies using a mixed-meal supplement,[332–334] Esmarck et al.[278] used a mixed supplement to produce a dramatic long-term (12-week) outcome (25% increase in mean muscle fiber area with no gain in muscle mass; see Section 15.7.2.5.2). The positive results may have been due to the immediate post-exercise timing of ingestion and the formula's higher protein-to-low CHO content ratio (10 g of protein and 7 g of CHO). These data would seem to support the notion that there is a solid application for AA supplementation in elderly athletes.

15.7.3.5.5   Athletes Engaged in High-Intensity or Volume Training

Overreaching is a short-term training phase in which the volume and intensity of training are far above normal. During an overreaching training phase, muscle strength and power generally decrease, due to the inability of the muscles to recover adequately between exercise bouts. Since AA supplementation can improve post-exercise MPS, Ratamess et al.[288] investigated the potential of AA supplementation to attenuate the usual strength reduction associated with overreaching. Subjects ingested 0.4 g/kg body weight daily of an AA supplement, divided into three doses consumed between meals. They found that the initial impact of overreaching did decrease muscle strength and power, and that AA supplementation did attenuate the reduction. However, there was no long-term ergogenic effect from continued use of the supplement, which is consistent with previous studies that have tested the effects of prolonged AA supplementation on strength increases[340,341] in resistance training subjects.

15.7.3.5.6   Hypertrophy and Performance

Andersen et al.[331] tested the effects of having healthy untrained young men consume 25 g of whey protein before and after resistance exercise, compared to having them consume 25 g of isoenergetic CHO, all other factors, including diet, remaining equal. The study involved measurement of performance and mass changes after 14 weeks. The principal findings were that resistance training combined with the protein supplement yielded gains in muscle performance similar to those observed with carbohydrate supplementation. However, only the protein-supplemented group demonstrated muscle hypertrophy, as determined through muscle biopsy sampling and analysis. The protein group had an 18% increase in type 1 fibers and a 26% increase in type 2, as opposed to no measurable changes in the carbohydrate group. Although this study provided protein rather than an AA mixture, the amounts provided were adequate to satisfy the EAA amounts (6 to 18 g) that have been shown to promote an acute increase in MPS.

Eccentric training is known to cause increased muscle damage while contributing to strength development,[342-346] often resulting in delayed-onset muscle soreness (DOMS). Sugita et al.[347] investigated the effects of two doses per day of an AA mixture containing L-glutamine (~14% by weight), L-ARG (~14%/w), BCAAs (~30%/w), L-threonine, L-lysine, L-proline, L-methionine, L-histidine, L-phenyl-alanine, and L-tryptophan, totaling 5.6 g/dose. They used a double-blind crossover design to determine if regular AA ingestion could reduce muscle damage and speed recovery. The AA mixture accelerated the rate of elbow extensor muscle recovery compared to the placebo. Additionally, the mixture produced higher muscle strength throughout the recovery period and subjects reported less DOMS.

In a long-term trial, using the same AA combination, the investigators attempted to identify an effective dose range for reducing muscle damage during sustained exercise for 2 to 3 h/day, 5 days/week, for 6 months.[348] Athletes consumed three doses per day of AA mix: 2.2, 4.4, and 6.6 g/dose. Each dose was consumed for a 1-month period, and each period was separated from the next changed dosage period by a 1-month washout period. Blood was drawn at the end of each dosage trial. With the 2.2-g dose, there were no significant effects on blood indices of muscle damage or oxygen-carrying capacity. The 4.4-g dose produced significant increases in serum albumin and reductions in serum iron and blood lactic acid concentrations. The 6.6-g dose produced the greatest improvements in all areas, including noticeable changes in physical condition (self-assessment) and measures of muscle damage and oxygen-carrying capacity (Table 15.8).

In another long-term trial, rugby players ingested the same 6.6-g formula two times daily for 3 months during intense training.[349] The investigators compared a variety of blood values following supplementation to presupplementation and 1 year postsupplementation in these continuously training athletes. Blood values following the supplementation period had significantly greater levels of red blood cells, hematocrit, and hemoglobin compared to presupplementation and 1 year postsupplementation, indicating potentially enhanced oxygen-carrying capacity of the blood. In addition, subjective reports of the athletes indicated a favorable effect on their physical performance; however, subject blinding was not possible in this study (Table 15.9).

As with the overreaching study by Ratamess et al.,[288] these studies seem to validate the use of AA supplementation during intense training. Many athletes, such as the track runners and rugby players in these studies, may always be close to overreaching or overtraining conditions for undesired or unknown periods. Based on these results, bodybuilders preparing for competition, star players that must play back-to-back games, practices, etc., or chronically overtrained athletes may all benefit from some sort of daily AA or high-quality protein supplementation.

TABLE 15.8
Effect of the 6.6 g/day Dose of the AA Mixture on Physical Parameters, Hematology, and Blood Biochemistry in Runners

	Pre-Test Period	Post-Test Period
Body weight, kg	60.4 ± 0.9	59.4 ± 0.9
Exercise load, % max	80 ± 4	90 ± 3
Physical condition (score range 1–5)	3.0 ± 0.1	3.7 ± 0.2*
Blood glucose, mg/dL	88 ± 1	93 ± 1*
Blood ammonia, µg/dL	79 ± 3	82 ± 6
Blood lactate, mmol/L	1.2 ± 0.1	1.2 ± 0.1
Hematocrit, %	44.9 ± 0.8	46.8 ± 0.6*
WBC, µL^{-1}	5300 ± 400	5400 ± 300
RBC, 10^4/µL	508 ± 12	528 ± 9*
Platelets, 10^4/µL	20.3 ± 0.9	20.2 ± 0.8
Hemoglobin, g/dL	15.2 ± 0.2	15.8 ± 0.3*
Serum HDL, mg/dL	65 ± 5	63 ± 4
Serum albumin, g/dL	5.0 ± 0.1	5.2 ± 0.1*
Serum TC, mg/dL	168 ± 7	161 ± 7
BUN, mg/dL	17.2 ± 15	16.6 ± 0.8
Serum iron, µg/L	114 ± 15	99 ± 12
Serum ferritin, µg/L	40 ± 6	43 ± 7
Serum CPK, U/L	366 ± 52	198 ± 22*
Serum GOT, U/L	32 ± 2	24 ± 1*
Serum GPT, U/L	28 ± 3	27 ± 5
Serum LDH, U/L	365 ± 19	361 ± 16
Serum γ-GTP, U/L	25 ± 4	25 ± 3

Note: Subjects (n = 13) consumed the 6.6 g/day AA mixture for 30 days; blood samples were taken just before and after the 30-day period. Data are means 6 SEM.

WBC = white blood cells; RBC = red blood cells; HDL = high-density lipoproteins; TC, total cholesterol; BUN = blood urea nitrogen; GOT = glutamate-oxaloacetate aminotransferase; GPT = glutamate-pyruvate aminotransferase; LDH = lactate dehydrogenase; γ-GTP = γ-glutamyltranspeptidase.

*p, 0.05 vs. pretest values.

Reproduced from Ohtani et al, *J. Nutr.*, 136(2), 538–543, 2006. With permission of American Society for Nutrition.

TABLE 15.9
Effect of Ingesting 6.6 g/d of the AA Mixtue for 90 d on Physical Parameters, Hematology, and Blood Chemistry in Elite Rugby Players

	Sampling Time[a]			Statistics[b]	
	Pre (A)	Post (B)	1-y Post (C)	A vs. B	B vs. C
Body weight, kg	93.6 ± 2.8	93.5 ± 2.7	93.2 ± 2.6		
BUN, mg/dL	16.4 ± 0.8	16.1 ± 0.6	17.7 ± 0.8		*
Creatine, mg/dL	1.09 ± 0.04	1.10 ± 0.03	1.14 ± 0.02		*
WBC, mm^3	5900 ± 200	5400 ± 200	6500 ± 300		*
RBC, 10^4/μL	505 ± 7	516 ± 13	490 ± 6	*	*
Hematocrit, %	44.5 ± 0.6	46.2 ± 0.5	43.4 ± 0.5	*	*
Hemoglobin, g/dL	15.3 ± 0.2	15.6 ± 0.2	14.8 ± 0.2	*	*
Serum iron, μg/L	101 ± 6	121 ± 7	109 ± 9		
Total protein, g/dL	7.1 ± 0.1	7.2 ± 0.1	7.1 ± 0.1		
Total cholesterol, mg/L	169 ± 5	191 ± 8	178 ± 6	*	*
High density lipoprotein, mg/dL	52 ± 2	52 ± 2	51 ± 1		
Low density lipoprotein, mg/dL	87 ± 6	109 ± 10	101 ± 8	*	
Triglyceride, mg/dL	148 ± 18	150 ± 12	129 ± 13		
GOT, U/L	28 ± 4	26 ± 2	28 ± 2		
GPT, U/L	23 ± 2	21 ± 2	27 ± 4		
γ-GTP, U/L	26 ± 2	29 ± 4	39 ± 6		*
Alkaline phosphatase, U/L	229 ± 16	171 ± 10	225 ± 22	*	*

[a] The 90-d study period occurred from June through August.
[b] An asterisk indicates a significant difference ($p < 0.05$).

BUN, blood urea nitrogen; WBC, white blood cell count; RBC, red blood cell count; GOT, glutamate-oxalacetate aminotransferase; GPT, glutamate-pyruvate aminotransferase; γ-GTP, γ-glutamyl transpeptidase.

Reproduced from Ohtani et al., *J. Nutr.*, 136(2), 538–543, 2006. With permission from the American Society for Nutrition.

15.7.4 Conclusion and Suggestions

Daily exercise-induced changes in human muscle are virtually unnoticeable. Measurable alterations in muscle fiber type and diameter require repeated and progressive stimuli and relatively lengthy training periods (6 to 8 weeks).[350–352] Also, it seems clear that it is the post-exercise period when the greatest changes in MPS and tissue structure occur.[256,257,353] MPS can be stimulated in many ways, and as the research presented here describes, the various mechanisms may interact and have additive effects. Other variables are involved besides providing the appropriate amounts and types of AAs to muscle cells at the best times. Examples are type and amount of exercise, hormonal changes, cell volume changes, and vasodilatation. All of these elements may contribute to MPS and related adaptations to training.

Present rationale for a nutritional strategy to avoid training plateaus centers around findings[354] that the extent of negative protein balance induced by exercise appears to remain constant throughout a prolonged training regimen. Consequently, repeated exercise sessions continue to provide opportunity or "open the door" for anabolism. When the benefits of training and diet on muscle mass/performance have stabilized, measures like properly timed ingestion of specific AAs may play a role in plateau avoidance and progressive development for some athletes.

The question that remains to be answered for serious athletes is: Given that diet and training are already as optimal as individually possible, can additional strategies incorporating supplementation with AAs further enhance performance and adaptations to training in sports? The following paragraphs summarize the current analysis on the subject.

15.7.4.1 AAs as Hormonal Secretagogues

At this time there is little convincing evidence to support the use of oral ingestion of AAs to increase hormone levels in healthy athletes in order to improve training outcomes.

15.7.4.2 AAs as Cell Volume Contributors in PS

Supplementing creatine and glucose can increase cell volume in athletes and improve performance under certain conditions. L-Glutamine, taurine, glycine, and alanine have been used under clinical conditions to improve PS by increasing cell swelling, which gives rise to the rationale for including them in sports supplements. There is little evidence to support the concept that the cell volume-enhancing effects of these AAs have any significant effect on MPS in athletes.

15.7.4.3 AAs as NO Boosters

Proper dosing of L-ARG may increase the production of NO, increasing blood flow to the muscles, certainly in the presence of vascular disease. Unpublished data and anecdotal reports appear to support a potential application for acute increases in strength. Nothing is known regarding long-term use, but short-term use (less than 8 weeks) appears to be safe. Although current popular use by strength athletes requires further study, a common practice is to take 4 g of L-ARG three times daily during the final 3-week period leading up to and including competition day.

15.7.4.4 AAs in Maximizing PS

The strongest arguments in support of AA supplementation by athletes can be made for those under special conditions, such as energy restricted, overtrained, advanced age, etc. The evidence supporting the use of AA supplementation to maximize PS for all athletes is not as convincing at this time. Even if one accepts the proposal that AA supplementation has the potential to benefit training adaptation and sports performance, further studies comparing AA supplementation with high-quality protein supplementation are warranted.

There appears to be a delicate balance between managing insulin and maximizing protein synthesis,[272,276,277] which obviates the possibility of making any perfect recommmendation that meets the needs of all individual athletes. In addition, a person's size (especially lean body mass) and the type, intensity, and extent of training involved should all be factored into any recommendations. Much remains to be learned about the best strategies for athletes involved in strength and power sports, as opposed to those involved in endurance sports.

Acknowledging that there are significant limitations to our current understanding of the potential benefits and risks of AA supplementation, evidence is growing to support well-timed use of EAA mixtures (pre- and post-workout) to create more constant exercise-induced anabolic environments to assist athletes in maximizing recovery and adaptation to training. Application of this growing knowledge to specific athletes is a complex problem and must be placed in the context of meeting other basic macronutrient and micronutrient needs with reasonable meal frequency.

15.8 AA SAFETY/TOXICITY

A risk assessment model is used to determine tolerable upper intake levels (ULs) of consumed nutrients.[355] Sufficient data do not exist at this time to allow use of the risk assessment model for determining ULs for any of the AAs. Furthermore, athletes are highly unlikely to indulge in chronic excessive use of individual AAs, inasmuch as the AAs have no perceived value to them at dangerous levels, plus the fact that there is potential for stomach distress and discomfort involved in that practice. Consequently, collecting data on AA toxicity is difficult and possibly unnecessary. Some valuable information on this topic was recently reviewed by Garlick[95] in a brief summary of available evidence on the safety of individual AAs when taken in excess. Also see Section 15.6 for some potential adverse events of individual AAs.

Reported adverse events from acute and chronic high-level intakes of AAs are extremely rare.[356] A notable exception is the observation of a potential link between tryptophan and EMS during the late 1980s and early 1990s. At that time, the U.S. Food and Drug Administration banned the sale of tryptophan products in the U.S. It has since been generally accepted that the cause of this problem was not the tryptophan itself, but a contaminated batch that led to the disease in users.

AA supplementation safety appears to have survived the test of time as it relates to use by athletes. Despite the lack of adverse events reported by athletes who use AA products, and the lack of UL values for AA, the safety of chronic high intakes of AAs is unknown. However, the risk–benefit ratio appears to be rather low.

15.9 PRACTICAL RECOMMENDATIONS FOR MEETING AA NEEDS

15.9.1 AA Recommended Dietary Allowances

Table 15.10 presents the adult U.S. Recommended Dietary Allowance (RDA) values for EAAs and total protein. These RDA values are the amounts considered to be adequate to meet or exceed the needs of practically all healthy adults (nonpregnant

TABLE 15.10
RDA Values for EAAs and Total Protein in Adults 19 Years of Age and Older

	RDA (mg/kg/day)	RDA (mg/day for 70-kg adult)
Histidine	14	980
Isoleucine	19	1330
Leucine	42	2940
Lysine	38	2660
Methionine + cysteine	19	1330
Phenylalanine + tyrosine	33	2310
Threonine	20	1400
Tryptophan	5	350
Valine	24	1680
Total EAAs	214	14,980
Total protein	800 (0.8 g)	56,000 (56 g)

From Food and Nutrition Board, Institute of Medicine, *Dietary Reference Intakes for Energy, Carbohydrates, Fiber, Fat, Fatty Acids, Cholesterol, Protein, and Amino Acids*, National Academy Press, Washington, D.C., 2005.

and not lactating).[355] Based on these values, approximately 25% of the AAs in dietary protein should be comprised of a properly balanced mixture of EAAs.

Extensive endurance or resistance (strength) exercise training may increase protein and AA needs of athletes significantly above the RDA values established for moderately active people. Typical recommendations for protein intake of athletes participating in high-volume training are about twice the RDA.[357] Most athletes typically consume this level of protein in their diets unless they are attempting to lose weight or they consume a diet that restricts protein sources. The effect of heavy training on the need for specific AAs is less clear. However, it is known that some specific AAs are utilized to a greater extent during various types of exercise and training conditions. Also, recovery from heavy training bouts may increase the need for some AAs more than others.

15.9.2 Limiting AAs in Specific Dietary Patterns

Meeting total protein and EAA needs is dependent upon:

1. Total dietary protein intake
2. Digestibility of protein food sources
3. Quality of protein food sources (adequate supply of EAAs)

Generally, if athletes are meeting their energy needs with a reasonably balanced dietary pattern that includes animal foods, then they meet their needs for total protein and EAAs. However, if animal foods are restricted, the diet is at risk of providing too little lysine. Strict vegetarian (vegan) diets with total protein intake equal to the RDA are unlikely to provide adequate lysine, unless the diet contains significantly high amounts of beans and other legumes.[355] Also, the digestibility of the protein in many beans and grains ranges from 0.70 to 0.85 per h, compared to 0.94 to 0.97 per h for most animal protein sources.[358] Consequently, vegetarian diets for athletes should provide about 10% more total protein than omnivorous diets[359] in order to adjust for lower digestibility, and they should emphasize legumes to provide adequate lysine.

15.10 FUTURE RESEARCH NEEDS AND DIRECTIONS

The recently established RDA values for indispensable AAs provide reference points for evaluating the AA intake of athletes. Studies indicating that athletes have increased needs for total protein form a foundation for further evaluation of the specific AA needs of athletes involved in various types of training programs. Studies indicating additive effects of EAA supplementation on post-exercise MPS provide indications that the EAA needs of athletes may be elevated similar to total protein needs during certain types of training programs and stages of adaptation to the stresses of increased training intensity or duration. Under these training conditions, do athletes have EAA needs that exceed the RDA values?

Studies are needed on the effects of supplementing athletes with various individual AAs. Many claims are made for ARG-based supplements for enhancing NO synthesis, but there is very limited evidence to support such a practice in healthy athletes. There may be a reasonable case for recommending lysine supplementation in athletes who consume vegetarian or near-vegetarian diets. Comparison of the lysine intakes of vegetarian athletes with the RDA for lysine could prove to be enlightening.

In addition to further study of individual AAs, exploring the effects of supplementation with various AA mixtures may prove to be a fruitful study area, because AAs function in combination as they become part of the AA pool. Similarly, studies are needed that compare supplementation with EAA mixtures to supplementation with high-quality proteins.

Although the use of AAs for their potential cell-volumizing effect is unlikely to have a major impact on athletes, studies combining substances that affect cell swelling with EAA mixtures or high-quality proteins could provide potentially valuable information. In short, there is no shortage of questions to explore regarding the use of AAs in sports.

REFERENCES

1. Garrett RH, Grisham CM. *Biochemistry*, 3rd ed. Belmont, CA: ThomsonBrooks/Cole, 2005, pp. 78–80.
2. Schmidt CLA. Chemical statics of amino acids and proteins. In *The Chemistry of the Amino Acids and Proteins*, Schmidt CLA, Ed. Springfield, IL: Charles C. Thomas, 1944, chap. 1.

3. *Ajinomoto's Amino Acid Handbook.* Japan: Ajinomoto, 2004.
4. Gropper SS, Smith JL, Groff JL. *Advanced Nutrition and Human Metabolism*, 4th ed. Belmont, CA: Wadsworth, 2005, pp. 205–206.
5. Liu Z, Barrett EJ. Human protein metabolism: its measurement and regulation. *Am J Physiol Endocrinol Metab* 2002;283:E1105–E1112.
6. Liu Z, Long W, Fryburg DA, Barrett EJ. The regulation of body and skeletal muscle protein metabolism by hormones and amino acids. *J Nutr* 2006;136(Suppl):212S–217S.
7. Castaneda C, Charnley JM, Evans WJ, Crim MC. Elderly women accommodate to a low-protein diet with losses of body cell mass, muscle function, and immune response. *Am J Clin Nutr* 1995;62:30–39.
8. Rennie MJ, Tipton KD. Protein and amino acid metabolism during and after exercise and the effects of nutrition. *Annu Rev Nutr* 2000;20:457–483.
9. Shils ME, Young VR. *Modern Nutrition in Health and Disease*, 7th ed. Philadelphia: Lea & Febiger, 1988, p. 4.
10. Linder MC. *Nutritional Biochemistry and Metabolism*, 2nd ed. New York: Elsevier, 1991, p. 93.
11. Wagenmakers AJ. Muscle amino acid metabolism at rest and during exercise: role in human physiology and metabolism. *Exerc Sport Sci Rev* 1998;26:287–314.
12. Mourtzakis M, Saltin B, Graham T, Pilegaard H. Carbohydrate metabolism during prolonged exercise and recovery: interaction between pyruvate dehydrogenase, fatty acids, and amino acids. *J Appl Physiol* 2006;June;100(6):1822–1830.
13. Pitkanen HT, Nykanen T, Knuutinen J, Lahti K, Keinanen O, Alen M, Komi PV, Mero AA. Free amino acid pool and muscle protein balance after resistance exercise. *Med Sci Sports Exerc* 2003;35:784–792.
14. Pitkanen H, Mero A, Oja SS, Komi PV, Pontinen PJ, Saransaari P, Takala T. Serum amino acid responses to three different exercise sessions in male power athletes. *J Sports Med Phys Fitness* 2002;42:472–480.
15. Venerando R, Miotto G, Kadowaki M, Siliprandi N, Mortimore GE. Multiphasic control of proteolysis by leucine and alanine in the isolated rat hepatocyte. *Am J Physiol* 1994;266:C455–C461.
16. Cynober LA. *Amino Acid Metabolism and Therapy in Health and Nutritional Disease.* Boca Raton, FL: CRC Press, 1995, p. 361.
17. Hunt SM, Groff JL. *Advanced Nutrition and Human Metabolism.* St. Paul, MN: West Publishing Co., 1990, pp. 134–154.
18. Aimaretti G, Corneli G, Razzore P, Bellone S, Baffoni C, Arvat E, Camanni F, Ghigo E. Comparison between insulin-induced hypoglycemia and growth hormone (GH)-releasing hormone + arginine as provocative tests for the diagnosis of GH deficiency in adults. *J Clin Endocrinol Metab* 1998;83:1615–1618.
19. Eto B, Le Moel G, Porquet D, Peres G. Glutamate-arginine salts and hormonal responses to exercise. *Arch Physiol Biochem* 1995;103:160–164.
20. Schaefer A, Piquard F, Geny B, Doutreleau S, Lampert E, Mettauer B, Lonsdorfer J. L-Arginine reduces exercise-induced increase in plasma lactate and ammonia. *Int J Sports Med* 2002;23:403–407.
21. McConell GK, Huynh NN, Lee-Young RS, Canny BJ, Wadley GD. L-Arginine infusion increases glucose clearance during prolonged exercise in humans. *Am J Physiol Endocrinol Metab* 2006;290:E60–E66.
22. Fahey JL. Toxicity and blood ammonia rise resulting from intravenous amino acid administration in man; protective effect of L-arginine. *J Clin Invest* 1957;36:1647.

23. Najarian JS, Harper HA. A clinical study of the effect of arginine on blood ammonia. *Am J Med* 1956;21:832.
24. Stevens BR, Godfrey MD, Kaminski TW, Braith RW. High-intensity dynamic human muscle performance enhanced by a metabolic intervention. *Med Sci Sports Exerc* 2000;Dec;32(12):2102–2108.
25. Buford BN, Koch AJ. Glycine-arginine-alpha-ketoisocaproic acid improves performance of repeated cycling sprints. *Med Sci Sports Exerc* 2004;36:583–587.
26. Colombani PC, Bitzi R, Frey-Rindova P, Frey W, Arnold M, Langhans W, Wenk C. Chronic arginine aspartate supplementation in runners reduces total plasma amino acid level at rest and during a marathon run. *Eur J Nutr* 1999;38:263–270.
27. Abel T, Knechtle B, Perret C, Eser P, von Arx P, Knecht H. Influence of chronic supplementation of arginine aspartate in endurance athletes on performance and substrate metabolism: a randomized, double-blind, placebo-controlled study. *Int J Sports Med* 2005;26:344–349.
28. Elam RP. Morphological changes in adult males from resistance exercise and amino acid supplementation. *J Sports Med Phys Fitness* 1988;28:35–39.
29. Calloway DH, Margen S. Creatine metabolism in men: creatine pool size and turnover in relation to creatine intake. *J Nutr* 1976;106;371:106.
30. Whitney EN, Rolfes SR, Eds. *Understanding Nutrition*, 7th ed. St. Paul, MN: West Publishing, 1996, pp. 197–226.
31. Berdanier CD. *Advanced Nutrition: Macronutrients*, 2nd ed. Boca Raton, FL: CRC Press, 2000, p. 177.
32. Rebouche CJ, Paulson DJ. Carnitine metabolism and function in humans. *Annu Rev Nutr* 1986;6:41–66.
33. Flodin NW. The metabolic roles, pharmacology, and toxicology of lysine. *J Am Coll Nutr* 1997;16:7–21.
34. Hall SL, Greendale GA. The relation of dietary vitamin C intake to bone mineral density: results from the PEPI study. *Calcif Tissue Int* 1998;63:183–189.
35. Civitelli R, Villareal DT, Agnusdei D, Nardi P, Avioli LV, Gennari C. Dietary L-lysine and calcium metabolism in humans. *Nutrition* 1992;8:400–405.
36. Oxlund H, Barckman M, Ortoft G, Andreassen TT. Reduced concentrations of collagen cross-links are associated with reduced strength of bone. *Bone* 1995;17(Suppl):365S–371S.
37. Torricelli P, Fini M, Giavaresi G, Giardino R, Gnudi S, Nicolini A, Carpi A. L-Arginine and L-lysine stimulation on cultured human osteoblasts. *Biomed Pharmacother* 2002;56:492–497.
38. McCarthy CF, Borland JL, Lynch HJ, Owen EE, Tyor MP. Defective uptake of basic amino acids and L-cystine by intestinal mucosa of patients with cystinuria. *J Clin Invest* 1964;43:1518–1524.
39. Merimee TJ, Lillicrap DA, Rabinowitz D. Effect of arginine on serum-levels of human growth-hormone. *Lancet* 1965;2:668–670.
40. Merimee TJ, Rabinowtiz D, Fineberg SE. Arginine-initiated release of human growth hormone. Factors modifying the response in normal man. *N Engl J Med* 1969;280:1434–1438.
41. Knopf RF, Conn JW, Falans SS, Floyd JC, Guntsche EM, Rull JA. Plasma growth hormone responses to intravenous administration of amino acids. *J Clin Endocrinol Metab* 1965;25:1140.
42. Monteleone P, Maj M, Iovino M, Steardo L. Evidence for a sex difference in the basal growth hormone response to GABAergic stimulation in humans. *Acta Endocrinol* (Copenh). 1988;119:353–357.

43. McCann SM, Vijayan E, Negro-Vilar A, Mizunuma H, Mangat H. Gamma aminobu-tyric acid (GABA), a modulator of anterior pituitary hormone secretion by hypotha-lamic and pituitary action. *Psychoneuroendocrinology* 1984;9:97–106.
44. McCann SM, Rettori V. Gamma amino butyric acid (GABA) controls anterior pitu-itary hormone secretion. *Adv Biochem Psychopharmacol* 1986;42:173–189.
45. Volpi R, Chiodera P, Caffarra P, Scaglioni A, Saccani A, Coiro V. Different control mechanisms of growth hormone (GH) secretion between gamma-amino- and gamma-hydroxy-butyric acid: neuroendocrine evidence in Parkinson's disease. *Psycho-neuroendocrinology* 1997;22:531–538.
46. Vankelecom H, Matthys P, Denef C. Involvement of nitric oxide in the interferon-gamma-induced inhibition of growth hormone and prolactin secretion in anterior pituitary cell cultures. *Mol Cell Endocrinol* 1997;129:157–167.
47. Alba-Roth J, Muller OA, Schopohl J, von Werder K. Arginine stimulates growth hormone secretion by suppressing endogenous somatostatin secretion. *J Clin Endo-crinol Metab* 1988;67:1186–1189.
48. McGilvery RW, Ed. *Biochemistry: A Functional Approach*, 2nd ed. Philadelphia: W.B. Saunders, 1979.
49. Nieper HA, Blumberger K. Electrolyte transport therapy of cardiovascular diseases. In *Electrolytes and Cardiovascular Diseases*, Vol. 2, Bajusz E, Ed. Basel: S. Karger, 1966.
50. Boszormenyl E, Farsang C, Debreczeni LA. Hemodynamic and cardiac effects of potassium magnesium aspartate in the dog. *Acta Physiol Acad Sci Hung* 1977;50:149–160.
51. Kuhn P, Probst P. Effect of potassium-magnesium aspartate on hemodynamics and myocardial metabolism of coronary disease patient during beta receptor stimulation. *Z Kardiol* 1975;64:616–624.
52. Saborowski F, Lang D, Albers C. Intracellular pH of cardiac muscle after administration of potassium-magnesium-aspartate. *Arzneimittelforschung* 1975;25:1897–1900.
53. Slezak J, Tribulova N. Morphological changes after combined administration of isoproterenol and K+,Mg2+-aspartate as a physiological Ca2+ antagonist. *Recent Adv Stud Cardiac Struct Metab* 1975;6:75–84.
54. Fedelesova M et al. Prevention by K+,Mg2+-aspartate of isoproterenol-induced met-abolic changes in the myocardium. *Recent Adv Stud Cardiac Struct Metab* 1975;6:59–73.
55. Fedelesova M, Ziegelhoffer A, Luknarova O, Dzurba A, Kostolansky S. Influence of K+,Mg++-(D,L)-aspartate on various ATPase activities of the dog heart. *Arzneimit-telforschung* 1973;23:1048–1053.
56. Yang JP, Zhang GL, Guo YS. Potentiated polarized liquid therapy and heart emer-gency. *Chung Hua Nei Ko Tsa Chih* 1992;31:617–618, 657–658.
57. Kuhn P, Oberthaler G, Oswald J. Anti-arrhythmia effectiveness of potassium-magne-sium-aspartate infusion. *Wien Med Wochenschr* 1991;141:64–65.
58. Aksel'rod LB, Arshinova LS, Gaidenko AI, Maksimovich IaB, Sukolovskaia DM. Comparative evaluation of cardiotropic effects of nicamag, panangin and asparkam. *Farmakol Toksikol* 1985;48:51–55.
59. Skotnicki AB, Jablonski MJ, Musial J, Swadzba J. The role of magnesium in the pathogenesis and therapy of bronchial asthma. *Przegl Lek* 1997;54:630–633.
60. Anonymous. The application of potassium magnesium aspartate in heart operation. *Zhonghua Xinxueguanbing ZaZhi* 1996;24:31–32.
61. Spath P, Barankay A, Richter JA. The influence of rapid potassium administration on hemodynamics and endogenous catecholamine production during extracorporeal cir-culation. *J Cardiothorac Anesth* 1989;3:176–180.

62. Sen Gupta J, Srivastava KK. Effect of potassium-magnesium aspartate on endurance work in man. *Indian J Exp Biol* 1973;11:392–394.
63. Trudeau F, Murphy R. Effects of potassium-aspartate salt administration on glycogen use in the rat during a swimming stress. *Physiol Behav.* 1993;54:7–12.
64. Marquezi ML, Roschel HA, dos Santa Costa A, Sawada LA, Lancha AH Jr. Effect of aspartate and asparagine supplementation on fatigue determinants in intense exercise. *Int J Sport Nutr Exerc Metab.* 2003;13:65–75.
65. Laborit H, Maynier R, Guiot G, Barow C, Niaussat P. Influence of various pharmacological agents on the swimming test of white rats. *Comput Rend Soc Biol* 1958;152:486.
66. Laborit H, Magnier R, Coirault R, Thiebault J, Guiot G, Niaussat P, Weber B, Jouany JM, Baron C. The place of certain salts of DL aspartic acid in the mechanisms of preservation of activity in reaction to the environment: summary of an experimental and clinical study. *Presse Med* 1958;66:1307.
67. Wesson M, McNaughton L, Davies P, Tristram S. Effects of oral administration of aspartic acid salts on the endurance capacity of trained athletes. *Res Q Exerc Sport* 1988;59:234–239.
68. Ahlborg B, Ekelund LG, Nilsson CG. Effect of potassium-magnesium-aspartate on the capacity for prolonged exercise in man. *Acta Physiol Scand* 1968;74:238–245.
69. Von Franz IW, Chintanaseri C. Uber die Wirkung des Kalium-Magnesium-Aspartates auf die ausdauerleistung unter besonder Berucksichtigung des aspartates. *Sportarzt Sportmed* 1977;28:37.
70. Nagle FJ, Balke B, Ganslen RV, Davis AW. The mitigation of physical fatigue with "Spartase." *US Civil Aeromed Res Inst Rep Civ Aeromed Inst US* 1963;Jul;94:1–10.
71. Fallis N, Wilson WR, Tetreault LL, Lasagna L. Effect of potassium and magnesium aspartate on athletic performance. *JAMA* 1963;185:129.
72. Consolazio CF, Nelson RA, Matoush LO, Isaac GJ. Effects of aspartic acid salts (Mg and K) on physical performance of men. *J Appl Physiol* 1964;19:257.
73. de Haan A, van Doorn JE, Westra HG. Effects of potassium + magnesium aspartate on muscle metabolism and force development during short intensive static exercise. *Int J Sports Med* 1985;6:44–49.
74. Hagan RD, Upton SJ, Duncan JJ, Cummings JM, Gettman LR. Absence of effect of potassium-magnesium aspartate on physiologic responses to prolonged work in aerobically trained men. *Int J Sports Med* 1982;3:177–181.
75. Maughan RJ, Sadler DJ. The effects of oral administration of salts of aspartic acid on the metabolic response to prolonged exhausting exercise in man. *Int J Sports Med* 1983;4:119–123.
76. Nakahara M, Yoshihara T, Tokita T, Nakanishi Y, Sakahashi H, Shibata N. Difference in action between D- and L-potassium and magnesium aspartates. *Arzneimittelforschung* 1966;16:1491–1494.
77. Lancha AH Jr, Recco MB, Abdalla DS, Curi R. Effect of aspartate, asparagine, and carnitine supplementation in the diet on metabolism of skeletal muscle during a moderate exercise. *Physiol Behav* 1995;57:367–371.
78. Crim MC, Calloway DH, Margen S. Creatine metabolism in men: urinary creatine and creatinine excretions with creatine feeding. *J Nutr* 1975;105:428–438.
79. Crim MC, Calloway DH, Margen S. Creatine metabolism in men, creatine pool size and turnover in relation to creatine intake. *J Nutr* 1976;106:371–375.
80. Kasai K, Kobayashi M, Shimoda SI. Stimulatory effect of glycine on human growth hormone secretion. *Metabolism* 1978;27:201–208.

81. Meister A, Anderson ME, Hwang O. Intracellular cysteine and glutathione delivery systems. *J Am Coll Nutr* 1986;5:137–151.

82. Smilkstein MJ, Knapp GL, Kulig KW, Rumack BH. Efficacy of oral N-acetylcysteine in the treatment of acetaminophen overdose. Analysis of the national multicenter study (1976 to 1985). *N Engl J Med* 1988;319:1557–1562.

83. Sen CK, Rankinen T, Vaisanen S, Rauramaa R. Oxidative stress after human exercise: effect of N-acetylcysteine supplementation. *J Appl Physiol* 1994;76:2570–2577.

84. Medved I, Brown MJ, Bjorksten AR, McKenna MJ. Effects of intravenous N-acetyl-cysteine infusion on time to fatigue and potassium regulation during prolonged cycling exercise. *J Appl Physiol* 2004;96:211–217.

85. Medved I, Brown MJ, Bjorksten AR, Murphy KT, Petersen AC, Sostaric S, Gong X, McKenna MJ. N-Acetylcysteine enhances muscle cysteine and glutathione availability and attenuates fatigue during prolonged exercise in endurance-trained individuals. *J Appl Physiol* 2004;97:1477–1485.

86. King MW. Introduction to Amino Acid Metabolism. IU School of Medicine, 2006. http://www.indstate.edu/thcme/mwking/amino-acid-metabolism.html#tyrosine.

87. Deijen JB, Orlebeke JF. Effect of tyrosine on cognitive function and blood pressure under stress. *Brain Res Bull* 1994;33:319–323.

88. Deijen JB, Wientjes CJ, Vullinghs HF, Cloin PA, Langefeld JJ. Tyrosine improves cognitive performance and reduces blood pressure in cadets after one week of a combat training course. *Brain Res Bull* 1999;48:203–209.

89. Owasoyo JO, Neri DF, Lamberth JG. Tyrosine and its potential use as a countermeasure to performance decrement in military sustained operations. *Aviat Space Environ Med* 1992;63:364–369.

90. Struder HK, Hollmann W, Platen P, Donike M, Gotzmann A, Weber K. Influence of paroxetine, branched-chain amino acids and tyrosine on neuroendocrine system responses and fatigue in humans. *Horm Metab Res* 1998;30:188–194.

91. Sutton EE, Coill MR, Deuster PA. Ingestion of tyrosine: effects on endurance, muscle strength, and anaerobic performance. *Int J Sport Nutr Exerc Metab.* 2005;15:173–185.

92. Chinevere TD, Sawyer RD, Creer AR, Conlee RK, Parcell AC. Effects of L-tyrosine and carbohydrate ingestion on endurance exercise performance. *J Appl Physiol* 2002;93:1590–1597.

93. Lieberman HR, Georgelis JH, Maher TJ, Yeghiayan SK. Tyrosine prevents effects of hyperthermia on behavior and increases norepinephrine. *Physiol Behav* 2005;84:33–38.

94. Yeghiayan SK, Luo S, Shukitt-Hale B, Lieberman HR. Tyrosine improves behavioral and neurochemical deficits caused by cold exposure. *Physiol Behav* 2001;72:311–316.

95. Garlick PJ. The nature of human hazards associated with excessive intake of amino acids. *J Nutr.* 2004;134(Suppl):1633S–1639S; discussion, 1664S–1666S, 1667S–1672S (review).

96. Graham TE, Sgro V, Friars D, Gibala MJ. Glutamate ingestion: the plasma and muscle free amino acid pools of resting humans. *Am J Physiol Endocrinol Metab* 2000;278:E83–E89.

97. Garattini S. Glutamic acid, twenty years later. *J Nutr* 2000;130(Suppl):901S–909S.

98. Watkins JC, Evans RH. Excitatory amino acid transmitters. *Annu Rev Pharmacol Toxicol* 1981;21:165–204 (review).

99. Walker R, Lupien JR. The safety evaluation of monosodium glutamate. *J Nutr* 2000;130:1049S–1052S.

100. Bruce M, Constantin-Teodosiu D, Greenhaff PL, Boobis LH, Williams C, Bowtell JL. Glutamine supplementation promotes anaplerosis but not oxidative energy delivery in human skeletal muscle. *Am J Physiol Endocrinol Metab* 2001;280:E669–E675.

101. Mourtzakis M, Graham TE. Glutamate ingestion and its effects at rest and during exercise in humans. *J Appl Physiol* 2002;93:1251–1259.

102. Yuan Y, So R, Wong S, Chan KM. Ammonia threshold: comparison to lactate threshold, correlation to other physiological parameters and response to training. *Scand J Med Sci Sports* 2002;12:358–364.

103. Eto B, Peres G, Le Moel G. Effects of an ingested glutamate arginine salt on ammonemia during and after long lasting cycling. *Arch Int Physiol Biochim Biophys* 1994;102:161–162.

104. Kriengsinyos W, Rafii M, Wykes LJ, Ball RO, Pencharz PB. Long-term effects of histidine depletion on whole-body protein metabolism in healthy adults. *J Nutr* 2002;132:3340–3348.

105. Johnson P, Hammer JL. Histidine dipeptide levels in ageing and hypertensive rat skeletal and cardiac muscles. *Comp Biochem Physiol B* 1992;103:981–984.

106. Guiotto A, Calderan A, Ruzza P, Borin G. Carnosine and carnosine-related antioxidants: a review. *Curr Med Chem* 2005;12:2293–2315 (review).

107. Begum G, Cunliffe A, Leveritt M. Physiological role of carnosine in contracting muscle. *Int J Sport Nutr Exerc Metab* 2005;15:493–514 (review).

108. Kraemer WJ, Gordon SE, Lynch JM, Pop ME, Clark KL. Effects of multibuffer supplementation on acid-base balance and 2,3-diphosphoglycerate following repetitive anaerobic exercise. *Int J Sport Nutr* 1995;5:300–314.

109. Suzuki Y, Nakao T, Maemura H, Sato M, Kamahara K, Morimatsu F, Takamatsu K. Carnosine and anserine ingestion enhances contribution of nonbicarbonate buffering. *Med Sci Sports Exerc* 2006;38:334–338.

110. Suzuki Y, Ito O, Mukai N, Takahashi H, Takamatsu K. High level of skeletal muscle carnosine contributes to the latter half of exercise performance during 30-s maximal cycle ergometer sprinting. *Jpn J Physiol* 2002;52:199–205.

111. Geliebter AA, Hashim SA, Van Itallie TB. Oral L-histidine fails to reduce taste and smell acuity but induces anorexia and urinary zinc excretion. *Am J Clin Nutr* 1981;34:119–120.

112. Askanazi J, Carpentier YA, Michelsen CB, Elwyn DH, Furst P, Kantrowitz LR, Gump FE, Kinney JM. Muscle and plasma amino acids following injury. Influence of intercurrent infection. *Ann Surg* 1980;192:78–85.

113. Sitren HS, Fisher H. Nitrogen retention in rats fed on diets enriched with arginine and glycine. 1. Improved N retention after trauma. *Br J Nutr* 1977;37:195–208.

114. Motil KJ, Thotathuchery M, Montandon CM, Hachey DL, Boutton TW, Klein PD, Garza C. Insulin, cortisol and thyroid hormones modulate maternal protein status and milk production and composition in humans. *J Nutr* 1994;124:1248–1257.

115. Miller RG, Keshen TH, Jahoor F, Shew SB, Jaksic T. Compartmentation of endogenously synthesized amino acids in neonates. *J Surg Res* 1996;63:199–203.

116. Huq F, Thompson M, Ruell P. Changes in serum amino acid concentrations during prolonged endurance running. *Jpn J Physiol* 1993;43:797–807.

117. van Loon LJ, Saris WH, Verhagen H, Wagenmakers AJ. Plasma insulin responses after ingestion of different amino acid or protein mixtures with carbohydrate. *Am J Clin Nutr* 2000;72:96–105.

118. van Loon LJ, Saris WH, Kruijshoop M, Wagenmakers AJ. Maximizing postexercise muscle glycogen synthesis: carbohydrate supplementation and the application of amino acid or protein hydrolysate mixtures. *Am J Clin Nutr* 2000;72:106–111.

119. Shaw K, Turner J, Del Mar C. Tryptophan and 5-hydroxytryptophan for depression. *Cochrane Database Syst Rev* 2002;1:CD003198 (review).
120. Davis JM, Alderson NL, Welsh RS. Serotonin and central nervous system fatigue: nutritional considerations. *Am J Clin Nutr* 2000;72:573S–578S.
121. Acworth I, Nicholass J, Morgan B, Newsholme EA. Effect of sustained exercise on concentrations of plasma aromatic and branched-chain amino acids and brain amines. *Biochem Biophys Res Commun* 1986;137:149–153.
122. Blomstrand E, Perrett D, Parry-Billings M, Newsholme EA. Effect of sustained exercise on plasma amino acid concentrations and on 5-hydroxytryptamine metabolism in six different brain regions in the rat. *Acta Physiol Scand* 1989;136:473–481.
123. Blomstrand E. Amino acids and central fatigue. *Amino Acids* 2001;20:25–34.
124. Fernstrom JD, Fernstrom MH. Exercise, serum free tryptophan, and central fatigue. *J Nutr* 2006;136:553S–559S.
125. Petruzzello SJ, Landers DM, Pie J, Blilie J. Effect of branched-chain amino acid supplements on exercise-related mood and performance. *Med Sci Sports Exerc* 1992;24:S2.
126. Krieder RB, Jackson CW. Effects of amino acid supplementation on psychological status during an intercollegiate swim season. *Med Sci Sports Exerc* 1994;26:S115.
127. Calders P, Pannier JL, Matthys DM, Lacroix EM. Pre-exercise branched-chain amino acid administration increases endurance performance in rats. *Med Sci Sports Exerc* 1997;29:1182–1186.
128. Farris JW, Hinchcliff KW, McKeever KH, Lamb DR, Thompson DL. Treadmill endurance of standard breed horses infused with tryptophan and/or glucose. *Med Sci Sports Exerc* 1996;28:S48.
129. Mittleman KD, Ricci MR, Bailey SP. Branched-chain amino acids prolong exercise during heat stress in men and women. *Med Sci Sports Exerc* 1998;30:83–91.
130. Segura R, Ventura JL. Effect of L-tryptophan supplementation on exercise performance. *Int J Sports Med* 1988;9:301–305.
131. Stensrud T, Ingjer F, Holm H, Stromme SB. L-Tryptophan supplementation does not improve running performance. *Int J Sports Med* 1992;13:481–485.
132. Patmas MA. Eosinophilia-myalgia syndrome not associated with L-tryptophan. *N Engl J Med* 1992;89:285–286.
133. Goda Y, Suzuki J, Maitani T, Yoshihira K, Takeda M, Uchiyama M. 3-Anilino-L-alanine, structural determination of UV-5, a contaminant in EMS-associated L-tryptophan samples. *Chem Pharm Bull* (Tokyo) 1992;40:2236–2238.
134. Remesy C, Fafournoux P, Demigne C. Control of hepatic utilization of serine, glycine and threonine in fed and starved rats. *J Nutr* 1983;113:28–39.
135. McDaniel MA, Maier SF, Einstein GO. "Brain-specific" nutrients: a memory cure? *Nutrition* 2003;19:957–975.
136. Jorissen BL, Brouns F, Van Boxtel MP, Ponds RW, Verhey FR, Jolles J, Riedel WJ. The influence of soy-derived phosphatidylserine on cognition in age-associated memory impairment. *Nutr Neurosci* 2001;4:121–134.
137. Monteleone P, Beinat L, Tanzillo C, Maj M, Kemali D. Effects of phosphatidylserine on the neuroendocrine response to physical stress in humans. *Neuroendocrinology* 1990;52:243–248.
138. Monteleone P, Maj M, Beinat L, Natale M, Kemali D. Blunting by chronic phosphatidylserine administration of the stress-induced activation of the hypothalamo-pituitary-adrenal axis in healthy men. *Eur J Clin Pharmacol* 1992;42:385–388.

139. Kingsley MI, Wadsworth D, Kilduff LP, McEneny J, Benton D. Effects of phosphatidylserine on oxidative stress following intermittent running. *Med Sci Sports Exerc* 2005;37:1300–1306.

140. Kingsley MI, Miller M, Kilduff LP, McEneny J, Benton D. Effects of phosphatidylserine on exercise capacity during cycling in active males. *Med Sci Sports Exerc* 2006;38:64–71.

141. Fukagawa NK, Galbraith RA. Advancing age and other factors influencing the balance between amino acid requirements and toxicity. *J Nutr* 2004;134(Suppl):1569S–1574S.

142. Trimble KC, Molloy AM, Scott JM, Weir DG. The effect of ethanol on one-carbon metabolism: increased methionine catabolism and lipotrope methyl-group wastage. *Hepatology* 1993;18:984–989.

143. Duranton B, Freund JN, Galluser M, Schleiffer R, Gosse F, Bergmann C, Hasselmann M, Raul F. Promotion of intestinal carcinogenesis by dietary methionine. *Carcinogenesis* 1999;20:493–497.

144. Humm A, Fritsche E, Steinbacher S, Huber R. Crystal structure and mechanism of human L-arginine:glycine amidinotransferase: a mitochondrial enzyme involved in creatine biosynthesis. *EMBO J* 1997;16:3373–3385.

145. Vaz FM, Wanders RJ. Carnitine biosynthesis in mammals. *Biochem J* 2002;361:417–429 (review).

146. Storch KJ, Wagner DA, Burke JF, Young VR. [1-13C; methyl-2H3]methionine kinetics in humans: methionine conservation and cystine sparing. *Am J Physiol* 1990;258:E790–E798.

147. Storch KJ, Wagner DA, Burke JF, Young VR. Quantitative study *in vivo* of methionine cycle in humans using [methyl-2H3]- and [1-13C]methionine. *Am J Physiol* 1988;255:E322–E331.

148. Kien CL, Young VR, Rohrbaugh DK, Burke JF. Increased rates of whole body protein synthesis and breakdown in children recovering from burns. *Ann Surg* 1978;187:383–391.

149. Yoshida A, Moritoki K. Nitrogen sparing action of methionine and threonine in rats receiving a protein free diet. *Nutr Rep Int* 1974;9:159–168.

150. Millward DJ, Rivers JP. The need for indispensable amino acids: the concept of the anabolic drive. *Diabetes Metab Rev* 1989;5:191–211 (review).

151. Yokogoshi H, Yoshida A. Some factors affecting the nitrogen sparing action of methionine and threonine in rats fed a protein free diet. *J Nutr* 1976;106:48–57.

152. Knopf RF, Conn JW, Fajans SS. Plasma growth hormone response to intravenous administration of amino acids. *J Clin Endocrinol* 1965;25:1140.

153. Chromiak JA, Antonio J. Use of amino acids as growth hormone-releasing agents by athletes. *Nutrition* 2002;18:657–661.

154. Harden LM, Neveling N, Rossouw F, Semple SJ, Marx FE, Rossouw J, Rogers G. The effects of an L-methionine combination supplement on symptoms of upper respiratory tract infections and performance in ultramarathon runners before, during, and after ultra-endurance exercise. *S Afr J Sports Med* 2004;16:10–16

155. Energy and Protein Requirements. Report of a joint FAO/WHO/UNU Expert Consultation. World Health Organization Technical Report Series 1985;724:1–206.

156. Borgonha S, Regan MM, Oh SH, Condon M, Young VR. Threonine requirement of healthy adults, derived with a 24-h indicator amino acid balance technique. *Am J Clin Nutr* 2002;75:698–704.

157. Kurpad AV, Raj T, Regan MM, Vasudevan J, Caszo B, Nazareth D, Gnanou J, Young VR. Threonine requirements of healthy Indian men, measured by a 24-h indicator amino acid oxidation and balance technique. *Am J Clin Nutr* 2002;76:789–797.

158. Dietary Reference Intakes for Energy, Carbohydrate, Fiber, Fat, Fatty Acids, Cholesterol, Protein, and Amino Acids (Macronutrients). Institute of Medicine, Food and Nutrition Board (FNB), Office of Disease Prevention and Health Promotion of the U.S. Department of Health and Human Services, 2005, p. 27. www.nap.edu.

159. Wolfe RR. Skeletal muscle protein metabolism and resistance exercise. *J Nutr* 2006;136:525S–528S.

160. Volek JS, Rawson ES. Scientific basis and practical aspects of creatine supplementation for athletes. *Nutrition* 2004;20:609–614 (review).

161. Lambert EV, Goedecke JH. The role of dietary macronutrients in optimizing endurance performance. *Curr Sports Med Rep* 2003;2:194–201.

162. Cynober L, Coudray-Lucas C. Ornithine and alpha-ketoglutarate administration in surgical, trauma and cancer-bearing patients. In *Nutritional Support in Cancer and Transplant Patients,* Latifi R, Marrell RC, Eds. Austin, TX: R.G. Landis Co., 2001, p. 145.

163. Berneis K, Ninnis R, Haussinger D, Keller U. Effects of hyper- and hypoosmolality on whole body protein and glucose kinetics in humans. *Am J Physiol* 1999;276:E188–E195.

164. Tapiero H, Mathe G, Couvreur P, et al. I. Arginine. *Biomed Pharmacother* (France) 2002;56:439–445.

165. Evain-Brion D, Donnadieu M, Roger M, Job JC. Simultaneous study of somatotrophic and corticotrophic pituitary secretions during ornithine infusion test. *Clin Endocrinol* (Oxf) 1982;17:119–122.

166. Corpas E, Blackman MR, Roberson R, Scholfield D, Harman SM. Oral arginine-lysine does not increase growth hormone or insulin-like growth factor-I in old men. *J Gerontol* 1993;48:M128–M133.

167. Lambert MI, Hefer JA, Millar RP, Macfarlane PW. Failure of commercial oral amino acid supplements to increase serum growth hormone concentrations in male bodybuilders. *Int J Sport Nutr* 1993;3:298–305.

168. Suminski RR, Robertson RJ, Goss FL, Arslanian S, Kang J, DaSilva S, Utter AC, Metz KF. Acute effect of amino acid ingestion and resistance exercise on plasma growth hormone concentration in young men. *Int J Sport Nutr* 1997;7:48–60.

169. Fogelholm GM, Naveri HK, Kiilavuori KT, Harkonen MH. Low-dose amino acid supplementation: no effects on serum human growth hormone and insulin in male weightlifters. *Int J Sport Nutr* 1993;3:290–297.

170. Fry AC, Kraemer WJ, Stone MH, Warren BJ, Kearney JT, Maresh CM, Weseman CA, Fleck SJ. Endocrine and performance responses to high volume training and amino acid supplementation in elite junior weightlifters. *Int J Sport Nutr* 1993;3:306–322.

171. Jorgensen JO, Pedersen SA, Thuesen L, Jorgensen J, Ingemann-Hansen T, Skakkebaek NE, Christiansen JS. Beneficial effects of growth hormone treatment in GH-deficient adults. *Lancet* 1989;1:1221–1225.

172. Degerblad M, Elgindy N, Hall K, Sjoberg HE, Thoren M. Potent effect of recombinant growth hormone on bone mineral density and body composition in adults with panhypopituitarism. *Acta Endocrinol* (Copenh) 1992;126:387–393.

173. de Boer H, Blok GJ, Van der Veen EA. Clinical aspects of growth hormone deficiency in adults. *Endocr Rev.* 1995;16:63–86.

174. Ahmad AM, Hopkins MT, Thomas J, Ibrahim H, Fraser WD, Vora JP. Body composition and quality of life in adults with growth hormone deficiency; effects of low-dose growth hormone replacement. *Clin Endocrinol* (Oxf) 2001;54:709–717.

175. Richelsen B, Pedersen SB, Borglum JD, Moller-Pedersen T, Jorgensen J, Jorgensen JO. Growth hormone treatment of obese women for 5 wk: effect on body composition and adipose tissue LPL activity. *Am J Physiol* 1994;266:E211–E216.

176. Rudman D, Feller AG, Nagraj HS, Gergans GA, Lalitha PY, Goldberg AF, Schlenker RA, Cohn L, Rudman IW, Mattson DE. Effects of human growth hormone in men over 60 years old. *N Engl J Med* 1990;323:1–6.

177. Frisch H. Growth hormone and body composition in athletes. *J Endocrinol Invest* 1999;22(Suppl):106–109 (review).

178. Taaffe DR, Jin IH, Vu TH, Hoffman AR, Marcus R. Lack of effect of recombinant human growth hormone (GH) on muscle morphology and GH-insulin-like growth factor expression in resistance-trained elderly men. *J Clin Endocrinol Metab* 1996;81:421–425.

179. Yarasheski KE, Zachwieja JJ, Campbell JA, Bier DM. Effect of growth hormone and resistance exercise on muscle growth and strength in older men. *Am J Physiol Endocrinol Metab* 1995;268:E268–E276.

180. Yarasheski KE, Campbell JA, Smith K, Rennie MJ, Holloszy JO, Bier DM. Effect of growth hormone and resistance exercise on muscle growth in young men. *Am J Physiol* 1992;262:E261–E267.

181. Yarasheski KE. Growth hormone effects on metabolism, body composition, muscle mass, and strength. *Exerc Sport Sci Rev* 1994;22:285–312.

182. Berggren A, Ehrnborg C, Rosen T, Ellegard L, Bengtsson BA, Caidahl K. Short-term administration of supraphysiological recombinant human growth hormone (GH) does not increase maximum endurance exercise capacity in healthy, active young men and women with normal GH-insulin-like growth factor I axes. *J Clin Endocrinol Metab* 2005;90:3268–3273.

183. Jorgensen JO, Moller J, Laursen T, Orskov H, Christiansen JS, Weeke J. Growth hormone administration stimulates energy expenditure and extrathyroidal conversion of thyroxine to triiodothyronine in a dose-dependent manner and suppresses circadian thyrotrophin levels: studies in GH-deficient adults. *Clin Endocrinol* (Oxf). 1994;41:609–614.

184. Wolthers T, Grofte T, Norrelund H, Poulsen PL, Andreasen F, Christiansen JS, Jorgensen JO. Differential effects of growth hormone and prednisolone on energy metabolism and leptin levels in humans. *Metabolism* 1998;47:83–88.

185. Lange KH, Isaksson F, Juul A, Rasmussen MH, Bulow J, Kjaer M. Growth hormone enhances effects of endurance training on oxidative muscle metabolism in elderly women. *Am J Physiol Endocrinol Metab* 2000;279:E989–E996.

186. Papadakis MA, Grady D, Black D, Tierney MJ, Gooding GA, Schambelan M, Grunfeld C. Growth hormone replacement in healthy older men improves body composition but not functional ability. *Ann Intern Med* 1996;124:708–716.

187. Zachwieja JJ, Yarasheski KE. Does growth hormone therapy in conjunction with resistance exercise increase muscle force production and muscle mass in men and women aged 60 years or older? *Phys Ther* 1999;79:76–82 (review).

188. Stoll B, Gerok W, Lang F, Haussinger D. Liver cell volume and protein synthesis. *Biochem J* 1992;287:217–222.

189. Lang F, Friedrich F, Paulmichl M, Schobersberger W, Jungwirth A, Ritter M, Steidl M, Weiss H, Woll E, Tschernko E, et al. Ion channels in Madin-Darby canine kidney cells (MDCK). *Ren Physiol Biochem* 1990;13:82–93.

190. Lang F, Ritter M, Volkl H, Haussinger D. The biological significance of cell volume. *Ren Physiol Biochem* 1993;16:48–65.

191. Weiss H, Lang F. Ion channels activated by swelling of Madin Darby canine kidney (MDCK) cells. *J Membr Biol* 1992;126:109–114.
192. Haussinger D, Lang F. Exposure of perfused liver to hypotonic conditions modifies cellular nitrogen metabolism. *J Cell Biochem* 1990;43:355–361.
193. Davis RJ. The mitogen-activated protein kinase signal transduction pathway. *J Biol Chem* 1993;268:14553–14556.
194. Haussinger D. The role of cellular hydration in the regulation of cell function. *Biochem J* 1996;313:697–710.
195. Hallbrucker C, Ritter M, Lang F, Gerok W, Haussinger D. Hydroperoxide metabolism in rat liver. K+ channel activation, cell volume changes and eicosanoid formation. *Eur J Biochem* 1993;211:449–458.
196. Saha N, Schreiber R, vom Dahl S, Lang F, Gerok W, Haussinger D. Endogenous hydroperoxide formation, cell volume and cellular K+ balance in perfused rat liver. *Biochem J* 1993;296:701–707.
197. Krippeit-Drews P, Lang F, Haussinger D, Drews G. H_2O_2 induced hyperpolarization of pancreatic B-cells. *Pflugers Arch* 1994;426:552–554.
198. Hallbrucker C, vom Dahl S, Lang F, Gerok W, Haussinger D. Inhibition of hepatic proteolysis by insulin. Role of hormone-induced alterations of the cellular K+ balance. *Eur J Biochem* 1991;199:467–474.
199. Hallbrucker C, vom Dahl S, Lang F, Gerok W, Haussinger D. Modification of liver cell volume by insulin and glucagon. *Pflugers Arch* 1991;418:519–521.
200. vom Dahl S, Hallbrucker C, Lang F, Gerok W, Haussinger D. Regulation of liver cell volume and proteolysis by glucagon and insulin. *Biochem J* 1991;278:771–777.
201. vom Dahl S, Hallbrucker C, Lang F, Haussinger D. Regulation of cell volume in the perfused rat liver by hormones. *Biochem J* 1991;280:105–109.
202. Haussinger D, Hallbrucker C, vom Dahl S, Decker S, Schweizer U, Lang F, Gerok W. Cell volume is a major determinant of proteolysis control in liver. *FEBS Lett* 1991;283:70–72.
203. Hallbrucker C, vom Dahl S, Ritter M, Lang F, Haussinger D. Effects of urea on K+ fluxes and cell volume in perfused rat liver. *Pflugers Arch* 1994;428:552–560.
204. al-Habori M, Peak M, Thomas TH, Agius L. The role of cell swelling in the stimulation of glycogen synthesis by insulin. *Biochem J* 1992;282:789–796.
205. Baquet A, Hue L, Meijer AJ, van Woerkom GM, Plomp PJ. Swelling of rat hepatocytes stimulates glycogen synthesis. *J Biol Chem* 1990;265:955–959.
206. Grant A, Tosh D, Burchell A. Liver perfusion with hyper-osmotic media stimulates microsomal glucose-6-phosphatase activity. *Biochem Soc Trans* 1993;21:39S.
207. Peak M, al-Habori M, Agius L. Regulation of glycogen synthesis and glycolysis by insulin, pH and cell volume. Interactions between swelling and alkalinization in mediating the effects of insulin. *Biochem J* 1992;282:797–805.
208. Haussinger D, Lang F, Bauers K, Gerok W. Control of hepatic nitrogen metabolism and glutathione release by cell volume regulatory mechanisms. *Eur J Biochem* 1990;193:891–898.
209. Low SY, Taylor PM, Rennie MJ. Responses of glutamine transport in cultured rat skeletal muscle to osmotically induced changes in cell volume. *J Physiol* (Lond) 1996;492:877–885.
210. Moran J, Maar TE, Pasantes-Morales H. Impaired cell volume regulation in taurine deficient cultured astrocytes. *Neurochem Res* 1994;19:415–420.
211. Law RO. Taurine efflux and the regulation of cell volume in incubated slices of rat cerebral cortex. *Biochim Biophys Acta* 1994;1221:21–28.

212. Faff-Michalak L, Reichenbach A, Dettmer D, Kellner K, Albrecht J. K(+)-, hypoosmolarity-, and NH4(+)-induced taurine release from cultured rabbit Muller cells: role of Na+ and Cl– ions and relation to cell volume changes. *Glia* 1994;10:114–120.

213. Kirk K, Kirk J. Volume-regulatory taurine release from a human lung cancer cell line. Evidence for amino acid transport via a volume-activated chloride channel. *FEBS Lett* 1993;336:153–158.

214. Schousboe A, Pasantes-Morales H. Role of taurine in neural cell volume regulation. *Can J Physiol Pharmacol* 1992;70(Suppl):S356–S361.

215. Fugelli K, Thoroed SM. Taurine transport associated with cell volume regulation in flounder erythrocytes under anisosmotic conditions. *J Physiol* (Lond) 1986;374:245–261.

216. Law RO. Taurine efflux and cell volume regulation in cerebral cortical slices during chronic hypernatraemia. *Neurosci Lett* 1995;185:56–59.

217. Goldstein L, Davis EM. Taurine, betaine, and inositol share a volume-sensitive transporter in skate erythrocyte cell membrane. *Am J Physiol* 1994;267:R426–R431.

218. Parry-Billings M, Bevan SJ, Opara E, Newsholme EA. Effects of changes in cell volume on the rates of glutamine and alanine release from rat skeletal muscle *in vitro*. *Biochem J* 1991;276:559–561.

219. Haussinger D, Hallbrucker C, vom Dahl S, Lang F, Gerok W. Cell swelling inhibits proteolysis in perfused rat liver. *Biochem J* 1990;272:239–242.

220. Fugelli K, Kanli H, Terreros DA. Taurine efflux is a cell volume regulatory process in proximal renal tubules from the teleost *Carassius auratus*. *Acta Physiol Scand* 1995;155:223–232.

221. vom Dahl S, Hallbrucker C, Lang F, Haussinger D. Role of eicosanoids, inositol phosphates and extracellular Ca2+ in cell-volume regulation of rat liver. *Eur J Biochem* 1991;198:73–83.

222. Baquet A, Maisin L, Hue L. Swelling of rat hepatocytes activates acetyl-CoA carboxylase in parallel to glycogen synthase. *Biochem J* 1991;278:887–890.

223. Baquet A, Lavoinne A, Hue L. Comparison of the effects of various amino acids on glycogen synthesis, lipogenesis and ketogenesis in isolated rat hepatocytes. *Biochem J* 1991;273:57–62.

224. Guzman M, Velasco G, Castro J, Zammit VA. Inhibition of carnitine palmitoyltransferase I by hepatocyte swelling. *FEBS Lett* 1994;344:239–241.

225. Graf J, Haddad P, Haeussinger D, Lang F. Cell volume regulation in liver. *Ren Physiol Biochem* 1988;11:202–220.

226. Lang F, Stehle T, Haussinger D. Water, K+, H+, lactate and glucose fluxes during cell volume regulation in perfused rat liver. *Pflugers Arch* 1989;413:209–216.

227. Meijer AJ, Baquet A, Gustafson L, van Woerkom GM, Hue L. Mechanism of activation of liver glycogen synthase by swelling. *J Biol Chem* 1992;267:5823–5828.

228. Rivas T, Urcelay E, Gonzalez-Manchon C, Parrilla R, Ayuso MS. Role of amino acid-induced changes in ion fluxes in the regulation of hepatic protein synthesis. *J Cell Physiol* 1995;163:277–284.

229. Felipe A, Snyders DJ, Deal KK, Tamkum MM. Influence of cloned voltage-gated K+ channel expression on alanine transport, Rb+ uptake, and cell volume. *Am J Physiol* 1993;265:C1230–C1238.

230. Kristensen LO, Folke M. Volume-regulatory K+ efflux during concentrative uptake of alanine in isolated rat hepatocytes. *Biochem J* 1984;221:265–268.

231. Wettstein M, vom Dahl S, Lang F, Gerok W, Haussinger D. Cell volume regulatory responses of isolated perfused rat liver. The effect of amino acids. *Biol Chem Hoppe Seyler* 1990;371:493–501.

232. Biolo G, Tipton KD, Klein S, Wolfe RR. An abundant supply of amino acids enhances the metabolic effect of exercise on muscle protein. *Am J Physiol* 1997;273:E122–E129.

233. Meijer AJ, Gustafson LA, Luiken JJ, Blommaart PJ, Caro LH, Van Woerkom GM, Spronk C, Boon L. Cell swelling and the sensitivity of autophagic proteolysis to inhibition by amino acids in isolated rat hepatocytes. *Eur J Biochem* 1993;215:449–454.

234. Kruppa J, Clemens MJ. Differential kinetics of changes in the state of phosphorylation of ribosomal protein S6 and in the rate of protein synthesis in MPC 11 cells during tonicity shifts. *EMBO J* 1984;3:95–100.

235. Roth E, Spittler A, Oehler R. Glutamine: effects on the immune system, protein balance and intestinal functions. *Wien Klin Wochenschr* 1996;108:669–676.

236. Varnier M, Leese GP, Thompson J, Rennie MJ. Stimulatory effect of glutamine on glycogen accumulation in human skeletal muscle. *Am J Physiol* 1995;269:E309–E315.

237. Wu G, Flynn NE. Regulation of glutamine and glucose metabolism by cell volume in lymphocytes and macrophages. *Biochim Biophys Acta* 1995;1243:343–350.

238. Smith RJ. Glutamine metabolism and its physiologic importance. *J Parenter Enteral Nutr* 1990;14(Suppl):40S–44S.

239. Hudson RL, Schultz SG. Sodium-coupled glycine uptake by Ehrlich ascites tumor cells results in an increase in cell volume and plasma membrane channel activities. *Proc Natl Acad Sci USA* 1988;85:279–283.

240. vom Dahl S, Stoll B, Gerok W, Haussinger D. Inhibition of proteolysis by cell swelling in the liver requires intact microtubular structures. *Biochem J* 1995;308:529–536.

241. Holen I, Gordon PB, Seglen PO. Inhibition of hepatocytic autophagy by okadaic acid and other protein phosphatase inhibitors. *Eur J Biochem* 1993;215:113–122.

242. Luiken JJ, Blommaart EF, Boon L, van Woerkom GM, Meijer AJ. Cell swelling and the control of autophagic proteolysis in hepatocytes: involvement of phosphorylation of ribosomal protein S6? *Biochem Soc Trans* 1994;22:508–511.

243. Strange K, Ed. *Cellular and Molecular Physiology of Cell Volume Regulation.* Boca Raton, FL: CRC Press, 1994, pp. 215–224.

244. Bianchini L, Grinstein S. In *Interaction of Cell Volume and Cell Function.* Lang F, Haussinger D, Eds. Heidelberg: Spinger Verlag, 1993, pp. 249–277.

245. Colclasure GC, Parker JC. Cytosolic protein concentration is the primary volume signal in dog red cells. *J Gen Physiol* 1991;98:881–892.

246. Maeda T, Wurgler-Murphy SM, Saito H. A two-component system that regulates an osmosensing MAP kinase cascade in yeast. *Nature* 1994;369:242–245.

247. Galcheva-Gargova Z, Derijard B, Wu IH, Davis RJ. An osmosensing signal transduction pathway in mammalian cells. *Science* 1994;265:806–808.

248. Lang F, Haussinger D, Eds. *Interaction of Cell Volume and Cell Function.* Heidelberg: Springer Verlag, 1993.

249. Slawinski M, Grodzinska L, Kostka-Trabka E, Bieron K, Goszcz A, Gryglewski RJ. L-arginine — substrate for NO synthesis — its beneficial effects in therapy of patients with peripheral arterial disease: comparison with placebo-preliminary results. *Acta Physiol Hung* 1996;84:457–458.

250. Ceremuzynski L, Chamiec T, Herbaczynska-Cedro K. Effect of supplemental oral L-arginine on exercise capacity in patients with stable angina pectoris. *Am J Cardiol* 1997;80:331–333.

251. Bradley SJ, Kingwell BA, McConell GK. Nitric oxide synthase inhibition reduces leg glucose uptake but not blood flow during dynamic exercise in humans. *Diabetes* 1999;48:1815–1821; erratum, 1999;48:2480.

252. Kingwell BA, Formosa M, Muhlmann M, Bradley SJ, McConell GK. Nitric oxide synthase inhibition reduces glucose uptake during exercise in individuals with type 2 diabetes more than in control subjects. *Diabetes* 2002;51:2572–2580.

253. Tipton KD, Rasmussen BB, Miller SL, et al. Timing of amino acid-carbohydrate ingestion alters anabolic response of muscle to resistance exercise. *Am J Physiol Endocrinol Metab* 2001;281:E197.

254. Campbell B, Baer J, Roberts M, Vacanti T, Marcello B, Thomas A, Kirksick C, Wilborn C, Rohle D, Taylor L, Rasmussen C, Greenwood M, Wilson R, Kreider R. Effects of Arginine Alpha-Ketoglutarate Supplementation on Body Composition and Training Adaptations. Paper presented at International Society of Sports Nutrition National Conference, June 17–18, 2004, Las Vegas, NV.

255. Vacanti T, Campell B, Marcello B, Thomas A, Kirksick C, Wilborn C, Rohle D, Taylor L, Rasmussen C, Greenwood M, Wilson R, Kreider R. Effects of Arginine Alpha-Ketoglutarate Supplementation on Markers of Catabolism and Health Status. Paper presented at International Society of Sports Nutrition National Conference, June 17–18, 2004.

256. Biolo G, Maggi SP, Williams BD, Tipton KD, Wolfe RR. Increased rates of muscle protein turnover and amino acid transport after resistance exercise in humans. *Am J Physiol* 1995;268:E514.

257. Chesley A, MacDougall JD, Tarnopolsky MA, Atkinson SA, Smith K. Changes in human muscle protein synthesis after resistance exercise. *J Appl Physiol* 1992;73:1383.

258. Phillips SM, Tipton KD, Aarsland A, Wolf SE, Wolfe RR. Mixed muscle protein synthesis and breakdown following resistance exercise in humans. *Am J Physiol* 1997;273:E99.

259. Yarasheski KE, Zachwieja JF, Bier DM. Acute effects of resistance exercise on muscle protein synthesis rate in young and elderly men and women. *Am J Physiol* 1993;265:E210.

260. Phillips SM, Tipton KD, Ferrando AA, Wolfe RR. Resistance training reduces the acute exercise-induced increase in muscle protein turnover. *Am J Physiol* 1999;276:E118.

261. Rasmussen BB, Tipton KD, Miller SL, Wolf SE, Wolfe RR. An oral essential amino acid-carbohydrate supplement enhances muscle protein anabolism after resistance exercise. *J Appl Physiol* 2000;88:386.

262. Tipton KD, Ferrando AA, Phillips SM, Doyle DJ, Wolfe RR. Postexercise net protein synthesis in human muscle from orally administered amino acids. *Am J Physiol* 1999;276:E628–E634.

263. Svanberg E, Möller-Loswick A-C, Matthews DE, et al. Effects of amino acids on synthesis and degradation of skeletal muscle proteins in humans. *Am J Physiol* 1996;271:E718.

264. Svanberg E, Ohlsson C, Hyltander A, Lundholm KG. The role of diet components, gastrointestinal factors, and muscle innervation on activation of protein synthesis in skeletal muscles following oral refeeding. *Nutrition* 1999;15:257.

265. Svanberg E, Jefferson LS, Lundholm K, Kimball SR. Postprandial stimulation of muscle protein synthesis is independent of changes in insulin. *Am J Physiol* 1997;272:E841.

266. Svanberg E. Amino acids may be intrinsic regulators of protein synthesis in response to feeding. *Clin Nutr* 1998;17:77.
267. Tipton KD, Wolfe RR. Exercise-induced changes in protein metabolism. *Acta Physiol Scand* 1998;162:377.
268. Bohe J, Low A, Wolfe RR, Rennie MJ. Human muscle protein synthesis is modulated by extracellular, not intramuscular amino acid availability: a dose response study. *J Physiol* 2003;552:315.
269. Carraro F, Stuart CA, Hartl WH, Rosenblatt J, Wolfe RR. Effect of exercise and recovery on muscle protein synthesis in human subjects. *Am J Physiol* 1990;259:E470–E476.
270. Biolo G, Fleming RYD, Wolfe RR. Physiologic hyperinsulinemia stimulates protein synthesis and enhances transport of selected amino acids in human skeletal muscle. *J Clin Invest* 1995;95:811–819.
271. Borsheim E, Tipton KD, Wolf SE, Wolfe RR. Essential amino acids and muscle protein recovery from resistance exercise. *Am J Physiol Endocrinol Metab* 2002;283:E648.
272. Miller SL, Tipton KD, Chinkes DL, Wolf SE, Wolfe RR. Independent and combined effects of amino acids and glucose after resistance exercise. *Med Sci Sports Exerc* 2003;35:449.
273. Tipton KD, Borsheim E, Wolf SE, Sanford AP, Wolfe RR. Acute response of net muscle protein balance reflects 24-h balance after exercise and amino acid ingestion. *Am J Physiol Endocrinol Metab* 2003;284:E76.
274. Bohe J, Low Aili F, Wolfe RR, Rennie MJ. Latency and duration of stimulation of human muscle protein synthesis during continuous infusion of amino acids. *J Physiol* 2001;532:575–579.
275. Volpi E, Kobayashi H, Sheffield-Moore M, Mittendorfer B, Wolfe RR. Essential amino acids are primarily responsible for the amino acid stimulation of muscle protein anabolism in healthy elderly adults. *Am J Clin Nutr* 2003;78:250–258.
276. Wojtaszewski JF, Nielsen JN, Richter EA. Invited review: effect of acute exercise on insulin signaling and action in humans. *J Appl Physiol* 2002;93:384–392.
277. Kimball SR, Farrell PA, Jefferson LS. Invited review: role of insulin in translational control of protein synthesis in skeletal muscle by amino acids or exercise. *J Appl Physiol* 2002;93:1168–1180 (review).
278. Esmarck B, Andersen JL, Olsen S, et al. Timing of postexercise protein intake is important for muscle hypertrophy with resistance training in elderly humans. *J Physiol* 2001;535:301.
279. Tarnopolsky MA, MacDougall JD, Atkinson SA. Influence of protein intake and training status on nitrogen balance and lean body mass. *J Appl Physiol* 1988;64:187–193.
280. Tarnopolsky MA, Atkinson SA, MacDougall JD, et al. Evaluation of protein requirements for trained strength athletes. *J Appl Physiol* 1992;73:1986.
281. Lemon PW, Tarnopolsky MA, MacDougall JD, Atkinson SA. Protein requirements and muscle mass/strength changes during intensive training in novice bodybuilders. *J Appl Physiol* 1992;73:767.
282. Walberg JL, Leidy MK, Sturgill DJ, Hinkle DE, Ritchey SJ, Sebolt DR. Macronutrient content of a hypoenergy diet affects nitrogen retention and muscle function in weight lifters. *Int J Sports Med* 1988;9:261–266.
283. Hoffer LJ, Bistrian BR, Young VR, Blackburn GL, Matthews DE. Metabolic effects of very low calorie weight reduction diets. *J Clin Invest* 1984;73:750–758.

284. Millward DJ, Bowtell JL, Pacy P, Rennie MJ. Physical activity, protein metabolism and protein requirements. *Proc Nutr Soc* 1994;53:223.

285. Millward DJ. *The Role of Protein and Amino Acids in Sustaining and Enhancing Performance*. Washington, DC: National Academy Press, 1999, p. 169.

286. Butterfield GE, Calloway DH. Physical activity improves protein utilization in young men. *Br J Nutr* 1984;51:171.

287. Gontzea I, Sutzescu P, Dumitrache S. The influence of adaptation to physical effort on nitrogen balance in man. *Nutr Rep Int* 1975;22:231.

288. Ratamess NA, Kraemer WJ, Volek JS, Rubin MR, Gomez AL, French DN, Sharman MJ, McGuigan MM, Scheett T, Hakkinen K, Newton RU, Dioguardi F. The effects of amino acid supplementation on muscular performance during resistance training overreaching. *J Strength Cond Res* 2003;17:250–258.

289. Phillips SM, Parise G, Roy BD, et al. Resistance-training-induced adaptations in skeletal muscle protein turnover in the fed state. *Can J Physiol Pharmacol* 2002;80:1045.

290. Todd KS, Butterfield GE, Calloway DH. Nitrogen balance in men with adequate and deficient energy intake at three levels of work. *J Nutr* 1984;114:2107.

291. Calloway DH, Spector H. Nitrogen balance as related to caloric and protein intake in active young men. *Am J Clin Nutr* 1954;2:405.

292. Zachwieja JJ, Ezell DM, Cline AD, et al. Short-term dietary energy restriction reduces lean body mass but not performance in physically active men and women. *Int J Sports Med* 2001;22:310.

293. Cox KL, Burke V, Morton AR, Beilin LJ, Puddey IB. The independent and combined effects of 16 weeks of vigorous exercise and energy restriction on body mass and composition in free-living overweight men — a randomized controlled trial. *Metabolism* 2003;52:107.

294. Kraemer WJ, Volek JS, Clark KL, et al. Influence of exercise training on physiological and performance changes with weight loss in men. *Med Sci Sports Exerc* 1999;31:1320.

295. Farnsworth E, Luscombe ND, Noakes M, et al. Effect of a high-protein, energy restricted diet on body composition, glycemic control, and lipid concentrations in overweight and obese hyperinsulinemic men and women. *Am J Clin Nutr* 2003;78:31.

296. Richardson DP, Wayler AH, Scrimshaw NS, Young VR. Quantitative effect of an isoenergetic exchange of fat for carbohydrate on dietary protein utilization in healthy young men. *Am J Clin Nutr* 1979;32:2217.

297. Phillips SM. Protein requirements and supplementation in strength sports. *Nutrition* 2004;20:689–695 (review).

298. Hellman A, Brummer K. Effect of dietary supplement on plasma hGH following exercise challenge. *Biolog Biomed Sci*, 2003; 1.

299. Fricker PA, Beasly SK, Copeland IW. Physiological growth hormone response of throwers to amino acids, eating, and exercise. *Aust J Med Sport* 1988;20:21.

300. Isidori A, Lo Monaco A, Cappa M. A study of growth hormone release in man after oral administration of amino acids. *Curr Med Res Opin* 1981;7:475–481.

301. Carlson HE, Gillin JC, Gorden P, Snyder F. Abscence of sleep-related growth hormone peaks in aged normal subjects and in acromegaly. *J Clin Endocrinol Metab* 1972;34:1102–1105.

302. Finkelstein JW, Roffwarg HP, Boyar RM, Kream J, Hellman L. Age-related change in the twenty-four-hour spontaneous secretion of growth hormone. *J Clin Endocrinol Metab* 1972;35:665–670.

303. Rudman D, Kutner MH, Rogers CM, Lubin MF, Fleming GA, Bain RP. Impaired growth hormone secretion in the adult population: relation to age and adiposity. *J Clin Invest* 1981;67:1361–1369.

304. Prinz PN, Weitzman ED, Cunningham GR, Karacan I. Plasma growth hormone during sleep in young and aged men. *J Gerontol* 1983;38:519–524.

305. Zadik Z, Chalew SA, McCarter RJ Jr, Meistas M, Kowarski AA. The influence of age on the 24-hour integrated concentration of growth hormone in normal individuals. *J Clin Endocrinol Metab* 1985;60:513–516.

306. Florini JR, Prinz PN, Vitiello MV, Hintz RL. Somatomedin-C levels in healthy young and old men: relationship to peak and 24-hour integrated levels of growth hormone. *J Gerontol* 1985;40:2–7.

307. Vermeulen A. Nyctohemeral growth hormone profiles in young and aged men: correlation with somatomedin-C levels. *J Clin Endocrinol Metab* 1987;64:884–888.

308. Ho KY, Evans WS, Blizzard RM, Veldhuis JD, Merriam GR, Samojlik E, Furlanetto R, Rogol AD, Kaiser DL, Thorner MO. Effects of sex and age on the 24-hour profile of growth hormone secretion in man: importance of endogenous estradiol concentrations. *J Clin Endocrinol Metab* 1987;64:51–58.

309. Tanaka K, Inoue S, Shiraki J, Shishido T, Saito M, Numata K, Takamura Y. Age-related decrease in plasma growth hormone: response to growth hormone-releasing hormone, arginine, and L-dopa in obesity. *Metabolism* 1991;40:1257–1262.

310. Pritzlaff CJ, Wideman L, Weltman JY, Abbott RD, Gutgesell ME, Hartman ML, Veldhuis JD, Weltman A. Impact of acute exercise intensity on pulsatile growth hormone release in men. *J Appl Physiol* 1999;87:498–504.

311. Sutton J, Lazarus L. Growth hormone in exercise: comparison of physiological and pharmacological stimuli. *J Appl Physiol* 1976;41:523–527.

312. Sutton J, Lazarus L. Effect of adrenergic blocking agents on growth hormone responses to physical exercise. *Horm Metab Res* 1974;6:428–429.

313. Gotshalk LA, Loebel CC, Nindl BC, Putukian M, Sebastianelli WJ, Newton RU, Hakkinen K, Kraemer WJ. Hormonal responses of multiset versus single-set heavy-resistance exercise protocols. *Can J Appl Physiol* 1997;22:244–255.

314. Kraemer WJ, Fleck SJ, Dziados JE, Harman EA, Marchitelli LJ, Gordon SE, Mello R, Frykman PN, Koziris LP, Triplett NT. Changes in hormonal concentrations after different heavy-resistance exercise protocols in women. *J Appl Physiol* 1993;75:594–604.

315. Kraemer WJ, Gordon SE, Fleck SJ, Marchitelli LJ, Mello R, Dziados JE, Friedl K, Harman E, Maresh C, Fry AC. Endogenous anabolic hormonal and growth factor responses to heavy resistance exercise in males and females. *Int J Sports Med* 1991;12:228–235.

316. Kraemer WJ, Marchitelli L, Gordon SE, Harman E, Dziados JE, Mello R, Frykman P, McCurry D, Fleck SJ. Hormonal and growth factor responses to heavy resistance exercise protocols. *J Appl Physiol* 1990;69:1442–1450.

317. Vanhelder WP, Radomski MW, Goode RC. Growth hormone responses during intermittent weight lifting exercise in men. *Eur J Appl Physiol Occup Physiol* 1984;53:31–34.

318. Kraemer RR, Kilgore JL, Kraemer GR, Castracane VD. Growth hormone, IGF-I, and testosterone responses to resistive exercise. *Med Sci Sports Exerc* 1992;24:1346–1352.

319. Ahlborg G, Felig P, Hagenfeldt L, Hendler R, Wahren J. Substrate turnover during prolonged exercise in man. Splanchnic and leg metabolism of glucose, free fatty acids, and amino acids. *J Clin Invest* 1974;53:1080–1090.

320. Kraemer WJ, Volek JS, Bush JA, Putukian M, Sebastianelli WJ. Hormonal responses to consecutive days of heavy-resistance exercise with or without nutritional supplementation. *J Appl Physiol* 1998;85:1544–1555.

321. Chandler RM, Byrne HK, Patterson JG, Ivy JL. Dietary supplements affect the anabolic hormones after weight-training exercise. *J Appl Physiol* 1994;76:839–845.

322. Spruce N, Titchenal A. *An Evaluation of Popular Fitness-Enhancing Supplements.* Thousand Oaks, CA: Evergreen Communications, 2001.

323. Sellini M, Fierro A, Marchesi L, Manzo G, Giovannini C. Behavior of basal values and circadian rhythm of ACTH, cortisol, PRL and GH in a high-protein diet. *Boll Soc Ital Biol Sper* 1981;57:963–969.

324. Jorgensen JO, Moller N, Lauritzen T, Christiansen JS. Pulsatile versus continuous intravenous administration of growth hormone (GH) in GH-deficient patients: effects on circulating insulin-like growth factor-I and metabolic indices. *J Clin Endocrinol Metab* 1990;70:1616–1623.

325. Laursen T, Jorgensen JO, Jakobsen G, Hansen BL, Christiansen JS. Continuous infusion versus daily injections of growth hormone (GH) for 4 weeks in GH-deficient patients. *J Clin Endocrinol Metab* 1995;80:2410–2418.

326. Macintyre JG. Growth hormone and athletes. *Sports Med.* 1987;4:129–142.

327. Quirion A, Brisson G, De Carufel D, Laurencelle L, Therminarias A, Vogelaere P. Influence of exercise and dietary modifications on plasma human growth hormone, insulin and FFA. *J Sports Med Phys Fitness* 1988;28:352–353.

328. Wolfe RR. Protein supplements and exercise. *Am J Clin Nutr* 2000;72(Suppl):551S–557S (review).

329. Paddon-Jones D, Sheffield-Moore M, Aarsland A, Wolfe RR, Ferrando AA. Exogenous amino acids stimulate human muscle anabolism without interfering with the response to mixed meal ingestion. *Am J Physiol Endocrinol Metab* 2005;288:E761–E767.

330. Paddon-Jones D, Sheffield-Moore M, Urban RJ, Sanford AP, Aarsland A, Wolfe RR, Ferrando AA. Essential amino acid and carbohydrate supplementation ameliorates muscle protein loss in humans during 28 days bedrest. *J Clin Endocrinol Metab* 2004;89:4351–4358.

331. Andersen LL, Tufekovic G, Zebis MK, Crameri RM, Verlaan G, Kjaer M, Suetta C, Magnusson P, Aagaard P. The effect of resistance training combined with timed ingestion of protein on muscle fiber size and muscle strength. *Metabolism* 2005;54:151–156.

332. Campbell WW, Crim MC, Young VR, Joseph LJ, Evans WJ. Effects of resistance training and dietary protein intake on protein metabolism in older adults. *Am J Physiol* 1995;268:E1143–E1153.

333. Fiatarone MA, O'Neill EF, Ryan ND, Clements KM, Solares GR, Nelson ME, Roberts SB, Kehayias JJ, Lipsitz LA, Evans WJ. Exercise training and nutritional supplementation for physical frailty in very elderly people. *N Engl J Med* 1994;330:1769–1775.

334. Welle S, Thornton CA. High-protein meals do not enhance myofibrillar synthesis after resistance exercise in 62- to 75-yr-old men and women. *Am J Physiol* 1998;274:E677–E683.

335. Volpi E, Ferrando AA, Yeckel CW, Tipton KD, Wolfe RR. Exogenous amino acids stimulate net muscle protein synthesis in the elderly. *J Clin Invest* 1998;101:2000–2007.

336. Volpi E, Mittendorfer B, Wolf SE, Wolfe RR. Oral amino acids stimulate muscle protein anabolism in the elderly despite higher first pass splanchnic extraction. *Am J Physiol* 1999;277:E513–E520.

337. Volpi E, Mittendorfer B, Rasmussen BB, Wolfe RR. The response of muscle protein anabolism to combined hyperaminoacidemia and glucose-induced hyperinsulinemia is impaired in the elderly. *J Clin Endocrinol Metab* 2000;85:4481–4490.

338. Fujita S, Volpi E. Amino acids and muscle loss with aging. *J Nutr* 2006;136(Suppl):277S–280S (review).

339. Volpi E, Sheffield-Moore M, Rasmussen BB, Wolfe RR. Basal muscle amino acid kinetics and protein synthesis in healthy young and older men. *JAMA* 2001;286:1206–1212.

340. Antonio J, Sanders MS, Ehler LA, Uelmen J, Raether JB, Stout JR. Effects of exercise training and amino-acid supplementation on body composition and physical performance in untrained women. *Nutrition* 2000;16:1043–1046.

341. Williams AG, Van den Oord M, Sharma A, Jones DA. Is glucose/amino acid supplementation after exercise an aid to strength training? *Br J Sports Med* 2001;35:109–113.

342. Singh M, Karpovich PV. Isotonic and isometric forces of forearm flexors and extensors. *J Appl Physiol* 1966;21:1435–1437.

343. Komi PV, Buskirk ER. Effect of eccentric and concentric muscle conditioning on tension and electrical activity of human muscle. *Ergonomics* 1972;15:417–434.

344. McNeil PL, Khakee R. Disruptions of muscle fiber plasma membranes. *Am J Pathol* 1992;140:1097–1099.

345. Warren GL, Lowe DA, Hayes DA, Farmer MA, Armstrong RB. Redistribution of cell membrane probes following contraction-induced injury of mouse soleus muscle. *Cell Tissue Res* 1995;282:311–320.

346. Byrd SK. Alterations in the sarcoplasmic reticulum: a possible link to exercise-induced muscle damage. *Med Sci Sports Exerc* 1992;24:531–536.

347. Sugita M, Ohtani M, Ishii N, Maruyama K, Kobayashi K. Effect of a selected amino acid mixture on the recovery from muscle fatigue during and after eccentric contraction exercise training. *Biosci Biotechnol Biochem* 2003;67:372–375.

348. Ohtani M, Maruyama K, Suzuki S, Sugita M, Kobayashi K. Changes in hematological parameters of athletes after receiving daily dose of a mixture of 12 amino acids for one month during the middle- and long-distance running training. *Biosci Biotechnol Biochem* 2001;65:348–355.

349. Ohtani M, Maruyama K, Sugita M, Kobayashi K. Amino acid supplementation affects hematological and biochemical parameters in elite rugby players. *Biosci Biotechnol Biochem* 2001;65:1970–1976.

350. Staron RS, Karapondo DL, Kraemer WJ, et al. Skeletal muscle adaptations during early phase of heavy-resistance training in men and women. *J Appl Physiol* 1994;76:1247.

351. Green H, Goreham C, Ouyang J, Ball-Burnett M, Ranney D. Regulation of fiber size, oxidative potential, and capillarization in human muscle by resistance exercise. *Am J Physiol* 1999;276:R591.

352. McCall GE, Byrnes WC, Dickinson A, Pattany PM, Fleck SJ. Muscle fiber hypertrophy, hyperplasia, and capillary density in college men after resistance training. *J Appl Physiol* 1996;81:2004.

353. Yarasheski KE, Pak-Loduca J, Hasten DL, et al. Resistance exercise training increases mixed muscle protein synthesis rate in frail women and men 76 yr old. *Am J Physiol* 1999;277:E118.

354. Tipton KD, Cocke TL, Wolf SE, Wolfe RR. Response of muscle protein metabolism to resistance training and acute resistance exercise during hyperaminoacidemia. *Am J Physiol* 2006; in press.

355. Food and Nutrition Board, Institute of Medicine. *Dietary Reference Intakes for Energy, Carbohydrate, Fiber, Fat, Fatty Acids, Cholesterol, Protein, and Amino Acids.* Washington, DC: National Academy Press, 2005.

356. Safety Information. Food and Drug Administration, 2006. http://www.fda.gov/medwatch/.

357. Maughan RJ, Burke LM. *Sports Nutrition: Olympic Handbook of Sports Medicine.* Oxford: Blackwell Publishing, 2002.

358. FAO/WHO. Protein Quality Evaluation. FAO Food and Nutrition Paper 51. Rome: FAO, 1991.

359. American College of Sports Medicine, American Dietetic Association, Dietitians of Canada. Joint position statement: nutrition and athletic performance. *Med Sci Sports Exerc* 2000;32:2130–2145.

360. Isidori A, Lo Monaco A, Cappa M. A study of growth hormone release in man after oral administration of amino acids. *Curr Med Res Opin* 1981;7(7):475–481.

361. Ohtani M, Sugita M, Maruyama K. Amino acid mixture improves training efficiency in athletes. *J Nutr* 2006;Feb;136(2):538S–543S.

362. Faber M, Benada AJ, Nutrient intake and dietary supplementation in bodybuilders. *S Afr Med J* 1987;72:831.

363. Roy BD, Tarnopolsky MA, MacDougall JD, Fowles J, Yarasheski KE. Effect of glucose supplement timing on protein metabolism after resistance training. *J Appl Physiol* 1997;82:1882.

364. Short SH, Short WR. Four-year study of university athletes' dietary intake. *J Am Diet Assoc* 1983;82:632.

Section IV

Recommended Intakes of the Energy-Yielding Nutrients

16 Recommended Proportions of Carbohydrates to Fats to Proteins in Diets

Henry C. Lukaski

CONTENTS

16.1 INTRODUCTION

Physically active people are concerned about their daily energy intake for various reasons. Individuals participating in endurance or resistance training, whose daily caloric intakes can exceed 5000 kcal (~21,000 MJ),[1] may be anxious not only to obtain an adequate amount of calories to match those expended in training, but also to consume the proportion of macronutrients to promote training and heighten performance. In contrast, sedentary men and women who seek to attain a healthy body weight by adopting healthful eating plans and increasing physical activity are anxious about limiting total energy intake and adjusting the mixture of macronutrients to optimize health and well-being.[2] Thus, the roles of dietary carbohydrate, fat, and protein, as well as the recommended intakes, remain topics of research interest not only to promote optimal performance among athletes, but also to support health and physical fitness in the general population.

The ability to perform mechanical work is a function of skeletal muscle, and factors that affect energy production in muscle directly impact the performance of physical activity. The immediate source of energy for muscle contraction is the hydrolysis of adenosine triphosphate (ATP) to yield energy. The ATP content in muscle is limited; it is estimated to be 5.5 mmol/kg, or ~3.4 g in 20 kg of skeletal muscle of a 70-kg man.[3] This amount of ATP would be exhausted in a few seconds of high-intensity activity; thus, ATP is rapidly replenished. Most physical activities rely on a combination of carbohydrate and fat metabolism to refill ATP stores by using aerobic pathways, principally mitochondrial oxidative phosphorylation. Anaerobic ATP production, however, is necessary when oxidative phosphorylation cannot provide ATP in adequate amounts needed to meet demands for muscle contraction. A number of factors influence muscle fuel selection, including the amount of stored substrates in muscle, the training status of the individual, exercise conditions (i.e., intensity and duration), environmental conditions, and nutrient intake during the activity. Among these factors, the pre-exercise endogenous fuel stores, particularly carbohydrate, are likely to limit physical performance.[3] Other dietary factors may influence performance and training. Adaptation to a high-fat diet is reported to promote endurance performance.[4] Consumption of high-protein diets also is thought to promote muscle accretion and strength gain during resistance training.[5]

This chapter succinctly describes the roles that the macronutrients play in facilitating exercise training and performance. Emphasis is placed on the relative amounts (percent daily energy intake and gram per kilogram body weight) of carbohydrate, fat, and protein consumed to promote optimal training and performance. A comparison of these guidelines (gram per kilogram body weight and percent energy) is provided.

16.2 CARBOHYDRATE AND PERFORMANCE

It is well accepted by sports dietitians and athletes that carbohydrate plays a key role in supporting physical activity because of the need to maintain blood glucose concentrations.[6] Although body stores of energy are variable, available carbohydrate is very limited (Table 16.1). The practical importance of stored carbohydrate or

TABLE 16.1
Estimated Energy Stores in Man[a]

	Weight, kg	Energy, kcal (KJ)
Blood glucose	0.02	80 (320)
Liver glycogen	0.1	400 (1670)
Muscle glycogen	0.4	1450 (6600)
Plasma fatty acids	0.0004	4 (16)
Plasma triacylglycerols	0.004	40 (167)
Intramuscular triacylglycerols	0.3	2620 (10,952)
Adipose fatty acids	10,500	92,940 (388,500)
Protein	12,000	48,800 (204,000)

[a] 70-kg man with 15% body fat.

Source: Adopted from Jeukendrup, A.E. et al., *Int. J. Sports Med.*, 19, 231–244, 1998.

glycogen is that, after hydrolyzed, it forms glucose, which is either used in muscle cells or transported from the liver for use by other cells. If glucose is fully oxidized to carbon dioxide and water (aerobic glycolysis or tricarboxylic acid cycle), more ATP is formed (39 vs. 4 moles of ATP per mole of glycosyl units consumed) than with anaerobic glycolysis and lactate formation. Another advantage of carbohydrate as an energy source is that it requires less oxygen for complete oxidation than fat (fatty acids) and protein (amino acids) because carbohydrate contains a higher ratio of oxygen to carbon and hydrogen. Thus, under conditions of limited oxygen availability, such as high-intensity work, carbohydrate is the preferential fuel source. A final benefit of carbohydrate is that its storage in skeletal muscle can be upregulated by diet and training regimens.[3] Dietary carbohydrate can be a limiting factor in promoting certain types of physical activity and performance.

16.2.1 USUAL CARBOHYDRATE INTAKE, MUSCLE GLYCOGEN, AND PERFORMANCE

Physically active men and women commonly report carbohydrate intakes similar to weight-matched inactive adults (45 to 55% of daily energy intake, or ~5 g/kg body weight/day).[8,9] In general, these intakes may be adequate to meet the carbohydrate needs of recreational or fitness athletes who participate in moderate levels of activity up to 1 h daily. In contrast, endurance athletes who train with more intense activities that deplete muscle glycogen may have greater carbohydrate needs to ensure adequate muscle glycogen concentrations.

Investigators generally agree that muscle glycogen stores limit physical work capacity and performance during prolonged, moderate- to high-intensity aerobic exercise (>70% peak VO_2 uptake). Thus, accumulation and maintenance of adequate skeletal muscle glycogen during training requires consumption of a carbohydrate-rich diet on a daily basis. Generally, skeletal muscle glycogen concentrations are

100 to 120 mmol/kg wet weight (ww). Consumption of a 45% carbohydrate diet did not maintain muscle glycogen concentrations during high-intensity training, as they declined from 110 to 88 to 66 mmol/kg during 3 days of intense running training.[10] In a comprehensive review, Sherman and Wimer[11] extended these findings in other groups of endurance athletes and concluded that more than 45% dietary carbohydrate was needed to replenish muscle glycogen stores during training and to avoid performance decrements. More recently, additional evidence shows that daily carbohydrate intake exceeding 50% total energy intake maintains muscle glycogen during training and performance of athletes participating in anaerobic sports.[12] Thus, amounts of dietary carbohydrate usually consumed by the population are inadequate to maintain muscle glycogen and performance of athletes.

16.2.2 PRE-EXERCISE CARBOHYDRATE INGESTION

The importance of a pre-event meal or snack is to compensate for a lack of adequate carbohydrate in the previous day's meals and ensure adequate glycogen stores in liver and muscle. Feedings are generally small but high in carbohydrate (200 to 300 g), moderate in protein, and low in fat and fiber. Findings of controlled studies reveal that 200 to 300 g of carbohydrate fed 3 to 4 h before testing improved various indices of cycling performance by 15 to 49%.[13]

In contrast, the effect on performance of carbohydrate feeding 30 to 60 min before exercise is unclear. Although blood glucose concentrations increased after ingestion of carbohydrate,[14] one study[15] reported improved and others[16,17] showed no effects on performance compared to controls. There was consensus of no adverse effects on performance. Sherman et al.[18] reported a 15% improvement in cycling performance when cyclists consumed ~300 g of carbohydrate 4 h before the performance test. Thus, exogenous carbohydrate fed before exercise may be beneficial to individuals who have low glycogen stores.

16.2.3 CARBOHYDRATE INGESTION DURING PHYSICAL ACTIVITY

Participation in moderate-intensity (65 to 80% peak VO_2 uptake) exercise for a prolonged duration (>90 min) leads to fatigue because of reductions in circulating glucose and tissue glycogen stores. Feeding carbohydrate during exercise delays fatigue by maintaining blood glucose levels, whereas the impact on muscle glycogen sparing is controversial.[19,20] Regardless of the mechanism, carbohydrate feeding during prolonged moderate- to high-intensity exercise was beneficial. Male cyclists who consumed 400 g of exogenous carbohydrate increased their endurance performance by 1 h compared to placebo.[19] Running trials with carbohydrate feedings also found improved performance. Men supplemented with 55 g of carbohydrate per hour had increased blood glucose concentrations and completed the last 5 km of a 40-km run faster than they did when running without carbohydrate.[21] In an endurance trial on a treadmill (80% peak VO_2 uptake), men fed 35 g of carbohydrate per hour ran 23 min longer than they did when running without carbohydrate.[22] Thus, consumption of exogenous carbohydrate during prolonged, intense physical activities benefits endurance performance.

The timing and rate of carbohydrate ingestion are also important considerations. If individuals wait until the onset of fatigue before consuming carbohydrate, they may not be able to absorb it quickly enough to avoid fatigue. Coggan and Coyle[23] found that the latest that an individual can consume carbohydrate and prevent fatigue is 30 min before the onset of fatigue. Ingestion of ~50 g of carbohydrate during the first 60 min of a bout of exhausting exercise improved endurance to exhaustion 14% compared to a water placebo.[24] Thus, consumption of carbohydrate during endurance exercise is recommended before the onset of subjective feelings of fatigue to enhance performance.

16.2.4 CARBOHYDRATE INTAKE DURING RECOVERY

Depletion of muscle glycogen content is a significant limitation to recovery from training and competition performance.[3] Muscle glycogen depletion can occur after prolonged (2 to 3 h), continuous (60 to 80% peak VO_2 uptake) training as well as brief, intense (90 to 120% peak VO_2 uptake), intermittent competition and training.[25] Thus, repletion of muscle glycogen stores is a target for recovery from strenuous physical activity.

Muscle glycogen replacement can occur at modest levels of carbohydrate intake. Some investigators report that a moderate carbohydrate intake of 5 to 6 g/kg body weight is adequate to maintain muscle glycogen concentration (~100 mmol/kg ww) during training.[26,27] Other findings indicate that a higher carbohydrate intake (10 vs. 5 g/kg/day) is needed to avoid a gradual depletion of muscle glycogen (33%) during repetitive endurance and sprint training with endurance athletes.[28] Other findings emphasize the importance of increasing dietary carbohydrate on muscle glycogen replenishment and key aspects of training and performance. During an 11-day period of intensive training, competitive athletes fed higher carbohydrate (8.5 compared to 5.4 g/kg/day) maintained physical performance and positive mood state and sustained higher rates of carbohydrate oxidation during exercise sessions.[29] These findings confirmed earlier observations of increased training intensity[30] when *ad libitum* carbohydrate intake increased from 6.5 to 9 g/kg/day during a 7-day period. In a study of competitive rowers during 4 weeks of training, increased dietary carbohydrate (10 vs. 5 g/kg/day) was associated with enhanced muscle glycogen (~155 vs. ~120 mmol/kg ww) and greater improvement in power out (11 vs. 2%) in time trials.[31] Overall, these findings demonstrate that trained athletes benefit from an increased carbohydrate intake during periods of intense training because of the maintenance or enhancement of muscle glycogen stores and an ability to sustain higher rates of carbohydrate oxidation during exercise.

16.2.4.1 Timing of Carbohydrate Intake

The optimal time for carbohydrate ingestion to replenish muscle glycogen stores is during the first hour after exercise.[32] Factors such as selective activation of glycogen synthase by glycogen depletion,[33] exercise-induced increases in insulin sensitivity,[34] and permeability of muscle cell to glucose facilitate glycogen synthesis and accumulation. Ivy et al.[32] found higher rates of glycogen storage (7.7 mmol/kg ww) when carbohydrate was fed during the first 2 h of recovery compared to more typical rates of storage (4.3 mmol/kg ww) without feeding. This finding is important in sports where time between competitions is brief (4 to 8 h).

Whereas it is important to consume carbohydrate as soon as practical after exercise to maximize glycogen repletion, there is little consensus about size of portions to accomplish this goal. Neither number nor size of meals or snacks during the 24 h after exertion significantly affected muscle glycogen storage.[35,36] However, rates of glycogen synthesis during the first 4 to 6 h of recovery were greater when a substantial amount of carbohydrate (10 g/kg) was fed in 16 hourly snacks compared to 4 large meals.[36] Thus, total carbohydrate intake, not a pattern of intake, is a key factor in facilitating muscle glycogen recovery. Issues related to the practicality and comfort of the individual athlete to avoid gastric discomfort should be considered.

16.2.4.2   Glycemic Index and Muscle Glycogen Replenishment

Another practical consideration in the restoration of muscle glycogen is the type of carbohydrate that promotes glycogen storage. Knowledge that glucose and insulin facilitate glycogen synthesis leads to the hypothesis that carbohydrate sources with high or moderate, compared to low, glycemic index enhance glycogen repletion during recovery from intense exercise training. Early studies, which used foods that were classified as containing starches and simple sugars to influence muscle glycogen stores after heavy training, provided conflicting results.[35,37] Burke et al.[38] fed foods with accepted glycemic index values to trained endurance athletes during a 24-h period of recovery after intense training. As hypothesized, the high-glycemic-index foods increased muscle glycogen storage 30% more than an identical amount of carbohydrate derived from low-glycemic-index foods. Subsequent studies have confirmed the benefit of high-glycemic-index carbohydrates in promotion of glycogen storage.[39,40]

16.2.5   Guidelines for Carbohydrate Intake in Athletes

Nutritional strategies to provide adequate amounts of carbohydrate to ensure optimal muscle glycogen replenishment in physically active people have been proposed.[25] It is recommended that a usual intake be 5 to 7 g/kg/day when training or activity is low or moderate intensity. To facilitate recovery after moderate to heavy endurance training, carbohydrate intake should be 7 to 12 g/kg/day. Under conditions of extreme training (i.e., in excess of 4 h daily), the target for carbohydrate intake is 10 to 12 g/kg/day. Regardless of workout intensity, the initial recovery period (0 to 4 h after exercise) should provide 1.0 to 1.2 g/kg/h at frequent intervals (15 to 30 min). The goal of this dietary regimen strategy is to achieve carbohydrate intakes to meet the fuel needs during physical training and to facilitate optimal levels of muscle glycogen stores between workout sessions and in preparation for competition.

16.3 DIETARY FAT AND PERFORMANCE

Participation in prolonged, moderate-intensity aerobic activities (i.e., running, cycling, swimming, etc.) requires both availability and oxidation of carbohydrate and fat regardless of training status. Body fat stores (blood lipids, adipose tissue, and intramuscular triglyceride depots) are a relatively abundant energy source, even among endurance athletes. Thus, factors that increase fat availability may promote endurance performance.[7] Catecholamines stimulate mobilization of fat stores and also increase the activity of lipoprotein lipase that promotes uptake of glycerol and fatty acids from the circulation into muscle cells after 15 to 20 min of moderate-intensity exercise.[41] Aerobic training impacts fuel metabolism by increasing fat oxidation while decreasing endogenous carbohydrate utilization, thus sparing glycogen, to meet energy needs.[42,43] Thus, factors that increase fat (fatty acid and glycerol) oxidation during exercise have been investigated.

16.3.1 FAT LOADING AND ENDURANCE PERFORMANCE

Consumption of diets with very high fat and low or no carbohydrate content leads to ketosis at rest and during activity. Adaptation to diets high in fat (>60% daily energy intake) in trained athletes has been associated with changes in time to exhaustion during endurance tests. In comparison to eucaloric, isonitrogenous diets high in carbohydrate and low in fat, consumption of low-carbohydrate, high-fat diets fed for periods of 1 to 3 days depleted muscle and liver glycogen stores and impaired work capacity and endurance performance.[3,44,45]

Other reports, however, indicate that a longer period (>7 days) of ingestion of a high-fat, low-carbohydrate diet promotes metabolic adaptations that significantly increase during exercise; these adaptations compensate for the relative lack of carbohydrate to meet the energy needs of the activity. Trained individuals consuming high-fat (>60% daily energy intake), low-carbohydrate diets for 5 to 30 days have significantly increased rates of fat oxidation and decreased rates of muscle glycogen utilization during submaximal exercise (50 to 70% peak VO_2 uptake) compared with isocaloric, isonitrogenous, high-carbohydrate diets. Importantly, time to exhaustion during laboratory tests significantly increased.[4,46-50] Although these findings have raised interest among competitive athletes, Burke and Hawley[51] have criticized many technical aspects of these studies, such as the findings being obtained in laboratory and not competitive conditions, and concluded that the suggestion that high-fat, low-carbohydrate diets are beneficial to endurance performance should be viewed cautiously. Their concerns are supported by other reports in trained[52] and untrained adults[53,54] who did not improve performance after eating high-fat, low-carbohydrate compared to high-carbohydrate, low-fat diets for periods up to 4 weeks. Thus, the performance benefits of long-term adherence to a high-fat, low-carbohydrate diet remain controversial.

16.3.2 Post-Exercise Diet and Intramuscular Triacyglycerol (IMTG)

Accumulating evidence indicates that IMTG is an important fuel source during prolonged moderate exercise (up to 85% peak VO_2 uptake) in trained individuals. Studies using histochemical assays[55,56] as well as proton magnetic resonance spectroscopy[57] showed a significant reduction in the IMTG of the upper and lower leg after prolonged exercise in endurance-trained athletes.

Controlled dietary studies revealed that the composition of the post-exercise diet affects the rate of repletion of the IMTG stores. Consumption of a high-fat (68% total energy) diet enhanced IMTG accumulation (33 to 45 mmol/kg) with no recovery (31 to 28 mmol/kg), compared to a low-fat (5%) diet during a 24-h recovery period.[44] Low-fat (20%), high-carbohydrate (65 to 70%) diets do not replete IMTG during 1 day of recovery after prolonged exercise in trained and untrained individuals.[58–61] Despite evidence that dietary fat intake positively influences IMTG levels, limited data indicate a detriment in endurance and sprint performance in cyclists.[62]

16.3.3 Dietary Periodization: Fat and Carbohydrate

Another nutritional strategy that seeks to simultaneously increase endogenous muscle fuel depots is dietary periodization. Endurance athletes adapt their muscles to a high-fat diet for 5 to 6 days, then switch to a very high carbohydrate diet (10 to 12 g/kg/day) and rest for 24 h to optimize glycogen content. The fat adaptation period results in a marked upregulation of muscle metabolic machinery to enhance fat oxidation and promote glycogen sparing in muscle. Unfortunately, there is no evidence that this dietary manipulation has any beneficial effects on physical performance.[63]

16.4 DIETARY PROTEIN NEEDS

Protein from food and beverages plays diverse roles in maintaining body structure and functions. These roles include formation of bone, muscle, connective tissue, hormones, and enzymes, maintenance of fluid and electrolyte balance, transport of micronutrients, and some contribution as an energy source during and after physical activity. Amino acids, which make up protein, are used as an energy source. During periods of energy deficit, amino acids, mobilized principally from endogenous protein stores in soft tissues, become substrates for gluconeogenesis to prevent hypoglycemia. Amino acids, specifically the branched-chain amino acids, can be oxidized directly by muscle and converted to Krebs cycle intermediates to increase acetyl-CoA oxidation.[64] Measurements of by-products of protein catabolism, such as urea and ammonia, in the blood and urine and *in vivo* assessments of oxidation of labeled amino acids, tyrosine and leucine, provide evidence that protein is used as an energy source during exercise. The contribution of protein and amino acids to total energy expenditure is relatively small (2 to 5%) during submaximal efforts but increases to 10% when carbohydrate is depleted during prolonged, intense activity.[65]

16.4.1 Effect of Physical Activity on Protein Requirements

The impact of physical activity on protein needs has been determined principally by using the nitrogen balance method. This approach requires measurements of nitrogen intake and losses (urine and feces) to determine individual protein requirements in response to stressors such as physical activity. A positive balance suggests protein accretion, whereas a negative balance suggests a net loss of body protein.

Studies of adults participating in resistance training highlight the need for increased protein. Lemon et al.[66] studied novice bodybuilders consuming two levels of dietary protein. The nitrogen balance was negative when protein intake was 0.99 g/kg/day, but positive with an intake of 2.62 g/kg/day. Regression analysis (nitrogen balance vs. protein intake) showed that an average protein intake of 1.43 g/kg/day was needed to achieve a 0 balance (i.e., no gain or loss of nitrogen); the apparent protein requirement (0 balance ± 2 SD) was calculated to be 1.6 to 1.7 g/kg/day. Other investigators reported similar estimates of protein needs during resistance training regardless of training status.[5,67] The increased protein requirement apparently is needed to promote accretion of muscle mass to enable strength gains.[5]

There are limited data of nitrogen balance in endurance athletes. Elite male endurance athletes required a protein intake of 1 to 2 mg/kg/day to produce a positive or 0 nitrogen balance during 12 weeks of intense training.[68] Similar protein intake estimates (1.5 to 1.8 g/kg/day) were reported for cyclists during a simulation of the Tour de France[69] and well-conditioned runners during training.[70] Tarnopolsky[65] compiled all of the nitrogen balance data for the subjects in these studies, performed regression analysis, and showed that an average protein intake of 1.09 g/kg/day was needed to achieve a 0 nitrogen balance; the apparent protein requirement (mean ± 2 SD) was determined to be 1.2 mg/kg/day for endurance athletes.

16.5 TRANSLATION OF DIETARY REFERENCE INTAKES (DRIS) FOR ENERGY TO PHYSICALLY ACTIVE PEOPLE

The DRIs contain categories of reference values for nutrients that are provided to promote the health and well-being of the public.[2] The Recommended Dietary Allowance (RDA) is the daily dietary nutrient intake sufficient to meet the nutrient requirement of nearly all (98%) healthy individuals of a particular sex and life stage group. The Adequate Intake (AI) is the recommended average daily intake level based on observed or experimentally determined estimates of nutrient intake by a group or groups of healthy people. The AI is used when an RDA cannot be calculated. The Estimated Average Requirement (EAR) is the average daily nutrient intake estimated to meet the requirement for half of the healthy individuals in a particular sex and life stage group. The Tolerable Upper Intake Level (UL) is the highest average daily nutrient intake that is likely to pose no risk of adverse health effects for almost all individuals in the general population. Although EAR and RDA values are available for carbohydrate and protein, Acceptable Macronutrient Distribution Ranges (AMDRs) for carbohydrate, fat, and protein, providing ranges of macronutrient intake expressed as a percentage of total energy intakes, were derived from inter-

TABLE 16.2
Examples of Macronutrient Content of Diets Containing Acceptable Macronutrient Distributions and Typical Intakes at Variable Energy Levels for Women (121 lb or 55 kg)

Energy, kcal/day	2000	2000	2000	2500	2500	2500	3000	3000	3000
Carbohydrate, %	45[a]	55[b]	65[a]	45[a]	55[b]	65[a]	45[a]	55[b]	65[a]
g/day	225	275	325	281	344	438	338	413	488
RDA, g/day	100	100	100	100	100	100	100	100	100
g/kg/day	4.1	5.0	5.9	5.1	6.3	7.9	6.1	7.5	8.9
Fat, %	35[a]	30[b]	20[a]	35[a]	30[b]	20[a]	35[a]	30[b]	20[a]
g/day	78	67	44	97	83	56	117	100	66
g/kg/day	1.4	1.2	0.8	1.7	1.5	1.0	2.1	1.8	1.2
Protein, %	35[a]	15[b]	10[a]	35[a]	15[b]	10[a]	35[a]	15[b]	10[a]
g/day	175	75	50	218	94	63	262	113	75
g/kg/day	3.2	1.4	0.9	3.9	1.7	1.1	4.8	2.1	1.4
RDA, g/kg/day	0.8	0.8	0.8	0.8	0.8	0.8	0.8	0.8	0.8

[a] Distributions.
[b] Intakes.

vention trials and epidemiological evidence that suggest a role in either prevention or increased risk of chronic disease.[2] Because macronutrients can be used, at least to some extent, interchangeably as sources of energy to support metabolism, ranges for macronutrients are recommended. The AMDRs for carbohydrate, fat, and protein are estimated to be 45 to 60, 20 to 35, and 10 to 35% of energy, respectively, for adults. The ADMR values are different for infants and children.

The challenge for physically active individuals is to translate nutritional guidelines into practical use. Examples of recommended intakes of macronutrients for adults are shown in Table 16.2 and Table 16.3. The RDAs for dietary carbohydrate and protein are far less than the AMDRs even at the lowest energy intake levels. Because of the key role that carbohydrate plays in facilitating training and performance, Burke and co-workers have emphasized the use of recommendations based on body weight rather than percentage total energy intake.[71] It is clear that athletes require flexibility to meet carbohydrate needs within the context of energy needs and training. During periods of general training, carbohydrate intakes of 5 to 7 g/kg/day are recommended and may be achieved at AMDR levels. However, when compensation of depleted muscle glycogen is needed, greater amounts of dietary carbohydrate are required (7 to 10 g/kg/day) without excessive increases in total energy intake. The challenge of an athlete consuming a very high carbohydrate diet (i.e., 65% energy) and energy in excess of his or her needs can lead to gradual weight gain and eventual performance deficits. This problem may be overcome if carbohydrate intake is based on weight and not total energy intake. Thus, recom-

TABLE 16.3

Examples of Macronutrient Content of Diets Containing Acceptable Macronutrient Distributions and Typical Intakes at Variable Energy Levels for Men (176 lb or 80 kg)

Energy, kcal/day	3000	3000	3000	4000	4000	4000	5000	5000	5000
Carbohydrate, %	45[a]	55[b]	65[a]	45[a]	55[b]	65[a]	45[a]	55[b]	65[a]
g/day	338	413	488	450	550	650	562	688	813
RDA, g/day	130	130	130	130	130	130	130	130	130
g/kg/day	4.2	5.2	6.1	5.6	6.9	8.1	7.0	8.6	10.2
Fat, %	35[a]	30[b]	20[a]	35[a]	30[b]	20[a]	35[a]	30[b]	20[a]
g/day	117	100	67	156	133	89	194	167	111
g/kg/day	1.5	1.3	0.8	1.9	1.7	1.1	2.4	2.1	1.4
Protein, %	35[a]	15[b]	10[a]	35[a]	15[b]	10[a]	35[a]	15[b]	10[a]
g/day	262	113	75	350	150	100	438	188	125
g/kg/day	3.3	1.3	0.9	4.3	1.7	1.25	5.5	2.1	1.5
RDA, g/kg/day	0.8	0.8	0.8	0.8	0.8	0.8	0.8	0.8	0.8

[a] Distributions.
[b] Intakes.

mendations based on body weight, compared to percentage of total daily energy intake, have practical advantages.

The RDA for protein (0.8 g/kg/day) is less than the AMDR, except at the lowest energy intakes (Table 16.2 and Table 16.3). It remains controversial if the protein needs to support endurance or resistance training exceed the RDA value.[2] If an individual selects a protein intake slightly exceeding the lowest AMDR value (i.e., >10% energy intake), there is an expectation that the protein intake, when normalized for body weight (i.e., >1.1 g/kg/day), will boost strength gain and muscle mass maintenance.[65] It is clear that protein intakes at the extreme levels of the AMDR are excessive and potentially a health hazard.

Recommendations for dietary fat have been proposed to avoid risks of future chronic disease. There is a paucity of data supporting an intake of fat that promotes performance. Assuming that the lowest level of the AMDR is healthful, dietary fat intakes of 1 to 1.5 g/kg appear to be adequate. Importantly, elite male cyclists consuming dietary fat at 30 to 50% total energy had increases in serum cholesterol and lipoprotein concentrations similar to those of sedentary adults.[72]

16.6 CONCLUSIONS

Experimental findings and practical outcomes emphasize the importance of an athlete's daily diet on performance. Because carbohydrate and fat are the principal sources of energy during physical training and competition, there has been an emphasis on the critical evaluation of dietary manipulations of these macronutrients on performance. There is consensus that increased carbohydrate intake before, during, and after exercise affects performance and recovery after training. In contrast, although high dietary fat may transiently enhance some aspects of physiological function during controlled laboratory studies, fat loading does not benefit endurance performance in the field. Protein, consumed at usual intakes, exerts no clear benefit in endurance or resistance training or performance. However, neutral or positive nitrogen balance is important in maintaining and increasing muscle mass. Consumption of excessive energy, regardless of macronutrient distribution, can limit performance and impair biomarkers of health.

Guidelines for macronutrient intakes of physically active people are complicated by the units used to express the recommended intakes. Individual macronutrient recommendations based on the percentage of total energy intake vary directly with the total calories consumed. Thus, alterations in daily energy intake affect the intake of the macronutrient. It is also confusing and tedious for individuals to consistently calculate carbohydrate needs when total energy intake is variable. A more practical approach is to use targeted amounts of carbohydrate based on body weight. Similarly, protein intake can be planned easily when intakes are designated on a body weight basis. For both carbohydrate and protein, desired intakes can be estimated from tables summarizing the macronutrient contents of foods, particularly foods desirable to the athlete. Thus, athletes should be instructed by sports dietitians to use standard food guides to estimate carbohydrate and protein intakes based on body weight. Fat intake should be flexible but not excessive.

16.7 FUTURE RESEARCH

The growing public health emphasis on increasing physical activity and consumption of a healthful diet to combat the epidemic of obesity demands renewed efforts to translate dietary recommendations into action. Although the DRI[2] and ADMR[2] provide guidelines for macronutrient intakes, there is a compelling need to develop, validate, and implement practical guidelines for these intakes. It is important to determine if the recommended intakes achieve better compliance based on percentage energy intake than on body weight. Also, the availability of the Dietary Guidelines for Americans 2005 (http://www.healthierus.gov/dietaryguidelines) with its implementation plan, Food Guide Pyramid, appears to be a possible tool to evaluate the ADMR. Overall, the challenge is to develop practical methods for general implementation of national nutritional guidelines for macronutrient intake among all segments of the population.

REFERENCES

1. Burke, L.M., Energy needs of athletes, *Can. J. Appl. Physiol.*, 26, S202–S219, 2001.
2. Food and Nutrition Board, Institute of Medicine, *Dietary Reference Intakes for Energy, Carbohydrate, Fiber, Fat, Fatty Acids, Cholesterol, Protein, and Amino Acids (Macronutrients)*, National Academy Press, Washington, DC, 2005.

3. Bergstrom, J., Hermansen, L., Hultman, E., and Saltin, B., Diet, muscle glycogen and physical performance, *Acta Physiol. Scand.*, 71, 140–150, 1967.

4. Phinney, S.D., Bistrian, B.R., Evans, W.J., Gervino, E., and Blackburn, G.L., The human metabolic response to chronic ketosis without caloric restriction: preservation of submaximal exercise capability with reduced carbohydrate oxidation, *Metabolism*, 32, 769–776, 1983.

5. Lemon, P.W.R., Do athletes need more dietary protein and amino acids? *Int. J. Sports Nutr.*, 5, S39–S61, 1995.

6. American College of Sports Medicine, American Dietetic Association, and Dietitians of Canada, Nutrition and athletic performance, *Med. Sci. Sports Exerc.*, 32, 2130–2145, 2000.

7. Jeukendrup, A.E., Saris, W.H.M., and Wagenmackers, A.J.M., Fat metabolism during exercise: a review — Part I, *Int. J. Sports Med.*, 19, 231–244, 1998.

8. Grandjean, A.C., Nutrition for swimmers, *Clin. Sports Med.*, 5, 65–76, 1986.

9. Hawley, J.A., Dennis, S.C., Lindsay, F.H., and Noakes, T.D., Nutritional practices of athletes: are they suboptimal? *J. Sport Sci.*, 13, S75–S87, 1995.

10. Costill, D.L., Flynn, M.J., Kirwin, J.P., Houmard, J.A., Mitchell, J.B., Thomas, R., and Park, S.H., Effects of repeated days of intensified training on muscle glycogen and swimming performance, *Med. Sci. Sports Exerc.*, 20, 249–254, 1988.

11. Sherman, W.M. and Wimer, G.S., Insufficient dietary carbohydrate during training: does it impair athletic performance? *Int. J Sports Nutr.*, 1, 28–44, 1991.

12. Walberg-Rankin, J., Dietary carbohydrate as an ergogenic aid for prolonged and brief competitions in sport, *Int. J. Sports Nutr.*, 5, S13–S28, 1995.

13. Wright, D.A., Sherman, W.M., and Dernback, A.R., Carbohydrate feedings before, during or in combination improve cycling performance, *J. Appl. Physiol.*, 71, 1082–1088. 1991.

14. Horowitz, J.P. and Coyle, E.F., Metabolic responses to preexercise meals containing various carbohydrates and fat, *Am. J. Clin. Nutr.*, 58, 235–241, 1993.

15. Neufer, P.D., Costill, D.L., Flynn, M.G., Kirwin, J.P., Mitchell, J.B., and Houmard, J., Improvements in exercise performance: effects of carbohydrate feedings and diet, *J. Appl. Physiol.*, 62, 983–988, 1987.

16. Alberici, J.C., Farrell, P.A., Kris-Etherton, P.M., and Shively, C.A., Effects of pre-exercise candy bar ingestion on glycemic response, substrate utilization and perform-ance, *Int. J. Sport Nutr.*, 3, 323–333, 1993.

17. Devlin, J.T., Calles-Escandon, J., and Horton, E.S, Effects of preexercise snack feeding on endurance cycle exercise, *J. Appl. Physiol.*, 60, 980–985, 1986.

18. Sherman, W.M., Brodowicz, G., Wright, D.A., Allen, W.K., Simonsen, J., and Dern-back, A., Effect of 4 h preexercise carbohydrate feedings on cycling performance, *Med. Sci. Sports Exerc.*, 21, 598–604, 1989.

19. Coyle, E.F., Coggan, A.R., Hemmert, W.K., and Ivy, J.L., Muscle glycogen utilization during prolonged strenuous exercise when fed carbohydrate, *J. Appl. Physiol.*, 61, 165–172, 1986.

20. Coggan, A.R. and Coyle, E.F., Metabolism and performance following carbohydrate ingestion late in exercise, *Med. Sci. Sports Exerc.*, 21, 59–65, 1989.

21. Millard-Stafford, M.L., Sparling, P.B., Rosskopf, L.B., Hinson, P.T., and Dicarlo, L.J., Carbohydrate-electrolyte replacement improves distance running performance in the heat, *Med. Sci. Sports Exerc.*, 24, 934–940, 1992.

22. Wilber, R.L. and Moffatt, R.J., Influence of carbohydrate ingestion on blood glucose and performance in runners, *Int. J. Sport Nutr.*, 7, 261–273, 1997.

23. Coggan, A.R. and Coyle, E.F., Reversal of fatigue during prolonged exercise by carbohydrate infusion or ingestion, *J. Appl. Physiol.*, 63, 2388–2395, 1987.
24. Tsintzas, O.K., Williams, C., Wilson, W., and Burrin, J., Influence of carbohydrate supplementation on endurance running capacity, *Med. Sci. Sports Exerc.*, 28, 1373–1379, 1996.
25. Burke, L.M., Kiens, B., and Ivy, J.L., Carbohydrate and fat for training and recovery, *J. Sport Sci.*, 22, 15–30, 2004.
26. Blom, P.C.S., Hostmark, A.T., Vaage, O., Kardel, K.R., and Maehlum, S., Effect of different post-exercise sugar diets on the rate of muscle glycogen synthesis, *Med. Sci. Sports Exerc.*, 19, 491–496, 1987.
27. Coyle, E.F., Substrate utilization during exercise in active people, *Am. J. Clin. Nutr.*, 61, S968–S979, 1995.
28. Sherman, W.M., Doyle, J.A., Lamb, D.R., and Strauss, R.H., Dietary carbohydrate, muscle glycogen, and exercise performance during 7-d of training, *Am. J. Clin. Nutr.*, 57, 27–31, 1993.
29. Achten, J., Halson, S.L., Moseley, L., Rayson, M.P., Casey, A., and Jeukendrup, A.E., Higher dietary carbohydrate content during intensified running training results in better maintenance of performance and mood state, *J. Appl. Physiol.*, 96, 1331–1340, 2004.
30. Millard-Stafford, M.L., Cureton, K.J., and Ray, C.A., Effect of glucose polymer supplement on responses to prolonged successive swimming, cycling and running, *Eur. J. Appl. Physiol.*, 58, 327–333, 1988.
31. Simonsen, J.C., Sherman, W.M., Lamb, D.R., Dernbach, A.R., Doyle, J.A., and Strauss, R.H., Dietary carbohydrate, muscle glycogen, and power output during rowing training, *J. Appl. Physiol.*, 70, 1500–1505, 1991.
32. Ivy, J.L., Katz, A.L., Cutler, C.L., Sherman, W.M., and Coyle, E.F., Muscle glycogen synthesis after exercise: effect of time of carbohydrate ingestion, *J. Appl. Physiol.*, 64, 1480–1485, 1988.
33. Wojtaszewski, J.P.F., Nielson, P., Kiens, B., and Richter, E.A., Regulation of glycogen synthase kinase-3 in human skeletal muscle: effects of food intake an bicycle exercise, *Diabetes*, 50, 265–269, 2001.
34. Richter, E.A., Mikines, K.J., Galbo, H., and Kiens, B., Effects of exercise on insulin action in human skeletal muscle, *J. Appl. Physiol.*, 66, 876–885, 1989.
35. Costill, D.L., Sherman, W.M., Fink, W.J., Maresh, C., Witten, M., and Miller, J.M., The role of dietary carbohydrates in skeletal muscle resynthesis after strenuous running, *Am. J. Clin. Nutr.*, 34, 1831–1836, 1981.
36. Burke, L.M., Collier, G.R., Davis, P.G., Fricker, P.A., Sanigorski, A.J., and Hargreaves, M., Muscle glycogen storage after prolonged exercise: effect of the frequency of carbohydrate feedings, *Am. J. Clin. Nutr.*, 64, 115–119, 1996.
37. Roberts, K.M., Noble, E.G., Hayden, D.B., and Taylor, A.W., Simple and complex-rich diets and muscle glycogen content of marathon runners, *Eur. J. Appl. Physiol.*, 57, 70–74, 1988.
38. Burke, L.M., Collier, G.R., and Hargreaves, M., Muscle glycogen storage after prolonged exercise: the effect of the glycemic index of carbohydrate feedings, *J. Appl. Physiol.*, 75, 1019–1023, 1993.
39. Jozsi, A.C., Trappe, T.A., Starling, R.D., Goodpaster, B., Trappe, S.W., Fink, W.A., and Costill, D.A., The influence of starch structure on glycogen resynthesis and subsequent cycling performance, *Int. J. Sports Med.*, 17, 373–378, 1996.

40. Rose, A.J., Howlett, K., King, D.S., and Hargreaves, M., Effect of prior exercise on glucose metabolism in trained men, *Am. J. Physiol. Endocrinol. Metab.*, 281, E766–E771, 2001.

41. Saltin, B. and Astrand, P.O., Free fatty acids and exercise, *Am. J. Clin. Nutr.*, 57, 752S–758S, 1993.

42. Karlsson, J., Nordesjo, L.-O., and Saltin, B., Muscle glycogen utilization during exercise after physical training, *Acta Physiol. Scand.*, 90, 210–217, 1974.

43. Kiens, B., Essen-Gustavsson, B., Christiansen, N.J., and Saltin, B., Skeletal muscle substrate utilization during submaximal exercise in man: effect of endurance training, *J. Physiol.*, 469, 459–478, 1993.

44. Starling, R.D., Trappe, T.A., Parcell, A.C., Kerr, C.G., Fink, W.J., and Costill, D.L., Effects of diet on muscle triglyceride and endurance performance, *J. Appl. Physiol.*, 82, 1185–1189, 1997.

45. Pitsiladis, Y.P. and Maughan, R.J., The effects of exercise and diet manipulation on the capacity to perform prolonged exercise in the heat and cold in trained humans, *J. Physiol.* 517, 919–930, 1999.

46. Lambert, E.V., Speechly, D.P., Dennis, S.C., and Noakes, T.D., Enhanced endurance in trained cyclists during moderate intensity exercise following 2 weeks adaptation to a high fat diet, *Eur. J. Appl. Physiol.*, 69, 287–293, 1994.

47. Muoio, D.M., Leddy, J.J., Horvath, P.J., Awad, A.B., and Pendergast, D.R., Effect of dietary fat on metabolic adjustments in maximal VO_2max and endurance in runners, *Med. Sci. Sports Exerc.*, 26, 81–88, 1994.

48. Goedecke, J.H., Christie, C., Wilson, G., Dennis, S.C., Noakes, T.D., Hopkins, W.G., and Lambert, E.V., Metabolic adaptations to a high-fat diet in endurance cyclists, *Metabolism*, 48, 1509–1517, 1999.

49. Lukaski, H.C., Bolonchuk, W.W., Klevay, L.M., Milne, D.B., and Sandstead, H.H., Interactions among dietary fat, mineral status, and performance of endurance athletes: a case study, *Int. J. Sport Nutr. Exerc. Metab.*, 11, 186–198, 2001.

50. Lambert, E.V., Goedecke, J.H., Zyle, C., Murphy, K., Hawley, J.A., Dennis, S.C., and Noakes, T.D., High-fat diet versus habitual diet prior to carbohydrate loading: effects on exercise metabolism and cycling performance, *Int. J. Sport Nutr. Exerc. Metab.*, 11, 209–225, 2001.

51. Burke, L.M. and Hawley, J.A., Effects of short-term fat adaptation on metabolism and performance of prolonged exercise, *Med. Sci. Sports Exerc.*, 34, 1492–1498, 2002.

52. Jacobs, K.A., Paul, D.R., Geor, R.J., Hinchcliff, K.W., and Sherman, W.M., Dietary composition influences short-term endurance training-induced adaptations of substrate partitioning during exercise, *Int. J. Sport Nutr. Exerc. Metab.*, 14, 38–61, 2004.

53. Helge, J.W., Richter, E.A., and Kiens, B., Interaction of training and diet on metabolism and endurance during exercise, *J. Physiol.*, 492, 293–306, 1996.

54. Helge, J.W., Wulff, B., and Kiens, B., Impact of a fat-rich diet on endurance in man: role of the dietary period, *Med. Sci. Sports Exerc.*, 30, 456–461, 1998.

55. Watt, M.J., Heigenhauser, G.F.J., and Spriet, L.L., Intramuscular triacylglycerol utilization in human skeletal muscle during exercise: is there a controversy? *J. Appl. Physiol.*, 93, 1185–1195, 2002.

56. Van Loon, L.J.C., Schauwen-Hinderling, V.B., Koopman, R., Wagenmakers, A.J.M., Hesselink, M.K.C., Schaart, G., Kooi, M.E., and Saris, W.H.M., Influence of prolonged endurance exercise cycling and recovery diet on intramuscular triglyceride content in trained males, *Am. J. Physiol. Endocrin. Metabol.*, 285, E804–E811, 2003.

57. Szczepaniak, L.S., Babcock, E.E., Schick, F., Dobbins, R.L., Garg, A., Burns, D.K., McGarry, J.D., and Stein, D.T., Measurement of intracellular triglyceride store by 1H spectroscopy: validation *in vivo*, *Am. J. Physiol. Endocrin. Metabol.*, 276, E977–E989, 1999.

58. Kiens, B. and Richter, E.A., Utilization of skeletal muscle triacylglycerol during postexercise recovery in humans, *Am. J. Physiol. Endocrin. Metabol.*, 275, E332–E337, 1998.

59. Decombaz, J., Schmitt, B., Ith, M., Decarli, B., Diem, P., Kreis, R., Hoppeler, H., and Boesch, C., Post-exercise fat intake repletes intramyocellular lipids but no faster in trained than untrained sedentary subjects, *Am. J. Physiol. Regul. Integrat. Compar. Physiol.*, 281, R760–R769, 2001.

60. Larson-Meyer, D.E., Newcomer, B.R., and Hunter, G.R., Influence of endurance training and recovery diet on intramyocellular lipid content in women: 1H NMR study, *Am. J. Physiol. Endocrin. Metabol.*, 282, E95–E106, 2002.

61. Kimber, N.E., Heigenhauser, G.J.F., Spriet, L.L., and Dyck, D.J., Skeletal muscle fat and carbohydrate metabolism during recovery from glycogen depleting exercise in humans, *J. Physiol.*, 548, 919–928, 2003.

62. Johnson, N.A., Stannard, S.R., Mehalski, K., Trenell, M.I., Sachinwalla, T., Thompson, C.H., and Thompson, M.W., Intramyocellular triacylglycerol in prolonged cycling with high- and low-carbohydrate availability, *J. Appl. Physiol.*, 94, 1365–1372, 2003.

63. Haverman, L., West, S., Goedecke, J.H., McDonald, I.A., St-Clair Gibson, A., Noakes, T.D., and Lambert, E.V., Fat adaptation followed by carbohydrate-loading compromises high-intensity sprint performance, *J. Appl. Physiol.*, 100, 94–102, 2006.

64. Felig, P. and Wahren, J., Amino acid metabolism in exercising man, *J. Clin. Invest.*, 50, 2703–2714, 1971.

65. Tarnopolsky, M., Protein metabolism in strength and endurance athletes, in *The Metabolic Basis of Performance in Exercise and Sport, Vol. 12, Perspectives in Exercise Science and Sports Medicine*, Lamb, D. and Murray, R., Eds., Cooper Publishing Group, Carmel, IN, 1999, pp. 125–164.

66. Lemon, P.W.R., Tarnopolsky, M.A., MacDougall, J.D., and Atkinson, S.A., Protein requirements and muscle mass changes during intensive training in novice bodybuilders, *J. Appl. Physiol.*, 73, 767–775, 1992.

67. Tarnopolsky, M.A., Atkinson, S.A., MacDougall, J.D., Senor, B.B., Lemon, P.W.R., and Schwarcz, H.P., Evaluation of protein requirements for trained strength athletes, *J. Appl. Physiol.*, 73, 1986–1995, 1992.

68. Tarnopolsky, M.A., MacDougall, J.D., and Atkinson, S.A., Influence of protein intake and training status on nitrogen balance and lean body mass, *J. Appl. Physiol.*, 64, 187–193, 1988.

69. Brouns, F., Stroecken, S.J., Thijssen, B.R., Rehrer, N.J., and ten Hoor, F., Eating, drinking and cycling. A controlled Tour de France simulation study. Part II. Effect of diet manipulation, *Int. J. Sports Med.*, 10, S41–S48, 1989.

70. Friedman, J.E. and Lemon, P.W.R., Effect of chronic endurance exercise on retention of dietary protein, *Int. J. Sports Med.*, 10, 118–123, 1989.

71. Burke, L.M., Cox, G.R., Cummings, N.K., and Desbrow, B., Guidelines for daily carbohydrate intake, *Sports Med.*, 31, 267–299, 2001.

72. Lukaski, H.C., Klevay, L.M., Bolonchuk, W.W., Milne, D.B., Mahalko, J.R., and Sandstead, H.H., Influence of type and amount of dietary lipid on plasma lipid concentrations in endurance athletes, *Am. J. Clin. Nutr.*, 39, 35–44, 1984.

Index

A

AAs. *See* Amino acids (AAs)
Acceptable Macronutrient Distribution Range
(AMDR), 75, 79, 366
N-Acetylcysteine, 298
Adrenic acid, 65. *See also* Omega-6 fatty acids
Alanine, 233
cell volume and release of, 308
chemical structure, 283
essentiality, 285
function, 291
hepatic uptake, 268
metabolism, 291–292
muscle, 294
oxidation, 112, 244
postexercise and, 300
pyruvate metabolism and, 271
serum, 294
supplemental, 330
synthesis, 112, 246
transamination and, 299
whey, 145
AMDR. *See* Acceptable Macronutrient
Distribution Range (AMDR)
Amino acids (AAs), 5, 118
absorption, 148
blends, 255, 320–321, 325
branch-chained, 112, 243–256, 280
chemical structure, 244
dietary and supplemental sources,
253–255
drinks, 255
energy metabolism and, 245
exercise performance and, 250–251
function, 243, 244
immune responses to exercise and,
252–253
metabolic functions, 244–249
muscle damaging exercise and, 252
oxidation, 112
soy, 147
toxicity and health risks associated with,
255–256
transamination, 112

whey, 144–145
drinks, 255, 320–321, 325
energy production, 290
in food commodities, 72–73
HMB and, 232, 233
metabolic pathway, 290
oxidation, 244
protein synthesis and supplementation with,
324–327
purified, 131–132
splanchnic handling, 149
whey, 144
Androstenedione, 228, 229, 230
Arachidonic acid, 63, 65, 66. *See also* Omega-6
fatty acids
body reserves, 69
composition of food commodities, 72–73
deficiency, 75
dietary sources, 73
fatty acid intake and, 75
fish oil supplementation and, 78
in formation of lipid mediators, 69
inflammatory disorders and, 75
metabolism, 74, 101
physical properties, 67
platelet aggregation and, 101
precursor, 64, 69
synthesis, 68, 71
Arginine, 110, 147, 167, 285, 292–294
ammonia levels and, 293
for cachexia, 232
chemical structure, 166
creatine synthesis and, 132, 166
exercise and, 293
growth hormone and, 292
HMB and, 232, 233
supplemental, 274, 292–293, 294
whey, 145
wound healing and, 233
Asparagine, 112, 145
aspartate and, 296
chemical structure, 284
essentiality, 285
isolation of, 282
supplemental, 296